Free Movement from the Very Start

VOLUME 1:
*Self-Initiated Movement and Sensorimotor Development
in the Growing Child*

JANE SWAIN

*The Waldorf Early Childhood Association of North America
Spring Valley, New York*

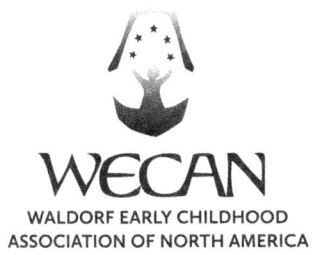

© 2025 Jane Swain

All rights reserved. No part of this book may be reproduced in any form without the written permission of the publisher, except for brief quotations embodied in critical reviews and articles.

ISBN 978-1-936849-64-2

Cover image courtesy of Jane Swain

Images on pages 11, 13, 56 courtesy of the Magyaroszági Pikler-Lóczy Társaság.

Image on page 138: New born baby at hospital with mother, © Select Stock, https://www.istockphoto.com/photo/new-born-baby-at-hospital-with-mother-gm1248789833-363809100

Image on page 219: New shoot of fern frond, © 7Michael, https://www.istockphoto.com/photo/new-shoot-of-fern-frond-on-new-zealand-tree-fern-gm1703245930-538939444

Drawings in chapters 2 and 7 courtesy of Robin Swain.

All images are used with permission and may not be reproduced.

Published in the United States by

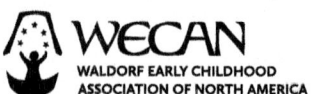

The Waldorf Early Childhood Association of North America
285 Hungry Hollow Rd.
Spring Valley, NY 10977
+1 845-352-1690
info@waldorfearlychildhood.org
www.waldorfearlychildhood.org

For a complete book catalog, contact WECAN or visit our online store at:
store.waldorfearlychildhood.org

This publication is made possible by a grant from the Waldorf Curriculum Fund.

Contents

Dedication 5

Preface 6

Acknowledgments 7

Introduction 8

1: The Life and Work of Dr. Emmi Pikler 11

2: Self-Initiated Gross Motor Development 22

3: Qualitative Movement Findings from Pikler's Research 36

4: Free Movement and Opportunities to Develop Self-Regulation 48

5: Aspects of Self-Initiated Movement 61

6: The Complexity of Baby Equipment 72

7: The Interplay Between Fine and Gross Motor Development 81

8: An Introduction to the Twelve Senses 97

9: Developmental Aspects of Sensing 111

10: Nourishing the Young Child's Sense Organs 121

11: The Forming of the Body Image 131

12: The Sense of Touch 137

13: The Sense of Life 148

14: The Sense of Self-Movement 163

15: The Sense of Balance 175

Appendix 1 193
    Supporting Free Movement through the Physical Environment

Appendix 2 201
    Toys to Support Free Movement

Appendix 3 212
    Pikler's Wooden Furnishings

Appendix 4 219
    The Outdoor Space

Endnotes 226

Bibliography 234

About the Author 239

Dedication

I dedicate this book to my brother, John.

Preface

I write this book out of my experiences as a pediatric physical therapist, movement therapist, adult educator, and mentor for early childhood professionals at Sophia's Hearth; and as a mother and grandmother. I have been profoundly influenced by the work of Rudolf Steiner, Emmi Pikler, Jaimen McMillan, A. Jean Ayres, and Berta Bobath. I bow to these remarkable innovators who have gone before me, and I acknowledge that I am standing on their shoulders. I reference their work throughout the book.

My work at Sophia's Hearth in Keene, New Hampshire has been an important part of my life. When our son was an infant, I stumbled across Waldorf education and the work of Rudolf Steiner, and couldn't study it enough! My husband and I committed to giving our son a Waldorf education, and we came to live in the Keene area. Susan Weber, who later founded Sophia's Hearth, was our son's kindergarten teacher for two years. Volunteering as the class parent, I got to know Susan. As fate would have it, we ended up working together for many years at Sophia's Hearth, where I taught with her in the teacher education program and consulted in the childcare.

Sophia's Hearth began in 1999 as a new initiative in the Waldorf early childhood movement. At that time, many held the belief that infants and young children should be home with a parent. Susan Weber recognized that this belief was not in line with the reality of the times, and she set out to explore how one could serve families with infants and young children. It didn't take long for her to discover the work of Dr. Emmi Pikler. Susan began facilitating parent-child groups and organizing adult education workshops. Soon, I began teaching about sensorimotor development in the infant and young child. Susan Weber, Nancy Macalaster (one of our first parent-child facilitators), and I all studied at the Pikler Institute in Budapest with Anna Tardos, the daughter of Emmi Pikler. In 2010 we built a brand-new building and opened our childcare, and this continues today. Our care of infants and young children at Sophia's Hearth is primarily based on the indications of Rudolf Steiner and the approach of Dr. Emmi Pikler.

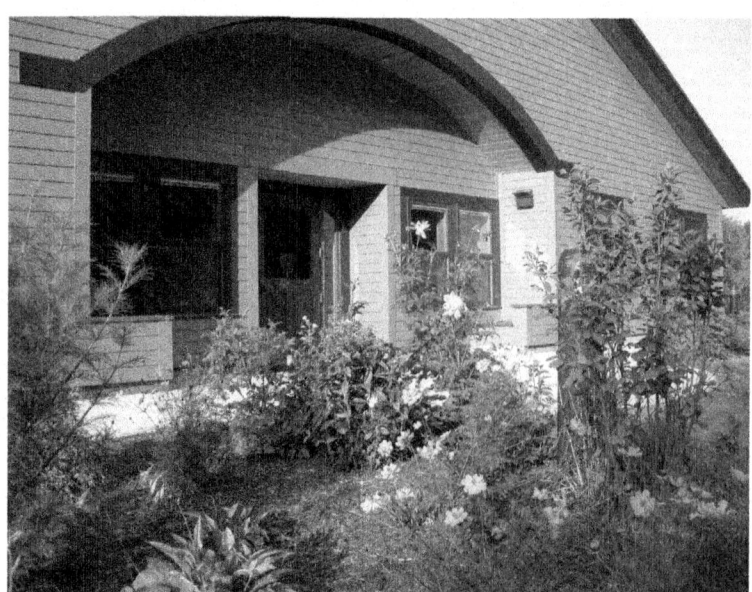

Sophia's Hearth in Keene, NH.

Today, Sophia's Hearth is internationally recognized as a leader in early childhood education. We offer both online and in-person educational opportunities for early childhood teachers. Additionally, our internship program provides the opportunity to study at Sophia's Hearth while applying the newfound knowledge in our year-round childcare setting.

Acknowledgments

I am deeply grateful to all the children and families with whom I have worked in my pediatric physical therapy practice over the years, as they have been my best teachers. I am especially filled with gratitude for my son and daughter-in-law, who embraced the Pikler approach (consisting of free movement and respectful caregiving) for their three children from the very start. I was always involved with my grandchildren, and then during the pandemic, I helped care for them in their home. It was here that I experienced firsthand how invaluable and how practical the Pikler approach can be in the home setting.

I am filled with deep appreciation for those who read portions of my manuscript and offered feedback. Jaimen McMillan's wise counsel added depth and refinement for several of the chapters in which I brought concepts from Spacial Dynamics. Liz Hagerman and Debbie Laurin were vitally important for the chapters dealing with the work of Dr. Emmi Pikler. I appreciate their nuanced discernment regarding the details of Pikler's work. Susan Howard offered warm support and guidance along the way for many of the chapters, as did Heather Church. Kyle Dunlap read the entire manuscript and introduced the idea of making the book into two volumes. Nancy Mellon gave me wise counsel at a crucial point in my writing.

I also thank my colleagues at Sophia's Hearth—both the childcare staff and the teacher education faculty—who encouraged and supported me in so many ways throughout my writing. Michelle Brooks was a touchstone for me when I needed to talk something over. I could count on her to bring illumination from her rich background of working with the very young child.

Words cannot express my gratitude to all of the people who combed through their existing photos or who took new, very specific photos that I requested, in order to provide a visual context through which to understand the text. These people will remain nameless in order to protect the privacy of the children, yet you know who you are, and please know how much this means to me. I am especially thankful to Cynthia Cote, who gave me endless advice regarding the artistic quality of the photos. Liz Hagerman also helped me select photos. She was steadfast in her willingness to give me her valuable insights.

I am ever grateful to my husband, Roy Swain, who just happens to have a degree in journalism! He diligently did the first round of editing for me. His many suggestions helped make the content more clear, concise, and organized. Roy is also a mechanical engineer, and he advised me on the physics of movement. It's also been my good fortune to work with my WECAN manuscript editor, Donna Miele, and my photo editor, Amy Thesing. Writing a book is a new adventure for me, and I appreciate their experience and perspective.

The staff at the Rudolf Steiner Library, especially Luke Stence, helped me with my research. I appreciate his goodwill and expertise.

Countless times while writing this book, I woke in the night or in the morning with ideas that "had come to me from out of the blue." Many times, too, I looked in a reference for one thing and stumbled across something else that was more important. More than once, I—seemingly randomly—found a book from my shelves and opened it to the exact passage that was needed. From all this help from across the threshold I have been sustained, and for it I am deeply grateful.

Introduction
Deborah Laurin PhD

This book establishes a foundation for responsive and ethical care of infants and young children. It is rooted in an approach that values slowing down, free movement, and responsive care at the heart of the caregiver-child relationship. Jane's reference to Henry David Thoreau in chapter 2 offers a fitting analogy of slower development for young children: Trees that grow more slowly at first develop a sound core, as if strengthened and solidified by avoiding an accelerated beginning.

In *Free Movement from the Very Start: Self-Initiated Movement and Sensorimotor Development in the Growing Child* (the first of a planned two volumes), Jane Swain successfully weaves insights from Dr. Emmi Pikler, Rudolf Steiner, and from the field of Spacial Dynamics. She imprints upon the reader a lasting image of the infant as a human being who feels, observes, remembers, and understands, if given the chance by their primary carers. Wisely, Dr. Emmi Pikler and Rudolf Steiner understood and valued an early developmental approach that was grounded in free movement and environments that supported a child's own time to come into being in a natural unfolding. Jaimen McMillan's approach to movement education through Spacial Dynamics is touched on frequently in describing the child's development through self-initiated movement, and will be explored more fully in volume 2.

While *Free Movement* describes key insights in the foundational development of children, it is also helpful for those working remedially with older children. It is filled with modern, up-to-date images depicting Pikler's self-initiated motor sequences and of children in the various stages of gross and fine motor development. Photos of caregiving moments capture the sacred relationship between the child and adult. There are also numerous photos illustrating key aspects of the four lower senses.

Free Movement is a clarion call, urging adults to allow babies and young children enough time to come into their own internal rhythm of development. It is about the child's deep need to move and to be in relationship with caring adults. Honed by her many years of observing babies' movements, Jane's approach brings us closer to the child's experiences, inviting us to be curious and allow for a child's inborn abilities to unfurl. How can we deepen our understanding of the unique needs of infants and toddlers?

Jane's insights illuminate the innate capacity of infants to self-initiate motor development, citing Dr. Emmi Pikler's groundbreaking documentation of the effects of responsive, reciprocal caregiving practices and self-initiated movement on the well-being and positive adjustment of children to life in and outside of institutionalized care. Chapters 1 through 7 offer a compelling picture of the sensorimotor development of infants through self-initiated movement and respectful, sensitive caregiving. As we read, we become observers feeling *with* the infants as Jane beautifully describes their journey of unfolding motor development, offering the reader a remarkable view of the child's innate capacities when they are given time to blossom. Exploring Pikler's core beliefs, we realize the integral relationship between the infant's free motor exploration and developing self-regulation. We also ask: How does the adult call forth the child's developing sense of Self? And in answer, *Free Movement* urges us to support the infant's access to self-initiated movement, which arises out of the healthy, secure relationship the infant feels with their primary caregiver. This allows the child, through their own efforts, to develop motor abilities, shaping the budding sense of Self.

In chapters 8 through 15, Jane probes Rudolf Steiner's lectures on the twelve senses as essential to our insights about infants and young children. Especially significant from birth are the four foundational senses of touch, balance, life, and movement. We learn that these four senses, which inform the child's developing sense of Self and weave together the child's body image (or scheme), cannot be taught to young children; the child must, on their own, come into relationship with their own body. Through respectful caregiving and creating a secure environment for free motor exploration, we support the conditions for the unfolding of the foundational senses.

Both Pikler and Steiner wrote extensively about the most favorable conditions to support the child's blossoming sensory motor system. Each child's sensory preferences are unique and require adult self-awareness of how we care for and interact with the infant. For example, during caregiving activities, the child absorbs and internalizes the experience of intimacy through the touch of the adult's hands. Vitally, the adult's hands convey the baby's first connection to the world and how the infant comes to see the world. These first connections powerfully shape, through repeated sensation, a general sense of well-being for the infant. Through touch, the child also comes to sense the border of their body, informing the proprioceptive sense or sense of self-movement, which will eventually allow the child to sense their body in space and how each body part moves in relation to another. In contrast, a hasty and mechanical approach to caregiving diminishes the child's sense of Self, misses opportunities for co-regulation and cooperative interactions between child and caregiver, and decreases chances for the child to experience a sense of their own rhythm.

Jane also examines the role of the adult gesture in being with and around young children, considering Steiner's views on the sense of life. She urges the adults to consider how the child responds to our touch, rather than considering only our own intentions in the way we are touching them. Are we observing the child's responses in the moment-to-moment encounter? Are the adult's actions congruent with their emotions? A child's access to free movement offers key moments to self-regulate. Imagine how the child moves freely, takes pauses, and may stop to rest when they get tired. The child is able to listen and act on their internal messages of fatigue. We learn that the healthy development of the life sense means the child has time and space to engage fully in movement and subsequently experience fatigue from giving it their all. The sense of life is supported through free movement!

To transform our approach with infants and toddlers requires a conscious rethinking and critical penetration of our perceptions and attitudes about young children. With intention, we slowly understand that healthy development is not about *what* the child can do. Instead, if given the time and space, we realize the importance of *how* young children do what they do as essential for them to thrive and flourish. This book is an antidote to the hurried pace of life. For all human beings who are interested in *how* to be with children, please ask yourself, what is the rush?

> Dr. Debbie Laurin
> Pikler Pedagogue Candidate
> Co-director, Early Childhood West Coast Institute of Anthroposophy

FREE MOVEMENT FROM THE VERY START

1: The Life and Work of Dr. Emmi Pikler

Emmi Pikler (1902–1984) was a groundbreaking pediatrician, author, and lecturer. Her work fundamentally changed the way infants and children were, and are, cared for in orphanages and childcare settings, as well as in private homes, throughout the world.

Vienna: A Reformist Medical Education

In the 1920s, when Emmi Madeline Reich studied medicine in Vienna, it was "the cradle of reformist ideas."[1] Two of her instructors in medical school, Professors Clemens von Pirquet and Hans Salzer, left lasting impressions on her. From them she learned about preventative medicine as well as about a holistic and respectful approach to caring for children. Professor von Pirquet stressed the importance of fresh air, play, and good nutrition for children. Under his direction, "It was forbidden to make a child eat one single spoonful more than the child wanted."[2] Professor Salzer, as a pediatrician, emphasized the importance of creating a relationship with the child so that the child could be at ease and cooperate during medical examinations and treatments. Salzer also taught his medical students to instruct parents about healthy lifestyles for their children.

During her training, Emmi Reich worked in an emergency room where she noticed that the children from lower socioeconomic groups seemed to have fewer trips to the emergency room. They also seemed to have fewer broken bones, lacerations, and concussions than the children from higher socioeconomic groups. The budding doctor researched the data, and indeed the statistics bore out her observation. It was common practice in those days for the children of lower socioeconomic levels to play freely outside on the streets, whereas the children from the homes with higher incomes were kept inside and were highly supervised by their nannies.[3] She also observed that all of the babies, rich and poor alike, were being propped to sit and placed into standing positions before they could assume these positions on their own. Additionally, all of the children had been assisted and encouraged to learn to walk. However, the "well-to-do families spent extra time manually exercising their babies' limbs in order to encourage physical development."[4] In other words, the adults in the well-to-do families were moving their babies' limbs, in a hand-over-hand manner, with the goal of teaching them to move.

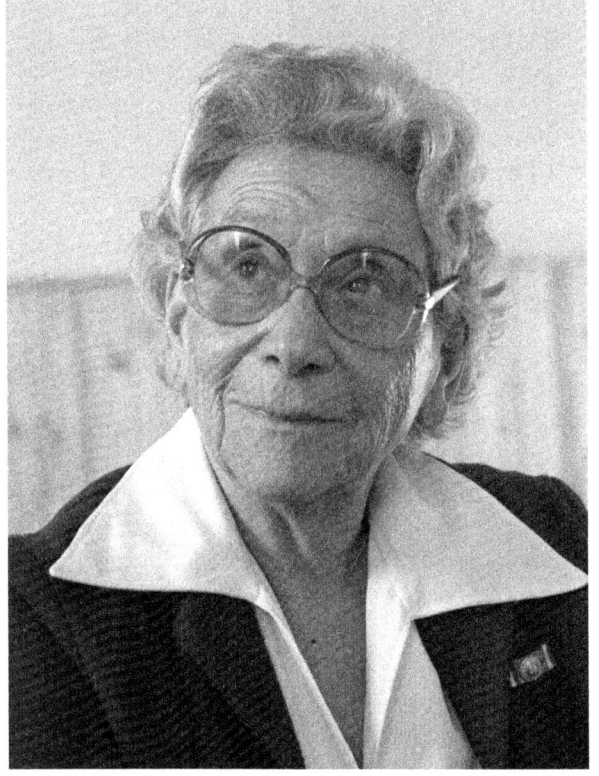

Dr. Emmi Pikler

Marriage and Parenthood

Emmi married György Pikler in 1930. György and Emmi saw eye to eye regarding how to support the development of children. György was teaching high school at the time, and he believed that "children should study at their own pace of development."[5] Their daughter, Anna, was born in 1931. Emmi and György decided to raise Anna according to their own beliefs, rather than according to the generally accepted child-rearing practices of the time. Baby Anna was allowed to progress from the horizontal positions up into verticality entirely though her own efforts and in her own time. Additionally, Anna was embedded into loving, respectful relationships with her parents. Baby Anna developed beautifully.

According to Dr. Judit Falk,* "Emmi Pikler had always doubted that infants needed adult intervention and stimulation—or that adult intervention speeded up a child's development. Assuming that development did occur more rapidly, she doubted that the effects on the child's overall life and development were opportune. . . . Naturally, Pikler would never have undertaken this 'experiment' if she had not been convinced of the validity of her hypothesis: that the child who is allowed to explore at [their] own pace learns to sit, stand, walk, speak and think better than the child who is encouraged to reach prescribed developmental stages."[6]

Impactful Experiences in Trieste, Italy

The young family moved to Trieste, Italy, for a year, where it was customary for families with young children to frequent the beaches. There, Pikler observed parents with their infants. Her observations illumined the tremendous importance of the parents' love for their child. Pikler also witnessed parents "teaching" their babies to sit, stand, and walk before the babies were able to do so on their own, causing the babies to do something different than they would have done if left to their own initiative.

Pikler saw this gesture of the adult as a distrust of the child's inborn abilities. Instead, she believed that infants—from day one—have an innate capacity to direct the unfolding of their motor capacities through self-initiated movement, if given the time and space to do so. Pikler believed that each child was uniquely qualified for this task—in fact, infinitely more qualified than any adult was. It follows, then, that infants should not be taught motor skills, but instead should be allowed to gradually come into the vertical positions of sitting and standing entirely through their own efforts. Dr. Judit Falk writes, "She asked the question, 'Does this communicate to the child that what [they are] doing is not good enough and that [they] should be doing something of which [they are] not yet capable?'"[7] Pikler's answer, essentially, was that the infant does exactly what they "should" be doing, and they do it at exactly the correct time in their development.

Settling in Budapest, Hungary

After a year in Trieste, the family moved to Budapest, Hungary. Dr. Pikler was not able to secure employment because she was Jewish, and so she went into private practice. Anna Tardos† relates that "She became well-known in Budapest, as an excellent pediatrician in the 1930s. The children she took care of—nearly one hundred families—were less ill, and had hardly a major disease. As a pediatrician, however, she was more interested in promoting healthy physical and psychological development than in preventing or curing illnesses. *Her vision of a healthy infant was an active, competent and peaceful infant, who lives in peace with themselves and their environment* [emphasis added]."[8]

---

* Judit Falk MD was a pediatrician who worked at Lóczy for 48 years. She succeeded Dr. Pikler as the director for twelve years between 1979 and 1991.
† Anna Tardos, daughter of Emmi Pikler, directed the children's home at Lóczy from 1998 until 2011. Tardos greatly expanded access to the Pikler approach to English speakers by giving Pikler trainings and lectures in English. She is a prolific author and editor regarding the Pikler approach.

In her medical practice, Dr. Pikler began making weekly house calls after a baby was born and this continued throughout the first year. In her visits, Pikler guided parents regarding the care of babies. She also gave concrete suggestions for how to provide optimal physical environments that would support the babies' motor development—even if they were living in a small apartment. Her support and recommendations helped the parents "learn to trust in the infant's inherent ability and to respect the path and rhythm of this development."[9]

Dr. Pikler's reputation spread in the community. When the parents in her practice took their children to the park to play, the public perceived that there was something unique about these children, and they became known as the "Pikler babies." At Sophia's Hearth, we have employed Dr. Pikler's approach since our inception. We take infants at three months old into our childcare program. When a child graduates from our program and goes on to other school settings, it is not uncommon for their new teachers to remark that they can tell that the child attended Sophia's Hearth. These teachers describe our graduates as exceedingly capable and resilient children. Our graduates also typically stand out as children who know how to play—something which is not always the case. In fact, one of the benefits of employing the Pikler approach from very early in the child's life is that when they are older, the children generally know how to occupy themselves. They have been given a multitude of opportunities to freely engage their wills and so they are used to this. They grow strong in their wills because they have exercised their wills.

Dr. Pikler was well loved by the families in her practice, so much so that some of them risked their own lives to protect her and her family from the Nazis during World War II. Several of the families took turns hiding the Pikler family in their basements.

Lóczy

After the war, Dr. Pikler was asked by the city of Budapest to organize and start a children's home (or orphanage) for infants and young children whose parents had been lost in the war or were in tuberculosis asylums. The children's home was founded in 1946, with Dr. Pikler as director from 1946–1978. After this, she continued her research there until her death in 1984.

Wanting the children to have ample access to the outdoors, she directed that the upstairs rooms have decks built with awnings for sun protection. Each deck had a large, fenced play area so the babies could play in the fresh air. For the older babies and children, structures were built in the yard for water play and climbing. Sand pits were constructed. Every morning the staff raked the sand into mounds to make the sand an inviting place for the children to play. The children took their naps out of doors, as was (and still is) the custom in Hungary; however, at night, they slept indoors.

Dr. Pikler's ten years of work in her private practice had served to help refine her vision of healthy practices for the caring of infants and young children.

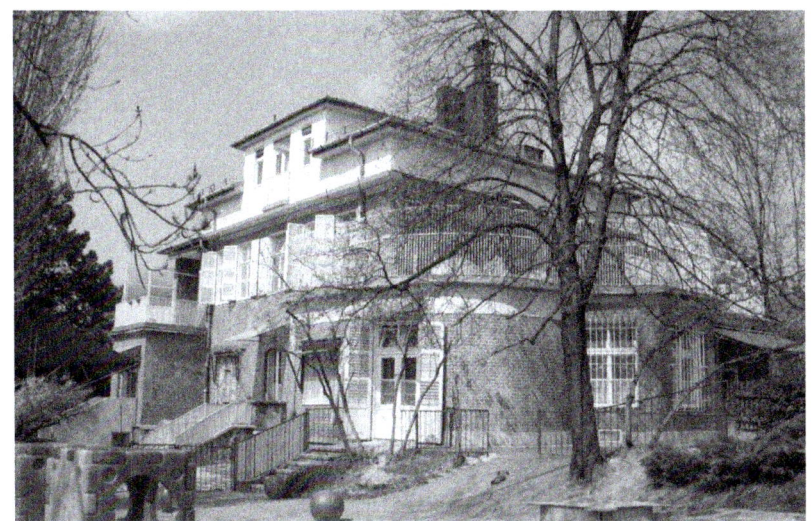

The city provided a house with a large yard in a residential area of Budapest, which was remodeled according to Dr. Pikler's specifications for the children's home.

She was an astute observer and was very detail oriented. Additionally, she taught the parents in her practice to make careful observations of their own children. Pikler and the parents then discussed their observations. In this way Pikler clarified and perfected her practices.

Directing the children's home gave Pikler the opportunity to expand the scope of her work. She was able to directly apply her approach in the care of the numerous children who attended the children's home. Additionally, an adult education program was begun at the children's home, where interested early childhood professionals from around the world came to learn and observe. They took Pikler's groundbreaking ideas back to their own facilities and implemented them. Pikler also made her ideas accessible through her many books and articles.

The children's home was originally called the National Methodological Institute for Infant Care and Education. Later its name was changed to the Pikler Institute, and the name underwent several other changes over the years. However, all along, the children's home was commonly known—both locally and abroad—as Lóczy (pronounced Loh-tsee), named for the street on which it is located. The children's home operated continuously for sixty-five years, and during this time over two thousand children lived there. It was originally established for children aged birth to three. However, over time, it served a variety of children from birth up to seven years, including those with histories of abandonment, abuse, and neglect. Also, a proportion of the children had special needs, including children with Down's and other syndromes, cerebral palsy, and orthopedic conditions.

Lóczy continues to operate today, although it ceased to be a residential nursery in 2011,[10] after the Hungarian government switched from an orphanage system to a foster care system. As a result, the manifestation of Pikler's work transformed to meet the needs of the time. Today, Lóczy hosts parent-infant classes and a childcare for local families. The adult education programs also continue.

Hospitalism Defeated

At the core of the Pikler approach is an understanding of the need to provide an environment in which children are nurtured, respected, and allowed free movement so that they may grow and develop into secure, confident, and fulfilled human beings. When the children's home was first established, there was an unfortunate, but widespread phenomenon known as hospitalism, whereby infants and young children who lived in orphanages generally did not progress well with regard to their physical, cognitive, and social-emotional development. Some children even died.

However, the children at Lóczy flourished. They were able to trust and develop a bond, built through respectful caregiving practices, with their primary caregivers. The child's ability to bond with their primary caregiver then transferred to the adoptive parents when the child was adopted. The children were able to finish school at the same rates as non-institutionalized children, hold jobs, get married, and take good care of their own children. Longitudinal research was carried out on the children raised at the Pikler Institute,

> including a landmark study funded by the World Health Organization in the 1960/70's looking at the social adjustment of the children reared at the Pikler Institute. ... The schooling level of the former boarders shows no unfavorable deviation from the age-group average. No vagrancy or criminal behavior emerged to date of the study. ... The results so far established indicate that former boarders of the institute are generally well adapted to society, and do not display the typical conspicuous signs generally considered characteristic of the subsequent development of children reared institutionally in their first years of life.[11]

In other words, Dr. Pikler broke the mold for young children who were institutionalized. These remarkable findings rather quickly became known and respected throughout the world. Pikler associations were founded in Europe, Asia, and North and South America. They continue today to serve as adult training centers for the practical application of Pikler's principles.

The Pikler Approach

When Dr. Pikler founded the children's home, she initially hired trained nurses to care for the infants and young children. However, Pikler was not satisfied with the manner in which the nurses interacted with the children. After three months she dismissed them all and "employed young [women] from the villages who had little education and no professional training but were interested in bringing up children."[12] Dr. Pikler invested considerable time and energy in educating the caregivers at Lóczy. For example, they were taught how to pick up, hold, and carry the infants, so that the infants could feel safe in the competent hands of their caregivers. The caregivers were taught to carry out similar sequences of care for each child. For example, when bathing, the parts of the body were washed in the same order. In this way, the babies could feel secure when a different caregiver took over.

However, the caregivers' lessons went far beyond learning techniques. Dr. Pikler did not give the caregivers rote phrases to say to the children when a certain type of situation occurred. The caregivers were not to care for the children in a routine manner. Dr. Pikler noted that "Movements that are repeated as part of a work routine usually become shorter, faster and slightly mechanical."[13] Pikler felt that this was an unfortunate setup, whereby the caregivers could potentially treat the children like objects. Instead, she wanted the adults to act out of their authentic selves in each individual situation with each individual child. This required that the adult stay fully present, observe in a finely tuned manner, and then act accordingly. This is not a minor task—it requires ego forces, artistry, and tact.

Dr. Pikler developed an *approach* to caring for infants and young children, rather than a *method*, and this is what she taught to the caregivers.

There are two fundamental pillars to the approach: (1) free motor exploration and (2) respectful, sensitive caregiving.

These two pillars are interdependent. The infant's ability to self-initiate movement is a function of the security of the relationship between the child and the primary adult. In fact, the healthy relationship is a *necessary* condition for the child's free movement to unfold. The child must have the feeling that they are important to and understood by someone, in order to be interested in the world and to want to explore it with self-initiated movements.

Similarly, free movement is a *necessary* condition for a healthy relationship to develop. During the free motor exploration, the child develops their motor abilities entirely through their own efforts, and this contributes to the development of their sense of Self.[14] In this way, they have more of their Self to bring to the relationship during the caregiving times. During the caregiving activities, also, the child is developing a sense of Self. The child comes to know their Self when they actively participate—to whatever degree they are able—in the tasks at hand. The child develops a feeling of agency because they can influence what happens to them in the caregiving activity. The adult reads the cues of the child and responds accordingly. There is a back and forth between adult and child. Caregiving is not done *to* the child, but rather, caregiving is done *with* the child. Dr. Maria Vincze speaks about the development of the Self during caregiving in greater detail later in the chapter.

At the children's home, every effort was made to maintain consistent caregivers for the children. Additionally, each child had one of their caregivers designated as their primary caregiver. The primary caregiver knew the child very well, took responsibility for consideration of the child's welfare and development, and recorded in-depth observations of the child on a regular basis. At the children's home, if an infant was experiencing challenges with their motor development, the first thing to consider was their relationship with their primary caregiver. Certainly, there could be other factors at play. However, if the relationship wasn't secure, then the child's movement would reflect this—the relationship was considered paramount.

Examples of Caregiving Activities in the Pikler Approach

Caregiving activities include feeding, dressing, bathing, diapering, cutting the fingernails, brushing the hair, putting on cream and sunscreen, and so on. In the Pikler approach, caregiving activities are viewed as opportunities for building and tending the relationship between child and caregiver. The changing table is seen as a place where the child's trust in the adult and in the world may develop—and may accompany them for the rest of their life. The infant is seen as a capable human being from the very start. The infant is viewed "as a person who feels, observes, remembers and understands—or will understand, if given the chance."[15]

Caregiving activities are important. Dr. Judit Falk states that "in early childhood the physical needs of the child and their satisfaction fundamentally determine the child's relation to [themselves] and to [their] environment."[16] Caregiving activities are also seen as opportunities for cooperative interactions between caregiver and child from the first day of the child's life. The adult must be alert and flexible as the child's development proceeds and their ability to participate changes over time. The child's ability to participate also varies from moment to moment, according to their level of hunger, fatigue, discomfort, and so on. It is the adult's responsibility to make the child feel welcome and safe, to read their cues, and to take into account their individual preferences; for example, with regard to feeding, does this child prefer the cereal lumpy or smooth? On one occasion an infant was not eating much, and so the caregivers at Lóczy experimented with various foods. They found that the child ate heartily if the food was sprinkled with a little bit of lemon juice![17]

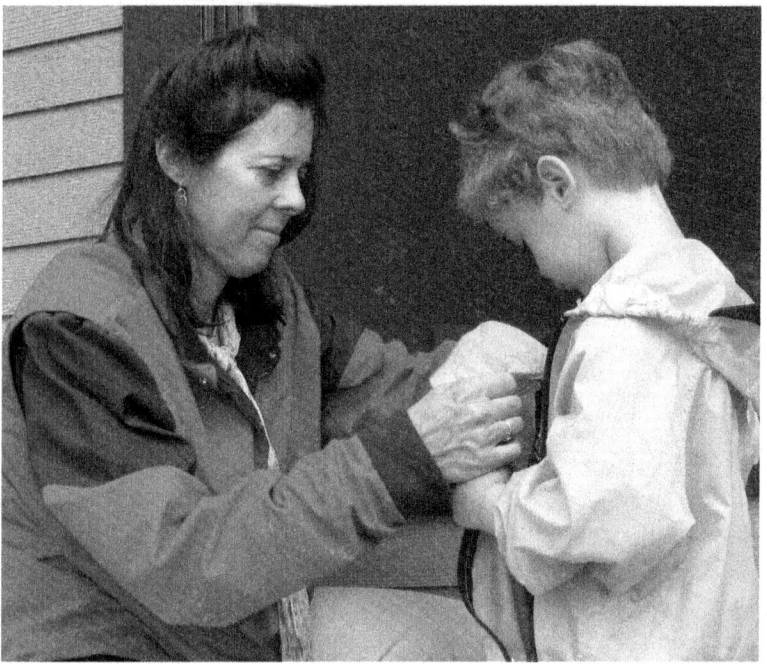

This caregiver is giving full attention to assisting the child with their rainsuit.

The children at the children's home became exceedingly capable in their self-care at an early age. However, the intention of the caregiver is not to promote independence. Rather, the goal is to make the caregiving activity a pleasant experience—to make the uncomfortable feelings (the hunger, the discomfort of a soiled diaper, feeling cold, etc.) go away. Initially, the newborn does not know that they are feeling hungry, thirsty, uncomfortable, cold, and so on. Over time, they come to recognize these states of being, and they also learn that it is they who are experiencing them. The infant comes to associate the adult with the subduing of the uncomfortable feelings, and this is an initial means of establishing the infant's bond with the adult. If the adult invites the baby to participate in the caregiving, and if the adult reads the cues of the baby, the child comes to feel empowered—the child recognizes that they too are making the uncomfortable feelings go away.[18]

A simple example of the reciprocity between adult and child may be seen during spoon-feeding a baby. If the baby turns their head away, the adult doesn't follow the turned head with the spoon. Rather, the adult waits until the child turns their head back to the midline (aligned between the right and left sides of the body) and opens their mouth. Here, the child learns that they will be fed when they place their head in midline and open their mouth. The baby also learns that they can indicate that they don't want any more food by turning their head away from midline. The goal of the adult is not that the baby "cleans their plate." Instead, the adult wants the baby to have a pleasurable feeding experience.

Calling Forth the Self

Dr. Mária Vincze[‡] explains the effect of this type of caregiving on the developing child, in that it serves to call forth the child's Self.

> For the healthy development of [the child's] personality, the kind words and gentle care are not enough. [The child] needs to feel that the friendly words are really addressed to [them], that the person bending over [them] really expects an answer with [their] eyes, [their] words and [their] hands, seeking [the child's] glance, attention, smile and [the child's] voice responding to [the adult's] voice. [The child] needs to feel that the hands touching [their] body are asking hands; and [they] can give an answer to the questions by relaxing, loosening [their] muscles and dissolving [the] tension, or—on the contrary—by increasing [their] tension, [their] resistance. This way the infant can experience that [their] signals are recognized and understood, that [their] needs are taken seriously and that [they are] able to respond effectively. In other words, [the child] thus experiences, from the very beginning, the sensation of being "competent," and can gradually recognize [their] "self" and [their] needs. This way [they] can reach to establishing a trust substantiating [their] personality.[19]

In this passage, Dr. Vincze summarizes one of Dr. Pikler's core beliefs, that for healthy development to ensue, each child needs to be treated as an individual and with respect. "Pikler affirmed that babies should never be treated mechanically nor handled like an object. She believed that the hands constituted the infant's first connection to the world and, depending on how these hands administered care, would result in how the infant would come to view the world."[20]

Free Motor Exploration

The child receives the adult's complete and continuous attention during the caregiving activities. As a result of the intimacy experienced during the respectful caregiving encounter, the child is "filled up," so to speak, so that when they are placed into the movement space, they are generally ready and happy to be on their own to move and play. In other words, they are in a well-regulated state. The child would not be "filled up" during this time if the adult was multitasking. Dr. Judit Falk elaborates, "We believe that, if the infant experiences affective security during care, [they] will be able to utilize the opportunities of activity after care, and will turn towards the external world with interest and pleasure without the intervention of an adult."[21]

During the periods of free movement, the child is embedded into the adult's loving presence—the adult is always willingly available to act should the child encounter a predicament that the child is unable to tolerate. However, during free play time, the adult's attention is more indirect and from farther away than it is during the caregiving activities. During free movement time, the adult is observing the play, but is holding back and refraining from "helping" the child. When the caregiver places the child into the play space, Dr. Pikler explained, it is most helpful for the child if the caregiver has the inner attitude of "now is your time to explore these nice toys" rather than "unfortunately, I must leave you now."

[‡] Dr. Vincze was a pediatrician at Lóczy who worked with Dr. Pikler.

In the Pikler approach, the adult sets up the movement space for the child, based on observations of the child's developmental needs and preferences. The goal is to safely provide the child with many possibilities for movement and play, and then the child is free to follow their interests. When the adult places the child into the movement space, the adult never places the child in a position out of which they cannot move—i.e., the child is never propped up into sitting, for example, or placed into "container" baby equipment. The clothes Dr. Pikler recommended were "designed to allow the greatest possible freedom of movement."[22] When setting up the movement space, the adult considers several factors: What is the baby's favorite toy, and which one do they no longer play with? Do they need a new toy? How many toys serve the child? (If there are too many toys, then the child may not play as well.) Which type of climbing structure is appropriate, if any? (For more on setting up the play space, please see the appendices.)

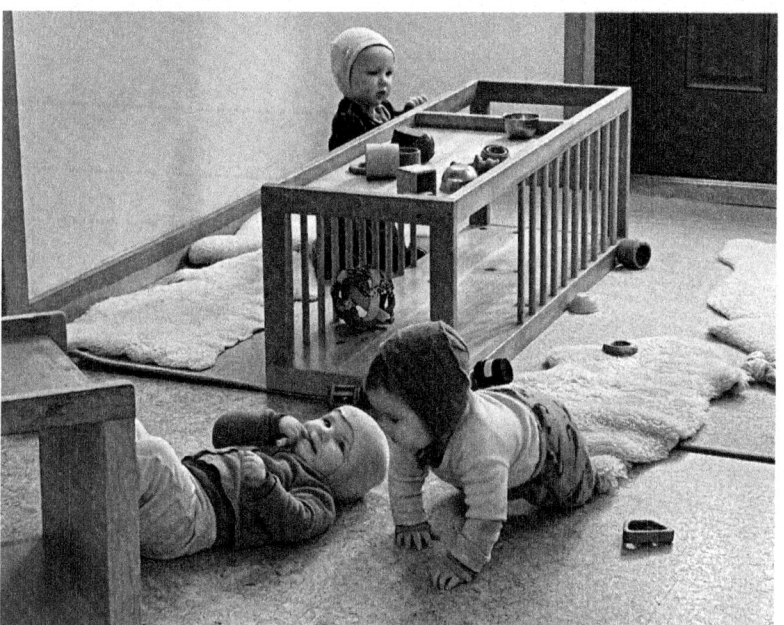

These babies are playing freely in the play space that has been carefully prepared for them by their early childhood educator.

The adult is interested in the child's accomplishments, but does not have an agenda for the child. Instead, the child is responsible for their own movements—which movements they perform, how they carry them out, and for how long. The child proceeds through the gross motor sequence from the horizontal positions up into standing and walking entirely through their own efforts and in their own time. The adult does not try to hurry up the child. The long, uninterrupted periods of free movement allow the child the freedom to start and stop any particular movement or activity as they see fit. They may stop and look around, rest, and then return to what they were doing—or not.

The child has opportunities to sense their state of being. They may perceive when they are tired or becoming frustrated and want to pause, and also when they are ready to proceed—they are learning to self-regulate. Similarly, no one is dictating when the child performs a fine motor activity or a gross motor activity. The child is free to switch back and forth between large motor movements and small motor movements. Dr. Pikler believed that children need opportunities for both, while inside and outside.

Babies and young children are incredibly perceptive to the attitudes of the adults around them. If the adult has a movement goal that they want the child to accomplish that day—even if it is unstated—the child may feel pressured. Children naturally want to please the important adults in their lives. If the child does not meet the adult's goal, the child may feel that they have "failed." Either way—whether the child meets or does not meet the adult's goal—the locus of control for the child is external. In contrast, if the baby sets their own goal—to reach for a toy—for example, and does not achieve it, the baby may not perceive this as a "failure" on their part. They are simply exploring and learning about the world.

Common Adult-Child Interactions and Practices

Thus far, we have explored Pikler's revolutionary approach for caring for babies and young children. In contrast, when the Pikler approach is not employed, it is not uncommon for the child to be viewed by the adult as behaving in an uncooperative manner during caregiving activities. For example, perhaps the adult expects the child to hold still in back-lying throughout a diaper change, and the child tries to move out of the position. The adult may respond by holding the child down and then rushing to complete the task—the adult may just want to get the job done. The idea of drawing the child into participation in the activity is foreign to the adult. The adult may also multitask during the caregiving activity—perhaps they are on a screen. The unfortunate result is that neither child nor adult may find the interaction satisfying.

During the child's motor exploration time, it is not uncommon for the adult to pay attention to the child and try to engage them. The adult may even feel an urge to entertain the child, and believe that this is the only way the child can be satisfied. The adult may also feel compelled to direct and encourage the child to achieve a particular goal of the adult's. For example, when the child is at the stage of pulling to standing, the adult may take the child's hands and "help" them to walk—something the child is not yet capable of doing independently. Later the adult may further encourage the child to walk. A common practice is for the adult to hold out their arms and tell the child to "come to me!" The child may receive praise and even a degree of cheerleading from the adult.

The adult may eventually tire of entertaining and teaching their child—the adult comes to need a break. However, the child has become used to the setup. If the adult stops giving the child so much attention, the child may react by becoming "clingy" or "demanding." This is often a challenging situation for the adult, who may be exhausted and feeling resentful. It is then that the adult may turn to "container" baby equipment or may give the child a screen, both of which have negative impacts on children (for more on this topic, see chapters 4 and 6). This scenario is preventable. Fortunately, the situation also can be turned around—with understanding, time, and patience.

The Pikler Approach Introduces Breathing into the Setup of the Day

The above-mentioned common adult-child interactions and practices may be described as lacking a quality of breathing. The adult and child are together in caregiving, but not in a satisfying manner. They are also together in the child's movement time, but not in a way where the child can achieve an authentic feeling of self-accomplishment.

In contrast, the Pikler approach affords time for more intimate togetherness during caregiving times, and time for more independent exploration during the child's free motor exploration periods. The latter periods give the child and the adult rhythmical times for a healthy degree of separation. Indeed, it is very beneficial for the child to have times when they are more on their own and may explore the extent of their abilities. In this way the child has an opportunity to develop a well-earned sense of self-confidence, because the child accomplishes something on their own—without help—although again, it is never intended that the child feel abandoned or be totally left alone. Additionally, the adult *contains* the motor exploration period by performing caregiving before and after it. A caregiving activity performed before free movement time prepares the child for it, and a caregiving activity afterward replenishes the child. As the old saying goes, absence makes the heart grow fonder—after having their more individual experiences, both parties are ready and happy to come back together again for another caregiving experience.

FREE MOVEMENT FROM THE VERY START

Careful Consideration of the Parents' Feelings

When early childhood professionals learn about Pikler's foundational concepts of self-initiated movement and respectful caregiving, sometimes they feel bad or even guilty if they have not followed this approach in their previous work or in raising their own children. In these situations, I respond by saying that it is important not to use one's knowledge as a weapon—against oneself or against any parent. Guilt is not a helpful emotion, as it interferes with the relationship between parent and child—and the relationship is paramount! It also must be mentioned that Dr. Pikler did not say that raising children according to the Pikler approach would guarantee problem-free development. Conversely, she also did not say that children not raised according to the Pikler approach would have problems.[23] Raising children is not this simple!

Today at Lóczy, in the childcare, a healthy, respectful relationship between caregiver and child continues to be essential. The staff also works directly with parents in the childcare and in the parent-child classes. The staff employs common sense and careful consideration in their approach to parents, so the parents are not made to feel inadequate in any way. The goal is to safeguard the relationship between each parent and their child. The staff seeks to support parents so that their day-to-day experiences with their infants and young children may be peaceful and rewarding, even amidst the many stresses of modern life.

Holding Space for the Child During Free Movement and Play Time

In her private practice, Dr. Pikler made house calls and worked closely with mothers. At this time in Budapest, the mothers were typically the ones at home caring for the babies. Pikler wanted the mothers to feel free to attend to their own work periodically throughout the day. The mother's work consisted primarily of housework, which had a degree of physicality to it; the mothers were not on screens and there were not as many gadgets then—no robot vacuum cleaners! According to Dr. Pikler's recommendations, the mother was to be ready and willing to attend to the child if needed. However, the mother was not to be overly involved with the child during their free movement time. The mother was not to "break the spell" of the child's play by unnecessarily speaking to the child or looking at the child for too long or with too much intensity. This is a way of honoring the sacredness of the child's play, which needs a degree of privacy. The child, for their part, was not to be encouraged to attend to the mother's activity, nor to think about the mother at all.[24]

Today, in the childcare at Lóczy, the adults attend to the meal cleanup while the children are playing. The adults work in the area that is gated off from the play area. They stack the dishes in a slow, ceremonious way. The work is orderly and it restores order. The dishes are not stacked too high on the tray—short cuts are not taken. The work is not rushed—there is no loud clanking of dishes.[25]

The adult's manner of working when around young children, as described above, is remarkably similar to that recommended by Rudolf Steiner. Let us consider Steiner's indications in this regard. It was very important to Rudolf Steiner that young children be surrounded by adults who are engaged in real work. In this way

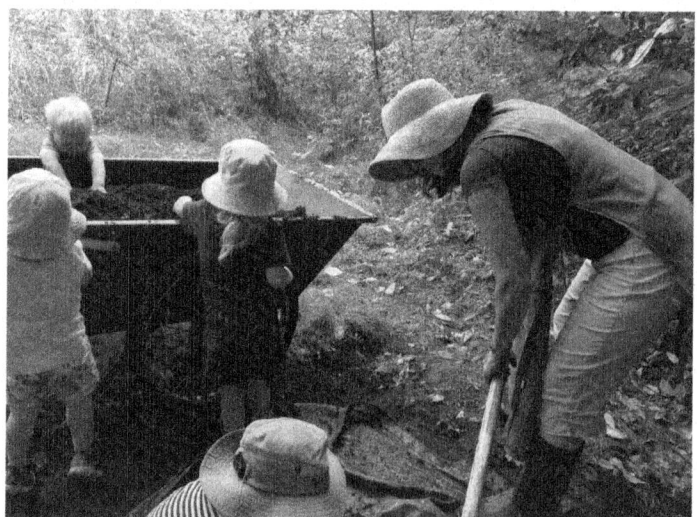

Here, the children are not imitating what the teacher is doing, yet they live into the manner in which she is working with the mulch.

the child is "held." The child is embedded into the adult's gesture of complete and devoted engagement with their work. The adult's actions are congruent with their emotions. The adult finds the work rewarding. They do not work begrudgingly. When the adult works with good body mechanics in an efficient, focused, purposeful, and confident fashion, it affords the child a chance to imitate a worthy gesture. The child will likely not imitate *what* the adult is doing, but they will imitate *how* the adult is doing it. In this way, the child can bring this same gesture to their own play activity.

When I care for my grandchildren, which I do on a regular basis, I often do some cleaning, during which time I consciously pay attention to my manner of working. I first make sure the children are cared for and settled in their play, and then I scrub the kitchen floor, for example. I personally enjoy cleaning. The children know that I am busy—that my work is important to me, that I take pride in it, and also that I am available should they need me. If they should want me, however, unless it is an urgent matter, I don't drop everything immediately. I tell them that I will finish a section of the floor, and then I will come to them. I don't rush. I am showing them that I care about what I am doing. After I finish my cleaning project, I again attend to the children's needs. I find that it goes well if I bookend my work activity with caregiving activities. If they want to help me, I give them a cloth to dry the floor with. I was recently visiting my grandchildren, and the older ones asked me if I would please scrub the floor, so that they could help me.

My Visit to Lóczy

In 2007, I travelled to Budapest for a two-week professional course at Lóczy, and also observed in the children's home, which was still in operation at that time. My visit was a life-changing experience. At Lóczy, the children did what they were capable of doing. They were not expected to do what was yet too difficult for them. As a result, the infants did not strain while moving, but rather their movements were extraordinarily fluid and graceful, and they moved a lot. They were deeply engaged with their movements and their play. As I watched the infants at Lóczy, I recognized that the environment and the practices there served to encourage the development and expression of the children's individual wills—from the very start of life. I wondered what the impact would be later in life for children who were raised in this manner. Would they have a better than average chance of avoiding obesity? Would they have less back pain and better posture because they had exercised their cores so thoroughly at the start of their lives? Would they have less incidence of depression (of which a major characteristic is compromised will activity) and other mental health issues because they had developed such feelings of agency early in life through their self-initiated activities?

During my visit, I felt a deep kinship with the Lóczy staff in our shared respect and love for the majesty of the infant's motor development. To me, there was a palpable understanding in the staff there that the self-initiated unfolding of motor development provides something essential to the process of becoming a human being.

2: Self-Initiated Gross Motor Development

Emmi Pikler's research

The previous chapter described how Dr. Emmi Pikler founded a children's home (or orphanage) for infants and young children in Budapest, Hungary, after World War II. Because the children who lived there were embedded into a stable, consistent environment, the children's home was an ideal setting for research on child development. Pikler's research differed from the usual infant research in its basic design. Typically, researchers try to prove or disprove a hypothesis. They look at an infant's behavior in a carefully crafted situation—they often consider what a child does in response to an adult's action or words, for example. Researchers rarely consider the child's spontaneous, independent deeds. In contrast, Pikler's research only involved activities self-initiated by the infants, performed over the normal course of their day. Pikler's method was purely observational, and the infants were not subject to contrived situations, as such. Pikler's desire was to simply observe, document, and study the findings in order to see what was revealed under these conditions.[1]

An extensive study, headed by Dr. Pikler, was conducted over a period of seventeen years, in which she observed the baby's self-initiated movement journey beginning with back-lying and progressing through all of the stages to standing and walking. The study involved typically developing infants and toddlers who were reared at the children's home. It explored the sequence and the timing of gross motor milestones when children are allowed free movement. The study was conducted under the uniform conditions practiced at the children's home, specifically: (1) The babies wore clothing that did not restrict their movements. (2) There was suitable space to allow for free movement. (3) They were provided with developmentally appropriate toys. (4) The adults did not teach the babies to move. (5) Building a healthy relationship between the child and the adult at the children's home was considered indispensable.[2]

Note that the results of Pikler's research may not necessarily transfer to infants raised in home settings today, because the conditions of the children's home and modern home environments are often very different. For example, in the children's home the children were rarely transported in cars, and it would be very difficult for a modern family to replicate this.

As Dr. Pikler describes the children in the study, "The 722 children stayed in the Institute between 1947–1964. They were admitted, in general, before three (premature ones four) months of age. They spent at least three months in the Institute. Of the 722 children, 393 arrived younger than two weeks of age. 199 stayed there at least till walking age. There were 591 children whose birthweights were above 2500 g (5.5 lb.), 131 under 2500 g (5.5 lb.) and 12 children's birthweights were unknown."[3] Pikler also states that "our research institute [was] founded in 1946 with [a] capacity for 70 children in residential care from 0 to 2 1/2 years of age."[4]

Dr. Pikler defined the recorded stages of the child's movement journey as follows:[5]

a) turns from back [to] the side and returns to back;

b) turns from supine [back-lying] to prone [tummy-lying]

c) turns from prone to supine, tumbles about

d) crawls [belly-crawls] (without lifting the trunk)

e) creeps [crawls] on hands and knees or hands and feet on level as well as on rising terrain

f) sits up by self[6]

g) kneels up by self and lets [self] down

h) stands up by self and lets [self] down

i) starts walking without clinging to objects

j) walks well, uses walking in everyday life for locomotion.

Note that I've revised "crawls" to "belly-crawls" and "creeps" to "crawls," above; in the Pikler literature, what we call belly-crawling is referred to as "crawling," and what we call crawling—on hands and knees—is referred to as "creeping."

Time to Reach Motor Milestones in Self-Initiated Motor Development

Let us look at the 591 children in the study whose birth weights were over 5.5 pounds. (Weights over 5.5 pounds were considered to be within normal limits.) Pikler recorded the average (mean) and the divergence (standard deviation) for each motor milestone in weeks. Pikler states that the "distribution in question approaches the normal distribution. About 70 per cent of all cases fall within one standard deviation of the mean: consequently this interval on either side of the mean indicates the characteristic time for the acquisition of each stage of motor ability."[7] As the lay reader in the United States may relate more to months than weeks, I have converted Pikler's findings into months, below, rounding ages to the nearest half month.

The research findings are organized below:[8]

- turns from back to side: 4 mos. average, with 70% from 3–5 mo.

- turns from supine to prone: 5.5 mos. average, with 70% from 4.5–6.5 mo.

- turns from prone to supine: 6.5 mos. average, with 70% from 5–8 mo.

- crawls [belly-crawls]: 9 mos. average, with 70% from 7–10.5 mo.

- creeps [crawls on hands and knees]: 10 mos. average, with 70% from 8.5–12 mo.

- sits up by self: 10 mos. average, with 70% from 9–11.5 mo.

- achieves kneeling by self: 10.5 mos. average, with 70% from 9–12 mo.

- stands up by self: 11 mos. average, with 70% from 9.5–13 mo.

- 1st steps without hanging onto furniture: 15.5 mos. average with 70% from 12.5–18 mo.

- walks with ease: 16.5 mos. average, with 70% from 14–19.5 mo.

FREE MOVEMENT FROM THE VERY START

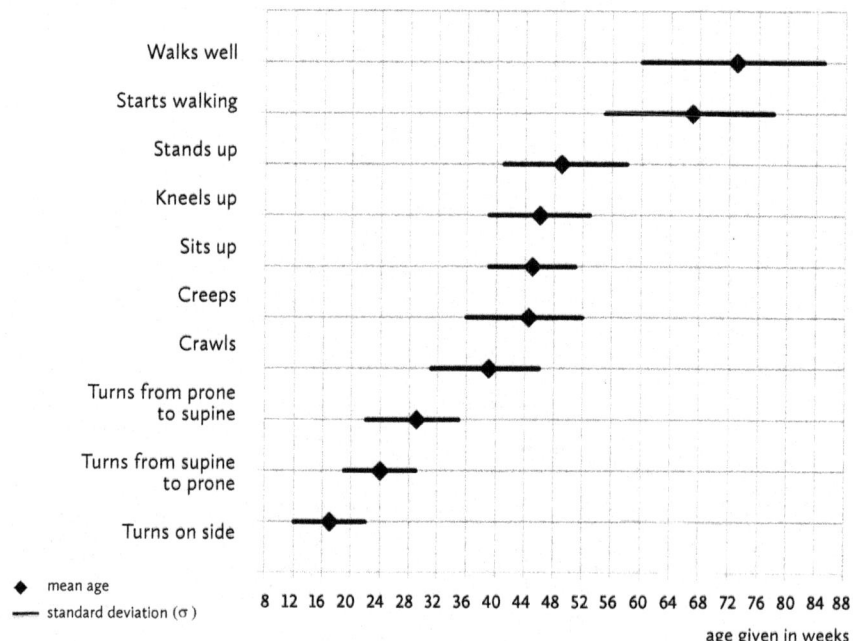

Mean age of attaining the principal stages of motor development
(591 children with normal birthweight)

Perhaps the most striking finding of Pikler's research is that if infants are allowed to negotiate the movement sequence under their own initiative, there is a wide range in the timing of each motor milestone for typically developing children. In our culture, we don't usually think of the acquisition of motor milestones in ranges. Instead, we tend to have more of a yes-no checklist mentality. For example, it is a generally held belief that infants should walk without hanging on to anything by twelve months. If this doesn't happen, many would advise intervention for the child. Pikler's research, however found that when children are allowed to reach their motor milestones through their own efforts and in their own time, on average, children take their first steps without hanging onto furniture at 15.5 months, with 70 percent of the children achieving this between 12.5 and 18 months. Note that the 70 percent range is 5.5 months—nearly half a year!

One might conclude, from initially looking at Pikler's findings, that it generally takes longer to achieve the motor milestones with the Pikler approach (where babies self-initiate their movements) than it does with the mainstream approach (adult-led, where babies are "taught" to move), but this would be like comparing apples to oranges. For example, Pikler studied and learned when the child sits up entirely through their own efforts. In the mainstream world, people count sitting up to be when a child placed in that position can maintain it. However, if you look at when a child achieves sitting by themselves, both groups of children attain the skill at the same time.

When one compares the timing of the actual skills of the two groups of children, they are remarkably similar. The children reared at Lóczy were delayed in only two stages of motor development compared to the mainstream group of children. The first stage was turning from prone (tummy-lying) to supine (back-lying). Dr. Pikler explains that the mainstream children basically had an adult-assisted head start—the mainstream children were placed on their tummies before they could get there on their own, and thus had early practice in learning to roll over onto their backs.[9]

Coming to stand was the second stage of development in which the children reared at Lóczy were delayed compared to the mainstream group of children. Dr. Pikler reasons, "The relative lateness of standing up may be related to the availability of adequate space and freedom for our children to move in it. According to our experience, children who spent practically no waking time in cots [or other restrictive devices] and have enough space for [crawling on hands and knees] show the tendency to get in vertical positions at a later time."[10] The children in Pikler's care had adequate space to crawl, and the space included interesting climbing and crawling structures (developed by Pikler and unique to the children's home at the time) along with developmentally appropriate toys for the children. These environmental factors likely played a role in the timing of the children's acquisition of standing up.

The Sequence of Self-Initiated Motor Development

In addition to the timing, Pikler's research also shows differences in the sequence between child-led and adult-led movement. In the adult-led model, as noted above, adults typically prop babies to sit before they can achieve the position by themselves. It is the general cultural expectation that babies sit at six months and crawl on hands and knees at eight months. However, according to Pikler's research—where babies are not placed into sitting but assume sitting on their own—babies may crawl before they sit up, or nearly simultaneously.

Pikler speaks specifically about the order of free motor development. She says that turning to the side and then turning from supine to prone always precede all of the other stages. She continues that there is variability, however, in the subsequent stages. "The sequence of the stages—[belly-crawling], [crawling], sitting up, kneeling up, standing up—is not stable, but kneeling up always precedes standing up; [crawling] and sitting up occur approximately at the same time. Sitting up precedes standing up in 90% of the cases. In the remaining 10%, standing up precedes sitting up or both occur at the same time."[11]

Movements Not Typically Seen in Free Movement

In self-initiated motor exploration, there are particular movement patterns that are considered atypical. Dr. Pikler noted that "Lying in [the] supine position and raising the head from the base, which is described in the majority of [conventional] publications, occurs only sporadically with us."[12] If this does occur, with the Pikler approach the caregivers try to ascertain where the movement is coming from and make the necessary adjustments in order to try and mitigate its expression. However, caregivers never force the child's head back down. It may be that the baby is not well supported when they are being picked up, carried, or held, and so they strain and lead with the head in an effort to stabilize themselves. It is particularly important to support the child's neck and head and all along their spine, so that they feel secure and do not strain or lose their balance.[13]

This pattern of leading with the head may also be seen when a baby lurches forward with their head when they are being fed on an adult's lap. The adult may need to adjust the height of their arm, so that the infant can relax into it. It may also be that when the baby is being fed, the baby is not receiving the spoon as fast as they would like, and so the child flexes their head forward. Each child has their own preferred pace, and this changes—even within one feeding. The pace often slows down as they become satiated. It is helpful to let the child determine the pace—the adult follows the child's cues for how fast they want to be fed. Another possible reason for the pattern of leading with the head is that the child is experiencing stress. In this case, one needs to explore the various factors of the child's life and try and attend to them appropriately so that the child can relax and feel more secure. When the child is lying supine, it could also be that the child is lifting their head off the surface in order to look at something. In this case, the baby can be repositioned on the floor, or the crib's placement in the room can be changed, so the baby can turn the head to their side in order to see, instead of lifting it up off the surface.[14]

Dr. Pikler describes another atypical movement. "It has also been rare for our infants to raise themselves into a sitting position from lying on [their] back by holding onto the [crib bars.]"[15] This was seen only in exceptional circumstances, such as when a child was confined to bed with an extended illness. The children typically come into sitting from the supine position by first turning to prone, transitioning to side-sit on extended arm, and then shifting into sitting on two sitz bones without supporting themselves with their hands.[16]

It is not uncommon for adults to take a baby's hands while the baby is lying on their back and pull them up to sitting in an effort to "exercise" their baby and teach them to do sit-ups.[17] Unfortunately, this is not a typical movement for babies or for young children. We can rest assured that the baby already is strengthening their abdominals in a multitude of developmentally appropriate ways through all of the free movement opportunities afforded them in the horizontal positions.

In the motor milestone literature at the time of the study, the stage of kneeling was not mentioned. However, Dr. Pikler describes that the children in her care regularly achieved kneeling and played in this position. Kneeling comes before standing up. Some children even walk on their knees, using it as a means of locomotion, however, this is not typical.

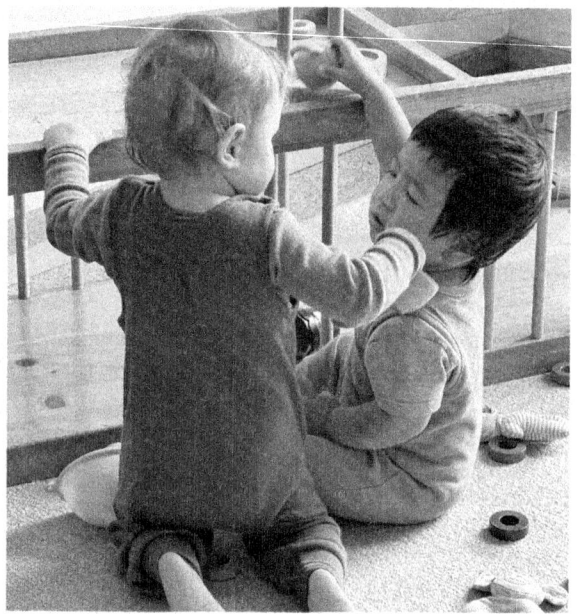

This baby is kneeling while holding on with one hand.

Reciprocal Crawling versus Sliding on the Bottom

Pikler's findings on reciprocal crawling were that "our children [crawl] regularly before walking, not only on level terrain but also climbing on stairs, on ladders, and up and down slopes."[18]

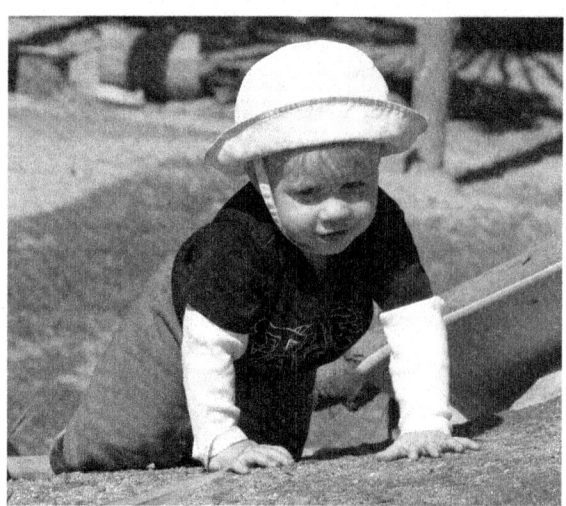

This baby is an experienced crawler, crawling long distances across the yard and up and down hills.

No children in the study performed "sliding on the bottom or sliding on bent legs in [the] sitting position."[19] This is a remarkable finding!

Pikler's study was published in 1971. When I travelled to Budapest in 2007 to study and observe at the children's home, I wondered if there was any new information regarding their experiences with crawling. When I inquired about the frequency of crawling in the children at Lóczy, I learned that typical infants who had been at Lóczy from early infancy did not always roll or belly-crawl as a means of locomotion, but they *all* crawled reciprocally on hands and knees. I explained that in the United States, it is common for children to skip reciprocal crawling and use compensatory patterns instead. My instructor, Anna Tardos, replied that there was one exception where they had had three children who used a compensatory bottom shuffling pattern exclusively. After trying to understand why, the staff realized that the floor was too slippery! Three coats of varnish had recently been applied to the wooden floor, and the infants' movements made sense in relationship to their environment. (After that, the floors got only one coat of varnish.)

I was impressed that the staff held true to their belief in the inherent capacity of the infants to direct their own motor development, and that the staff did not intervene with hands-on therapy or try to teach these children to crawl. Instead, they collectively questioned, observed, and reflected until, over time, the solution became clear.[20]

Why Do So Many Children Today Skip Reciprocal Crawling?

According to Pikler's findings, a typically developing baby who has free movement will self-initiate reciprocal crawling if they have sufficient opportunity and the environment supports this. As noted in the scenario above, the slipperiness of the floor is one determining environmental factor regarding whether a child crawls. Another factor which decreases the incidence of crawling is simply that the child is not given ample time on the floor. Additionally, there must be sufficient space and reason to crawl, e.g., in order to get something. If the space is very small and the toys are all within reach, there is no reason to crawl. Another interesting consideration is the type of footwear worn by the infant. High-top shoes that cover the ankle and have hard soles can interfere with crawling. In order to understand the effect on a baby of wearing these types of shoes, imagine yourself trying to crawl with skis on, versus crawling barefoot. Skis would not work so well for crawling. Similarly, because high top shoes limit ankle motion and are more awkward for crawling, the baby would likely proceed to pulling to stand and walking as soon as they could. The ideal situation is for babies to be barefoot at this stage of development, as this allows the most flexibility at the ankle joint. If warmth is an issue, they can wear thin, flexible, well-formed, non-slip footwear, such as socks with grippers. (For more on the footwear of babies, please see appendix 1.)

Thus far, we have discussed Dr. Pikler's work. Now, we will discuss various aspects of crawling based on the author's observations and study of crawling over many years.

Simply put, children typically skip crawling because they have skipped the stages before crawling. In order to crawl reciprocally, babies need opportunities to prepare their bodies for this complex and sophisticated movement. Babies don't have sufficient occasions for such preparation when they are not afforded free movement in the stages before crawling. This often happens because babies are placed in baby equipment that restricts their movements. When children are able to navigate their motor journey from back-lying up into standing and walking, each stage along the way, in and of itself, is valuable. In the adult-led model, some stages are considered more valuable than others, especially the vertical stages of sitting, standing, and walking. What is not generally understood is that it is not the end points of verticality that are important, but rather the means by which they are achieved. During each stage of motor development the child is developing the foundations for more sophisticated later patterns. During each stage the child is also exercising their will. When they do master a particular movement, we can imagine that they experience a feeling of satisfaction. In this way they may build up a true, well-earned self-confidence in their abilities. Their confidence comes from an inner knowing that they can accomplish something out of their own efforts, without external instruction or interventions—they come to trust themselves.

Each stage of child-led motor development is preparatory for the subsequent stages. Let us look at the preceding foundational stages for reciprocal crawling. In the Pikler approach the infant starts out in back-lying, the position which offers the most free movement. Here, the infant develops a degree of stability, and then, after they have had enough preparation, they venture into uncharted waters when they turn to their side at approximately three to five months. They may accomplish this maneuver in different ways. I have observed the following scenario to be common: the baby is lying on their back, holding onto their feet. They shift their weight slightly to the side—just enough to lose their stability—and they plop over into side-lying. In other words, initially, they may achieve side-lying with a fall, in which the body typically moves to the side as a unit—without any rotation in the spine. This type of rolling—which has no spinal rotation—is known as log-rolling. The baby practices log-rolling until they can perform it with control and with ease.

Over time, they roll to prone and back again. The next qualitative type of rolling that develops—in both supine to prone and prone to supine—is segmental rolling, a mature type of rolling involving rotation around the central axis of the spine. The baby may reach across the body with an arm or with a leg, rotating the spine in either case.

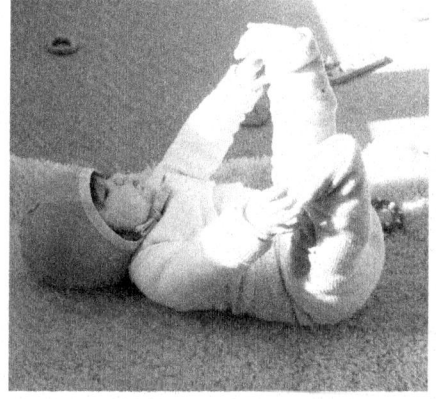 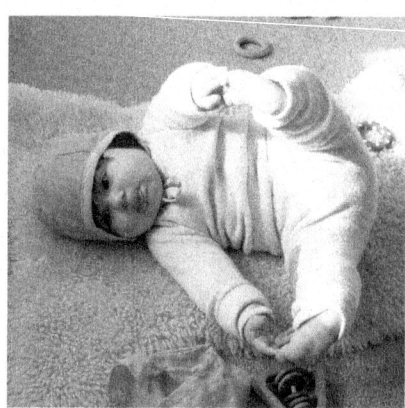

Here is an example of log-rolling, where the trunk moves as a unit, i.e., the shoulder and the hip move at the same time.

Some babies progress to rolling all the way across the floor, i.e., they use rolling as a means of locomotion. However, not all babies use rolling in this way.

As babies get more and more acclimated to the prone position, they gain stability in this position. After a while, they venture forth with belly-crawling. There are many variations of belly-crawling; for one example, the baby might pull symmetrically with the arms—both sides of the body moving in the same way—while pushing symmetrically with the toes.

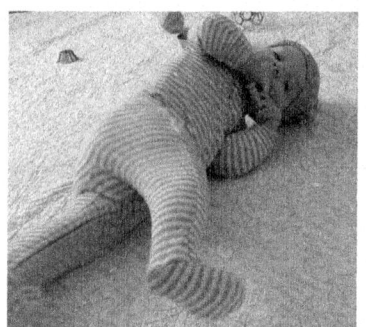 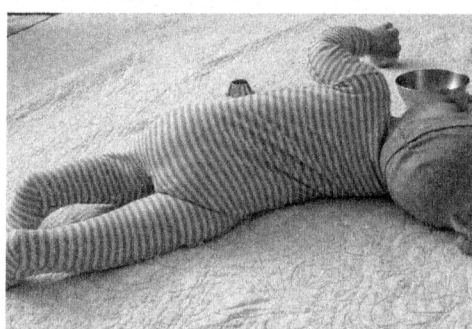

Above, left: This baby is rolling from back to tummy, leading with one leg, which causes the hip to move before the shoulder, thus employing rotation in the trunk.
Above, right: The same baby is rolling from tummy to back, leading with the head and shoulder. Note the rotation in the trunk.

For another example, the baby might pull with one arm repeatedly (an asymmetrical pattern) or they might alternate arms (a reciprocal pattern). Similarly, with the legs, they might push with one leg repeatedly or alternate legs. Over time, the child may coordinate alternating, opposing use of the arms with the legs. When this happens, the trunk has achieved counter-rotation. This is a very complex movement, whereby an

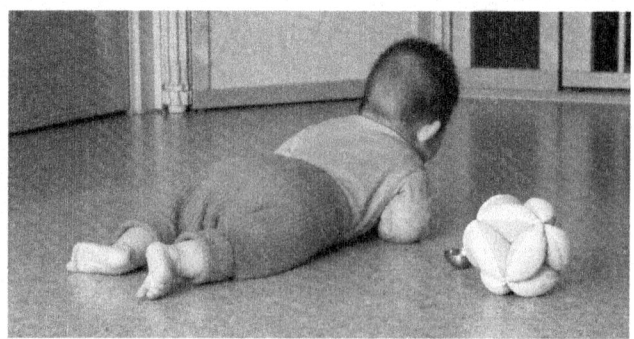

Symmetrical belly-crawling. This baby is pulling symmetrically with the arms as they belly-crawl across the floor.

arm coordinates its pulling with the opposite leg's pushing, thus integrating the arms with the legs. What is happening at the spine is also a sophisticated movement. The upper spine on one side rotates forward as the lower spine on the same side rotates backward. The upper spine moves counter to the lower spine, in a sort of "wring-out-the-dishrag" motion. This movement is also referred to as counter-rotation, or the cross-crawl pattern.

The baby progresses higher up off the surface to hands and knees, and they do so in a variety of ways. They typically start out in heel-sitting, gradually rocking forward and backward in larger excursions, until they can achieve the hands and knees position. The rocking serves to develop stability in the position.

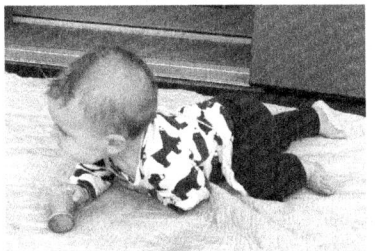 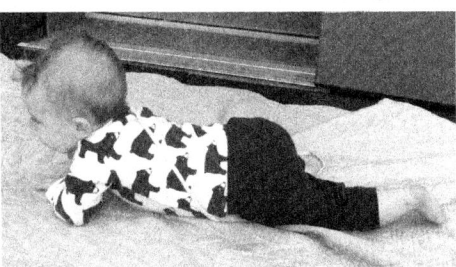

This baby is belly-crawling with a sophisticated counter-rotation pattern, where the opposite arm and leg work together.

Babies also assume the hands and knees position by rotating from side-lying on one arm into hands and knees.

After babies gain enough stability in the hands and knees position, they start to crawl. They may experiment briefly with a homolateral pattern of crawling (using the same side arm and leg together) before mastering the reciprocal pattern of crawling. About the same time that they start to crawl, they also transition from hands and knees into high side-sitting (side-sitting on an extended arm.) From high side-sitting they move into long-sitting (sitting symmetrically with the legs extended out in front.) During both of these transitions, the baby is rotating around the central axis of the spine. Here, they are perfecting the spinal rotation that they began when they first started to roll seg-

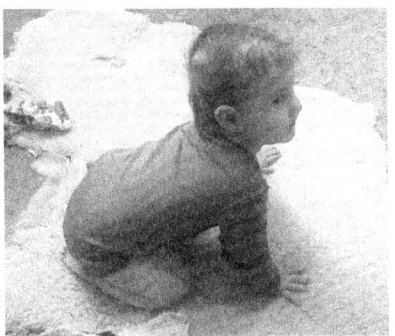 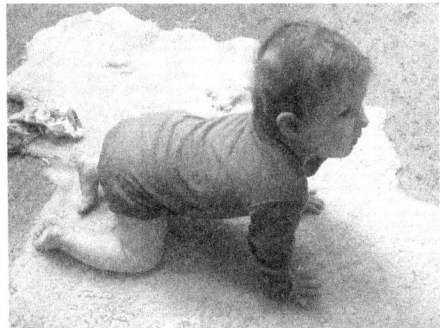

This baby is rocking forward and backward as they explore coming into the hands and knees position. They had only been rocking for a couple days when this photo was taken.

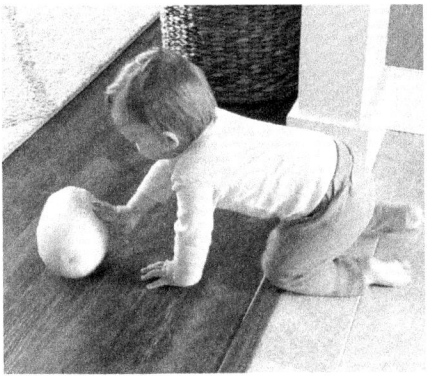 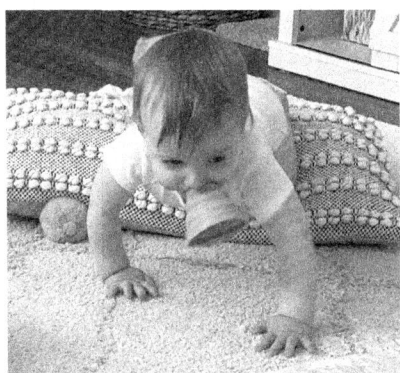

Left: This baby is an experienced crawler and is further developing their motor capacities—it takes more core stability to push the squash across the room than to simply crawl across it. Right: Crawling over firm pillows further develops the child's core stability and coordination.

mentally from back-lying to tummy-lying; now, they are up off the surface, and so the task is more challenging because it requires more balance. They also perfect their reciprocal crawling—crawling throughout the house for longer distances and typically with great speed.

FREE MOVEMENT FROM THE VERY START

During free motor exploration, by the time the baby achieves crawling, they have had a plethora of opportunities to exercise their spines in the lower horizontal positions of supine, side-lying, prone, in all of the transitional movements between these positions, and in rolling and belly-crawling. These increasingly complex motor activities have afforded the child opportunities to strengthen, elongate, and coordinate the musculature of the spine and trunk, so that when the child reaches hands and knees, they are well prepared to learn to crawl.

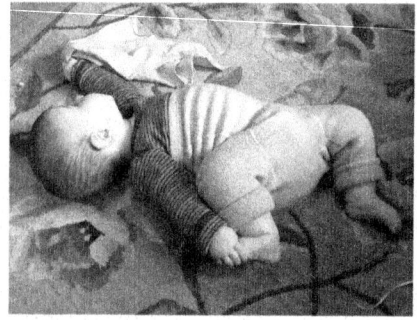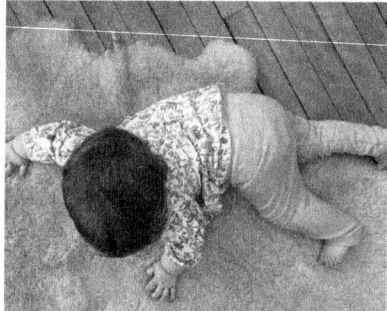

Above left: This baby is elongating the left side of the trunk as they shorten the right side.
Above right: Here, they are doing the opposite—elongating the right side of their trunk as they shorten the left side. These are just two of the many ways the trunk is exercised and developed when the child has opportunities for free movement.

If a child has not had such experiences in the lower positions, they are not well equipped to crawl, and they will likely use compensatory means of locomotion—such as bottom-sliding, side-sliding, and also bunny-hopping. In bottom-sliding, the child propels themself by sitting on their bottom with the legs bent in front of them, pressing into the floor with their heels, and symmetrically pulling themself forward.

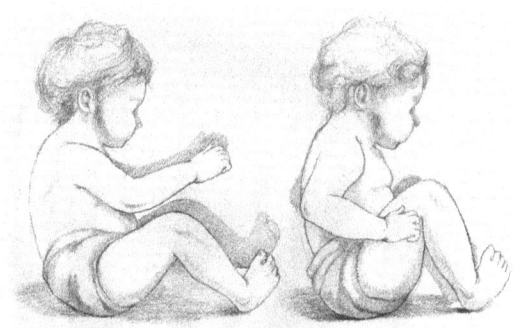

Bottom-sliding.

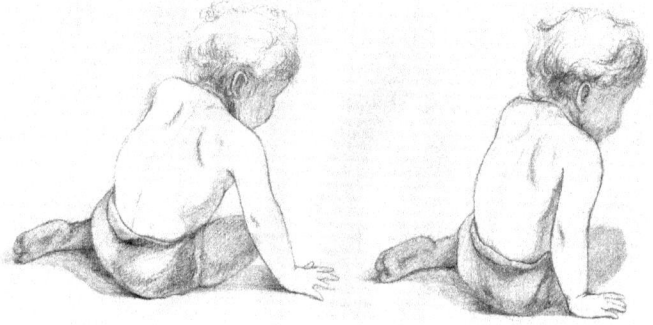

Side-sliding.

In side-sliding, the child sits on the floor with their legs flexed to the side and pulls themself to the side with an extended arm.

Bunny-hopping is a two-part motion. The child is in a crouched hands-and-knees position. First, they reach both extended arms out in front of the body and place their hands on the floor. Then they pull with the arms to draw the legs up to meet the arms. It is a sort of symmetrical hopping motion—hence the name, bunny-hopping.

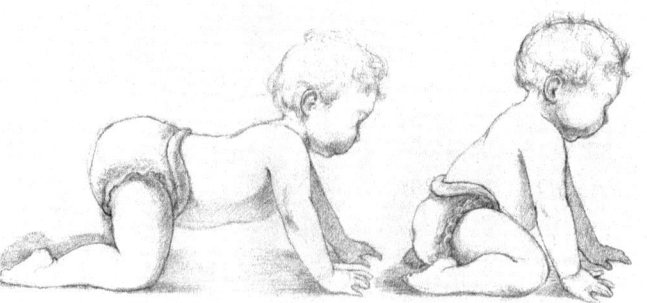

Bunny-hopping.

Chapter 2: Self-Initiated Gross Motor Development

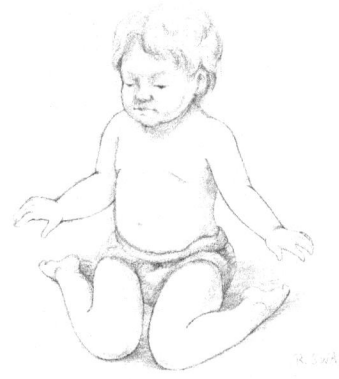

This is a classic W-sitting posture.

In all of these compensatory types of locomotion, the spine is straight—there is no rotation or counter-rotation.

When a child has skipped the lower horizontal stages, the preparatory patterns of spinal rotation and counter-rotation have not been incorporated into the child's underlying movement habits. Therefore, the child is not neurologically ready to reciprocally crawl—those patterns have not become familiar to the child. Instead, they will likely use one of the compensatory sliding or hopping patterns mentioned here. Those who use bunny-hopping are likely to have a stronger propensity to "W-sit," with the bottom placed between the legs and the legs flexed with the feet to the sides of the hips, rather than long-sit (with the legs out in front), heel-sit (with the bottom on top of the feet), or side-sit.*

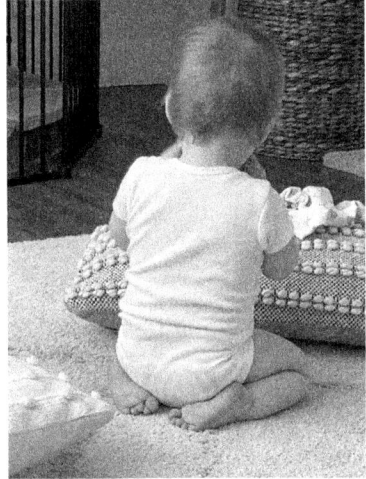 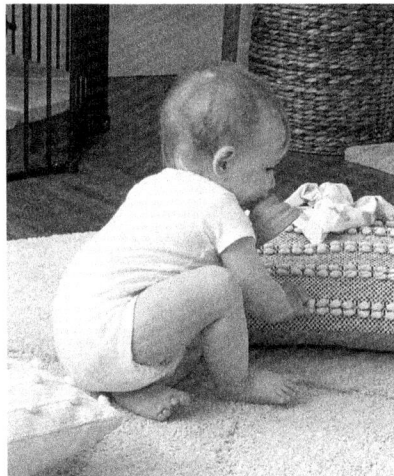 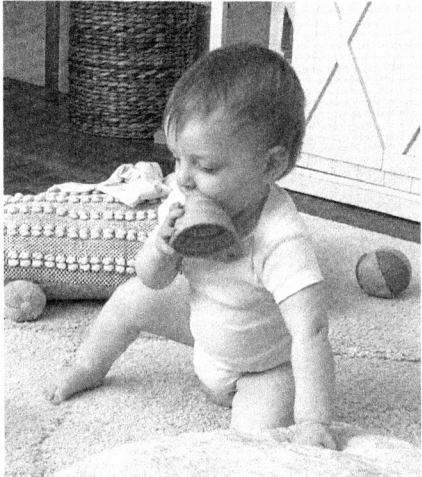

Above, left: This baby is in a narrow W-sitting position. As this is not a habitual position for them, it is not of concern. They use a variety of other positions, as depicted in the next two photos. Center: Shortly after W-sitting, this child transitioned into sitting with their feet out in front. Right: Soon after that, they assumed a low half-kneel position.

Crawling: Many Positive Aspects

In many ways, crawling paves the way for later learning. When crawling, it is very common for a child to look out across the room and then to look down at their hands. Perhaps they have a toy in one hand, or in both hands. Here, the eyes are focusing from far to near, a skill that is necessary for catching a ball or copying from the blackboard to the desk in school. The child will also look from one hand to the other as

---

* Every typically developing child will W-sit. However, there can be orthopedic concerns at the knees and hips if the child exclusively W-sits. With W-sitting, the ligaments on the inside of the knees are subject to excessive forces, and this can result in overstretching them. Additionally, in W-sitting, the position of the hips is not optimal. The hip sockets are not completely formed at birth, and the positions most conducive to proper hip formation have just the opposite pattern to that of W-sitting. The more developmentally advantageous position is called tailor sitting, often referred to in the care setting as "crisscross applesauce" sitting, where the child sits on their bottom with the knees out to the sides and the ankles crossed. We can provide the child prone to W-sitting with a small stool to sit on, as a good option. However, it is not a good idea to get into a battle of wills with the child over how they sit. If the child is exclusively W-sitting, then a referral to a pediatric physical therapist may be warranted. The W-sitting position is ultimately the result of lack of control and stability at the core, and the therapist can support the child to remedy this underlying cause.

they crawl. Here, the eyes are crossing the right-left midline, a skill that is necessary for reading, where the eyes track across the page and back again. The counter-rotation pattern of reciprocal crawling serves to integrate the upper body with the lower, the front of the body with the back, and the right side of the body with the left. The movements are registered in the brain and influence the developing anatomical pathways in the brain, ultimately serving to integrate the different parts of the brain. Also, the transitional movements from crawling to sitting serve to enhance balance. Reciprocal crawling is a unique portal for sensory integration. Specifically, when a child crawls across the floor, they are looking at objects in the room as they pass them, they are sensing the movements of their bodies, and they are keeping their balance as they do this. In this way, integration occurs between the sense of proprioception, the vestibular sense, and the sense of vision. Thus, brain development is positively impacted. Chapters 8 through 15 describe the foundational senses and sensory integration in greater detail.

Crawling and transitioning between sitting and crawling are key stages for fine motor development (described in detail in chapter 7). Like the arches of the foot, the arches of the hand are not developed at birth. Crawling serves to enliven the finer muscles of the hand and helps create its arches. When babies crawl and transition between crawling and sitting, they shift their body weight over the various parts of the hands. Bearing weight through the hands increases the proprioceptive and tactile sensory input in the hands, thus increasing the child's body scheme in this part of their body. Initially, the infant does not have a good sense of their body parts and what those body parts are doing. Crawling, especially, increases the child's awareness and subsequent coordination of their thumb. This helps the development of thumb opposition and the more complex manipulative functions of the hand. Crawling also supports the integration of several of the primitive reflexes, including the palmar grasp and the symmetrical tonic neck reflexes. (The primitive reflexes are discussed in detail in volume 2.)

All Is Not Lost if a Child Skips Crawling

Clearly, crawling is an important and unique stage of motor development. However, as Anna Tardos noted, "it is not a catastrophe if the child does not crawl."[21] Working as a pediatric physical therapist, I rarely ask a parent whether their older child crawled. I do not want a parent to feel guilty if their child did not crawl. Guilt can negatively impact the relationship between parent and child, and the relationship is paramount! I also do not want an older child to think they did something wrong when they were a baby. Indeed, knowing whether an older child crawled or not does not provide all the necessary information. I need to observe the child to see if they are currently employing the healthy movement patterns that are typically incorporated during the stage of reciprocal crawling. Perhaps the child did crawl but not long enough to sufficiently establish the movement patterns. Or perhaps the child did initially establish the movement patterns, but their movements have regressed due to excessive stress in their lives. In an older child I look to see, for example, if they are using the cross-crawl pattern, if they are focusing their eyes between near and far positions, and how they are using their hands. My emphasis is on the present—what can I do now to contribute positively to the child's motoric abilities?

If the child did skip the stage of crawling, crawling activities can be offered later, if they are developmentally appropriate. I encourage teachers and parents of preschooler and kindergarteners to get down on the floor and play crawling games with the children. A favorite children's game is London Bridge. This game can be altered such that two adults kneel and create an arch, and the children crawl through the arch instead of walking through it. We can also create inviting spaces in nature for older children to crawl through and climb on. Sculpting forsythia bushes into tunnels and caves for crawling through, and growing rhododendron "forests" for climbing create lovely outdoor living structures. Indoors, chairs, tables, and blankets can be made into tunnels for the children to crawl through. One can incorporate crawling rhythmically into the day. For example, preschool and kindergarten children can crawl down the hall to their classroom when coming in from outdoor play.

An older child may no longer be interested in crawling, and interest is vital for learning to move in a new way. For these children who skipped the stage of crawling, the components of crawling can be achieved later through other means. For example, there are other ways for a child to establish the counter-rotation pattern. Cross-country skiing, climbing, and negotiating monkey bars are excellent activities for this. Long walks can also help. One can observe that the cross-crawl pattern is taking hold when a reciprocal arm swing develops. If the family is so inclined, I encourage families to have hiking outings once a week or so, and to park at the back of the parking lot whenever they take their child shopping, to get in as much walking as possible.

Self-Initiated Motor Development in Children with Low Birth Weights

In her research paper, Dr. Pikler concluded that "The motor development of the group of children with birthweight under 2.5 kg (5.5 lb.) follows the same sequence as that of the group with higher birthweight but shows delay in time."[22] For the children whose weight was 2–2.5 kg (4.4–5.5 lb.), the delay was approximately 4–6 weeks, and it was consistent over time. "In the group with birth weight under 2 kg (4.4 lb.), the delay [was] greater and [grew] with increasing age." In other words, as development progressed, the more complex motor skills took longer for the child with the lowest birth rates to learn.[23] In general, Pikler deemed the Pikler approach to be "especially valuable" for those children with lower birth weights who were born prematurely.[24]

Faster Development Is Not Necessarily Better

Activity that takes place in the horizontal plane, before verticality is achieved, lays a strong foundation for later life. There is no need to rush the child in these stages. Dr. Pikler observed that if an infant spends a longer amount of time in a particular stage of motor development, the child explores more nuanced variations of movement in that position than does the infant who spends a shorter amount of time there and moves on to the next position more quickly. In other words, if an infant develops more slowly, they tend to penetrate the stages more deeply. Could there be good explanations for each individual child's rate of motor development that we are not aware of?

An astute observation made by Emmi Pikler illustrates this point beautifully. Pikler observed that the infants in her care whose parents had previous histories of back pain spent longer in the horizontal positions of supine, side-lying, and prone before coming into the vertical positions of sitting and standing. Indeed, these infants had more variety and more nuanced control of their movements in the horizontal positions than did the infants who moved into verticality more quickly. Movement in the horizontal plane provides abundant opportunities to strengthen the many muscles of the spine and trunk and to coordinate their use with each other—opportunities not possible in the vertical positions. One could speculate that the infants, who may have been predisposed to back pain because of their family histories, were working to prevent such pain in the future!

I have also witnessed that infants who had an especially strong manifestation of one of the primitive reflexes stay longer in lower stages of motor development. It is as if they are taking care to fully reap the benefits of a stage of development that is optimal for integrating that reflex. (The primitive reflexes will be explored further in volume 2.) Agnes Szanto-Feder, in her book *Moving with Pleasure from the Beginning*, explains that "it *varies greatly at what age different children reach the individual stages*; and furthermore, the *development pace of any given child is not necessarily steady* [emphasis in original]."[25] In other words, each stage of development does not necessarily take the same amount of time for a particular child. The child may linger in one or more of the stages.

The Pikler Approach and Slowly or Differently Developing Children

Szanto-Feder discusses the importance of free movement when a child is developing outside of the usual timetable of the gross motor milestones:

> For Pikler, autonomous activity plays an equally or even more important role in the case of slowly or differently developing children than with others. Autonomous activity in this context means that accommodating the specific child's skills and potentials ensures that they can find pleasure in moving, just like any other child; and through this, they can also gain self-confidence and learn to trust their skills and potential. ... Pikler highlighted that slowly developing children need free movement even more than their peers who are developing more quickly, in order to be able to acquire the appropriate positions to stay active in pursuing their interests.[26]

Dr. Pikler explicitly mentions the importance of the transitions for slowly or differently developing children. She says, "The transitional stages are of vital importance as they provide the preliminary conditions necessary to move on to the next stage, exactly like in the case of all the other children."[27] Dr. Pikler explained that slowly developing children were "in particular danger"—not because they were developing slowly—but because we are more likely to *hurry up* their motor development by putting them into positions that they are not yet ready for and asking them to do things for which they are not yet capable. In Pikler's experience, children who would otherwise have developed well at a slower pace and were not allowed free movement became uncertain and even clumsy in their motor skills.[28] I have witnessed similar occurrences.

Henry David Thoreau expresses this same idea in his beautiful, poetic style. He says, "I am struck by the fact that the more slowly trees grow at first, the sounder they are at the core, and I think that the same is true of human beings. We do not wish to see children precocious, making great strides in their early years like sprouts, producing a soft and perishable timber, but better if they expand slowly at first, as if contending with difficulties, and so are solidified and perfected. Such trees continue to expand with nearly equal rapidity to extreme old age."[29]

In this passage, Thoreau describes the slower development of very young trees as if they were "contending with difficulties." This is remarkably similar to the situation of young infants. At birth they are essentially bound to the face of the earth—they are subject to the unyielding forces of gravity, for which they initially have very little means of coping. In their unique motor journeys to reach verticality, they engage in an archetypal battle with gravity. Along the way they develop capacities that can only be garnered by overcoming the resistance of the earth's gravity. We do not want to take away this challenge from the baby, for when we allow them to do this important work on their own, they will emerge victorious and strengthened for life.

When I observed at Lóczy in 2007, I witnessed a couple of children who had special needs. I spoke at length with the head pediatrician about them. She told me they had been admitted to the children's home as very young infants and were reared according to the Pikler approach—just like any other child at Lóczy—but perhaps with even more attention to detail and adherence to the fundamental principles of the Pikler approach. One of the children had Down's syndrome. Though he was developing slowly, I have never seen a child with Down's syndrome developing so beautifully. His posture and the quality of his movements and alignment were remarkable, and he was very active in his play. I did not see the typical low muscle tone, with resultant wide base of support and sprawling postures, that are so characteristic of children with this condition. I asked the head pediatrician about previous children who had Down's syndrome and had been reared at Lóczy. She told me that their movements were of similar quality to those of this child.

The children reared at Lóczy were not hurried to develop in any way. Pikler states, "Let us not force the infant. Let us provide well for [them], but let us not disturb the slow, steady process that has its own rhythm and course with every child." She also explains, "the most essential is not 'what' the baby can already do, but 'how' [they do] what [they do.]"[30] The leisurely, unpressured pace permeating the atmosphere of Lóczy was beautifully expressed by Anna Tardos when she said, "What's the rush? We have our whole lives to be vertical!"[31]

When Is Intervention Warranted?

Pikler trusted that infants inherently know what they need to do, how they need to do it, and how fast they need to proceed. Pikler's trust in the wise infant was not blind trust, however; she also relied on her ability to make nuanced qualitative observations of the child's movements. There are times when intervention is indicated, including when a child is manifesting obvious asymmetry, abnormal muscle tone, perseveration of movement without subtle changes in the movement, or when the child's movements are not progressing over time. For example, if the child's motor development is clearly not progressing, it might be that the child doesn't have the cardiac capacity to do so—perhaps they have an underlying heart condition. If the child is showing asymmetry in the legs or not using one leg, it could be that there is a congenital hip condition. If there is spasticity (high muscle tone), there may be neurological involvement. In my experience, if there is neurological involvement, intervention is warranted. I would recommend a referral to a pediatric physical therapist, although one often needs to start with the primary care provider, depending on the insurance.

Other Experts Speak about Motor Development Timing

Dr. Michaela Glöckler and Dr. Wolfgang Goebel offer interesting commentary regarding the timing of normal development: "The question is often put to us as to what is 'best' in terms of a normal development. This we cannot answer in a general way even if we wished to, because all human beings, unlike animals, go through an individual personal development. This development, seen spiritually, always swings between a too early and a too late. To do the right thing at the right time is the highest art of living, and every human being inclines towards this ideal whether consciously or unconsciously."[32]

It is interesting to ponder why the human being's development is so extended, compared to that of animals. In another passage, Glöckler and Goebel state, "When we compare the rate of development of different animals, we discover that the faster an animal develops, the more its abilities are bound to its physical organs. The slower the development, the more these abilities can be extended by processes of learning. Because the human being has to learn everything that makes an individual into a human being, there is potential to extend all these attributes."[33] They go on to say that as a result of the extended process of human development, we acquire "the ability to keep learning all through life, that is to say, to become freer."[34]

3: Qualitative Movement Findings from Pikler's Research

Dr. Pikler's extensive research on self-initiated movement conducted over a seventeen-year period at the orphanage (or children's home) in Budapest was the topic of the previous chapter. The timing and sequence of the milestones of unhindered motor development along with movements that are not typically seen in this type of motor development were explored. In this chapter, we will delve into some of the study's more nuanced qualitative movement findings. We will explore the sensory component of sensorimotor development; the development of the child's sensing capacities is a crucial factor for the manifestation of coordinated, fluid movement. We will also address tummy time and plagiocephaly (misshapen heads). Much of this chapter's discussion is supported by *Moving with Pleasure from the Beginning* by Agnes Szanto-Feder, who was, herself, a "Pikler baby" and became an expert in the Pikler approach.

Harmonious Movement

In perhaps the most notable finding of her research, Dr. Pikler describes the children as having *harmonious movement*. In 2007, I visited the children's home, and I saw this harmonious movement firsthand. When I observed the babies and very young children, I was in awe of the grace, beauty, and efficiency of their movements. I found their balance, coordination, and posture to be extraordinary. Their movement possibilities were vast; they were very active and well acquainted with transitional movements—that is, they did not remain in a few static positions, but instead moved in and out of positions easily. They appeared to move with joy. I did not see nearly the degree of drooling, low tone in the trunk, wide bases of support, compensatory high shoulders and stiffness, retention of primitive reflexes, delayed balance, and other movement challenges that I so often see in "typically developing" children in the United States.

Describing harmonious movement in more detail, Pikler says:

> In this way, the infant is generally able to move and coordinate all [their] muscles with dynamic balance while learning new motor skills. Harmonious movement is typical for [them; they] do not move rigidly or spasmodically. This is contrary to the customary course of motor development in which the children first learn to keep a new posture which they are unable to adopt yet and keep it but with an inappropriate coordination. When they learn to move in a new way, they do it spasmodically, rigidly, with the aid of the adult or instrument. Only later are they able to correct, more or less, the inappropriate performances.[1]

When we place babies into positions that they are not yet ready for—which is the typical practice in the United States—we set them up to move rigidly and stiffly, rather than with ease and grace. Then, later, they must overcome their initial stiffness and awkwardness. In other words, placing babies into positions that they cannot yet achieve on their own creates an avoidable hindrance for the child.

Dr. Pikler reports the manner in which the babies progress through the gross motor sequence when they are given opportunities to self-direct their movements. She says that the children "first learn to assume a new posture, and only after this to stay in it or, starting from it, to experiment with movements."[2] As they experiment with movements within the new position, they master that position and prepare themselves for the next position. In fact, "The child practices preparatory motor actions for several weeks. [They] practically [prepare themself] for the new movement before trying to attain a new posture or perform a new motion."³ In this way, the baby feels safe as they progress through the motor sequence.

Let us consider a specific scenario. Perhaps the baby rolls from supine (or back-lying) to their side for the first time. At this point the child is not yet comfortable or acclimated to side-lying, and so they do not remain in the position for long. Instead, they return to the previous position of supine where they can move freely and feel more comfortable. However, they do return to side-lying—infrequently at first, and then more frequently. They gradually develop the motor skills to stay in the position for longer periods. Over time, they develop ease of movement within the new side-lying position, and they will stay there and play. The child has sole control over how frequently and for how long they negotiate the new position.

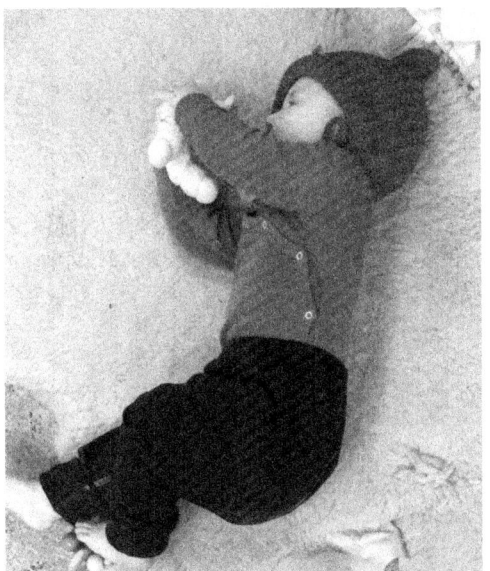 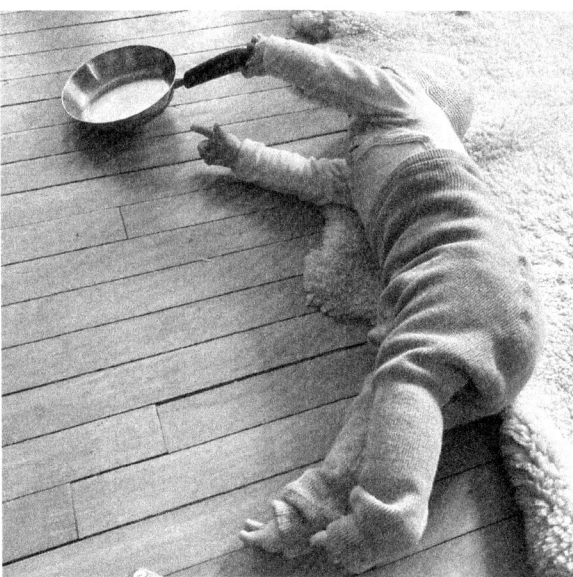

Above, left: This child is relatively new to the side-lying position. They are practicing maintaining the position and moving in and out of it. Above, right: Here, the same child is older and more experienced in the side-lying position. Their legs are straighter and more in line with the trunk. Thus, they have a narrower base of support, which requires a higher level of balance. They maintain the position for an extended period and play with a relatively large and heavy skillet. This takes considerable motor control and core stability. They are aligning the level of difficulty of activity with their level of ability.

When they first assume a new position, they are essentially *moving at the edge of their ability*, and so it makes sense that they would initially only want to be there infrequently and for short periods. For example, it is not uncommon for a baby who is primarily playing in prone on elbows and starting to belly-crawl to momentarily assume the higher position of prone on extended arms, and then go right back down to play in prone on elbows. When I was learning to ride the unicycle several years ago, I too was at the edge of my ability. I practiced as long as I felt comfortable, and then I stopped. I was listening to the sensations from my body, and responding accordingly. When I got tired, I didn't feel as secure in my ability to balance, and I stopped. If I had been forced to practice longer than my tolerance level, it would have likely been an unfortunate and unpleasant experience for me. Perhaps I would not have wanted to ride the unicycle any longer. Having someone else dictate the duration of my practicing on the unicycle would have likely taken away my joy in learning to ride it.

The Baby Seeks Out Comfortable and Economical Positions

When the baby is mastering a new position or learning a new motor skill, they are similarly receiving sensations from their bodies, *perceiving* those sensations at an unconscious level, and using those sensations to inform their movements. Dr. Pikler observes that babies who are allowed to direct their own movements "accompany play activity with manifold postures and motions, always trying to attain the most comfortable and economical one."[4] In other words, they use the sensations from their bodies to achieve comfortable and biomechanically sound positions, and they adjust their postures very frequently in order to do this. In fact, as Agnes Szanto-Feder states, "When a young child is happy and satisfied, and has the opportunity, they *move almost constantly* during their waking hours! This is only possible if they are not [restrained with baby equipment] and not confined to a seat, if their clothing does not restrict the free movement of their limbs, and if they have enough space. If they have the opportunity to do what they want, they will be active in their own way, in accordance with their taste, mood, current shape, and age."[5] I have also observed that children who are self-directed in their movements "move almost constantly" when they are awake, and, I might add, they often then go to sleep easily and peacefully afterward.

The baby's sensory systems are still developing, and so it is even more important that the baby attends to their bodily sensations than it is for a mature adult. When we place a child in a position that they cannot get out of, we hamstring this developing sensory feedback loop for the child. They are stuck in the "too difficult" position. They feel uncomfortable in it, but are unable to do anything about their discomfort. They strain to maintain the new position, and they learn to move with excessive tension—without a balanced, harmonious muscle tone. Unfortunately, this becomes "normal" movement for them, and, as Pikler states above, "Only later are they able to correct, more or less, the inappropriate performances."[6]

Feeling Safe—An Essential Condition of Free Movement

In the Pikler approach, the periods of free movement are preceded by caregiving activities in which there is a respectful dance of warm, affirming interaction between child and adult. The adult is attuned to the child's needs and communications—whether verbal or nonverbal. The child feels seen and met and therefore is increasingly expressive. There is a sensitive connection developing between child and adult.

These types of qualitative interactions are optimal situations, whereby the child can come into a state of regulation known in polyvagal theory as the *ventral vagal state*. In the ventral vagal state, the person feels safe. They are calm, regulated, able to connect with others, and ready to engage.[7] Thus, the caregiving activity prepares the child neurologically for the more independent period of free movement. A child who has been cared for in this manner will be able to play, whereas a child who has been handled more roughly will be less able to play, because they have not been neurologically prepared. Successful free play is dependent upon respectful, sensitive caregiving. Similarly, self-initiated movement periods support the caregiving activities. In free movement periods, the child explores what they can

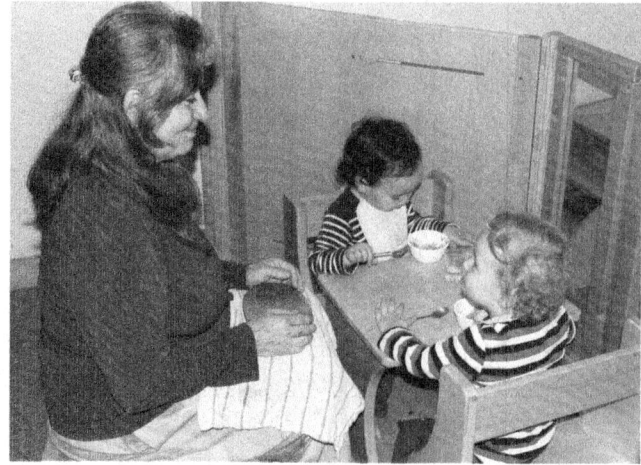

During this caregiving experience at the feeding bench, one can perceive the developing relationship between the caregiver and child, as seen by the gaze between them.

do on their own. They develop their own capacities as an independent being. In this way they are strengthened, and then more able to participate during the caregiving activities as a unique and distinct partner.

Because of the caregiving experience, the child enters into free play time feeling safe. They continue to feel safe while they are moving, because they do what they are capable of doing. The adult does not ask them to perform a motor activity of which they are not yet capable; for example, the adult does not place the child into a position that they have not yet achieved through their own efforts. Children feel unsafe in these positions that are too difficult for their current stage of balance, where they are at risk of falling. As noted earlier in the chapter, the child engages in preparatory movements before they proceed to a new position, and they alone are the best judge of when they are sufficiently prepared and ready to move on to a new position. Thus, babies who are allowed to self-initiate their own motor development move into a new position *when* they are safe in that position, and also when they *feel* safe in it. They come to rely on their own sensations, and to trust their own judgement.

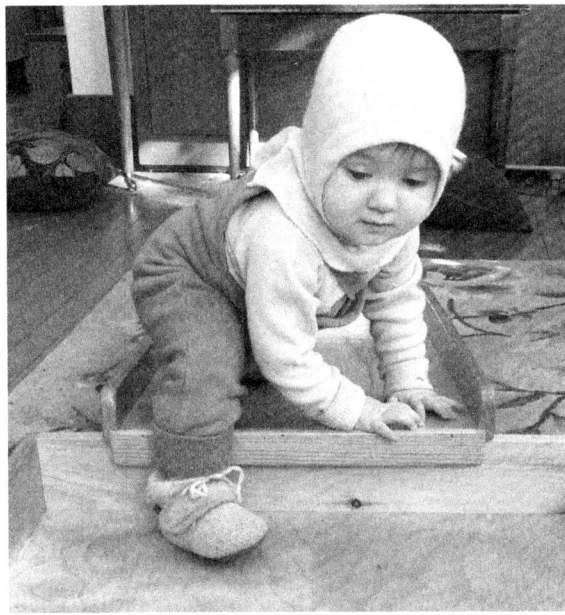

This child is a beginning walker. They successfully walked up the incline that was placed next to the Pikler box, but then got down on hands and knees to crawl into the box. Here, they sensed that they did not yet have sufficient balance in standing to be able to step down off the incline into the box. They were safe and appeared to feel safe throughout the maneuver.

Agnes Szanto-Feder describes children who are reared with the Pikler approach as "skillful, harmonious, careful, and safe."[8] She continues, "At their own level of development, they can be considered competent insofar as they are able to be active since they continuously feel in control of their own movements; and *before, during, and after the movement, they feel perfectly safe* [emphasis added]. One direct consequence of this is that the child has the opportunity to play continuously, persistently, and attentively."[9]

An essential feature of self-directed movement is that the child be given the conditions to be able to complete any initiated movement at any stage of their motor development without losing their sense of security; they should not feel they are in danger as they progress through any motor sequence.[10] Furthermore, Szanto-Feder writes, "If children's motor development took place freely, i.e., based on their own initiative, no 'disruption' will be experienced in their *need to perceive a safe posture*, not even after having learned to walk. This means that the adoption of postures and the performance of movements will remain harmonious and secure: *the children will want to feel safe*. ... They will remain cautious when discovering new things and will not forget to be careful [emphasis added]."[11]

A. Jean Ayres and Feeling Safe

From our discussion of the child's feelings of safety during the caregiving activities and during free motor periods, we can infer that, under the Pikler approach, the child's ability to perceive that they are safe is crucial for the development of harmonious movement. Now let us turn our attention to the relationship between feeling safe and the child's developing sense of balance. According to A. Jean Ayres, founder of the sensory integration movement:

> *Our relationship to gravity is our most important source of security* [emphasis added]. The gravitationally insecure child probably feels that any body movement might send [them] hurling off into [outer] space. A little bit of movement may make [them] feel 'spacey' or 'all spaced out.' One person, after a movement experience that most people would not find uncomfortable, said, 'I felt as though I were leaving the earth and I would never get back!' There is no more primal threat. . . . If the child-earth relationship is not secure, then all other relationships are apt to be less than optimal.[12]

When we experience this "primal threat" of being at risk of losing our balance, as Dr. Ayres describes it, we go into a neurological condition of fight or flight. When we are in this self-protective state, we are dysregulated, and our capacities for successful, pleasant encounters with the world are drastically reduced. This is not what we want for our babies!

Agnes Szanto-Feder also comments on balance, and her thoughts concur with those of Dr. Ayres. Szanto-Feder says, "We only act when we are balanced (mostly without even being aware of it); more precisely, we simply cannot act if we are not or do not feel we are balanced."[13] We can infer that human beings have a fundamental need to feel balanced *in order* to move and act freely in the world.

How Do We Support the Child to Feel Safe During Their Movements?

If, as Dr. Ayres claims, "Our relationship to gravity is our most important source of security," and we want our babies to feel secure, then it makes sense that we wouldn't place them in positions where they do not have the ability to balance.[14] The child is capable of balancing in a position if they have acquired that position through their own initiative; they have prepared themselves for the new position during the slow buildup to achieving it. As a result of this self-directed process, they are ready to come into the new position and can do so without feeling insecure.

The adult must use common sense in providing an environment for the baby that is safe. We don't want them to get hurt! However, this does not mean that we should "overprotect" the child so that they never fall. If we were to do this, we would short-circuit the child's sensory feedback loop. Dr. Pikler advises that it is best if we let the infant learn from their own movement experiences. If the infant experiences a bump two or three times, they will naturally prevent a subsequent bump. It is not helpful to protect them from every bump. "If we were to protect our children at this young age from all the little but uncomfortable bumps we would really bring them into much greater danger in the future."[15]

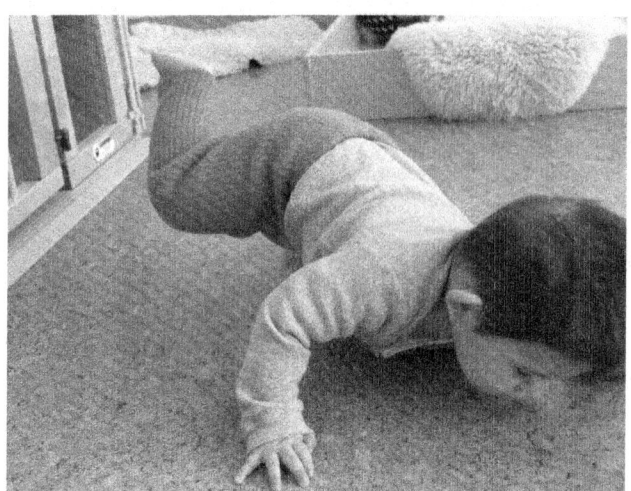
This child took a tumble when crawling. This is an example of a fall that is common and of low risk.

The child needs to learn how to fall safely. "Though the children are very mobile and courageous and fall fairly often, only one fracture has occurred in the Institute since its establishment in 1946. This happened to a child who did not go through [their] gross motor development at the Institute as [they] could walk when admitted."[16] The ability to fall safely contributes to the child's feeling of security during movement.

A Balance between Flexor and Extensor Muscle Groups

We opened this chapter with Dr. Pikler's observations about the harmonious movements of the children in her care. Now, from my point of view as a pediatric physical therapist, let us examine some additional observations about harmonious movements.

A characteristic of harmonious movement is that there is a synergistic relationship between opposing muscle groups. As an example, let us consider the two main opposing muscle groups of the trunk. The flexor muscles are located on the front side of the body. When the arms, fingers, legs, and toes flex, they bend or curl—as in a biceps curl. When the trunk flexes, it tucks up into a ball. The extensor muscles are on the back side of the body. When the trunk extends, it arches back. When the arms, fingers, legs, and toes extend, they straighten out.

The extensors on the backside of the body are an inherently larger group of muscles, and so they have an advantage over the flexors at birth. For example, in the newborn, the head is characteristically extended (and rotated to either side.) Here, the extensors of the neck are dominating, and so the head is tilted back. Thus, the flexors must play catch-up in order to balance out the body's initial bias toward using the extensors. The head of an infant is relatively large and heavy. Initially, it is difficult for them to control their head in the vertical positions. Because the head is supported in supine (or back-lying), the best position for the infant to exercise and develop the strength of the flexors is in supine. Here, the baby learns to tuck the chin and to hold the head in the middle of the body. Thus, in supine, the head has good opportunity to come into a balanced position, with neither too much extension nor too much flexion. The baby continues to experiment with balancing out the activity of the neck musculature in all of the subsequent developmental positions.

In the young infant, in addition to the neck, the trunk is also predisposed to extension, because the extensor muscles on the back side are bulkier than are the flexors (abdominal muscles) on the front side. We see this dominance of extensor activity when the baby arches their back in back-lying and side-lying.

The photo below is a classic example of a baby employing a pattern of total trunk extension: Two babies were playing in the same part of the room. One baby started banging a toy on a nearby wooden structure. The second baby was positioned facing away from the first baby, and noticed this unusual sound. As she hadn't yet begun to roll, she arched her back in a total extension pattern in order to look behind her. This was a good strategy for this situation and for this stage of development. It is commonly seen. When she gains more flexor control and is faced with a similar situation, she will very likely roll over to look instead of arch.

The best position for the abdominals to become activated and strengthened is supine. We can recognize the activity of the abdominals when the baby lifts their arms up in the air in supine, waves them around, and plays with toys there. The abdominals are activated to a higher degree when the feet come up in the air in supine. Kicking also activates the abdominals. Babies kick with their legs high in the air—symmetrically and reciprocally—and they kick with their legs down closer to the surface. They hold

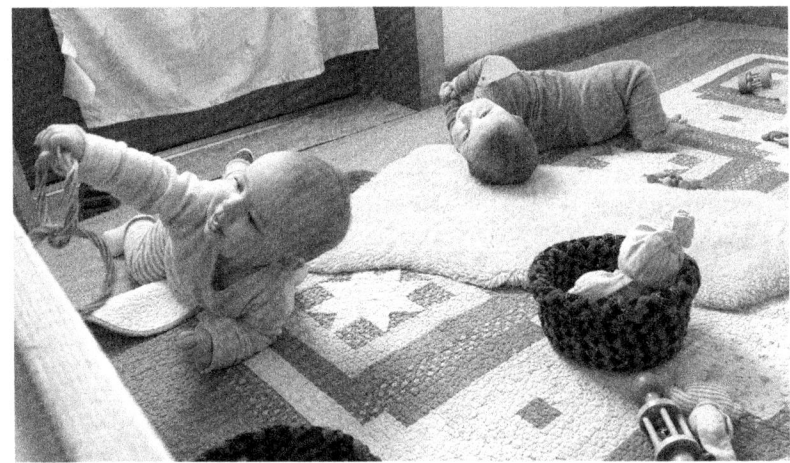

The baby on the right is in total trunk extension.

their legs in the air with and without hanging on to their feet with their hands. They hold toys between their feet and move them around. They leave their feet in the air for extended periods of time, and shift their weight from side to side. I have also seen babies lift their legs in the air, moving them symmetrically out to the side and back to center again, in a clapping sort of maneuver. All of these activities in supine are strengthening the abdominals. The baby looks like they are doing a Pilates core workout!

The next position in the developmental sequence is side-lying, where there are excellent opportunities for the flexors and extensors to begin to work together. Later, rolling necessitates a more sophisticated coordination of the flexors and the extensors. In the first part of the roll, the flexors initiate the roll. Then the flexors must back off and work evenly with the extensors during the side-lying portion of the roll. The extensors finish off the roll. Here we see the exquisitely choreographed interplay between these two muscle groups.

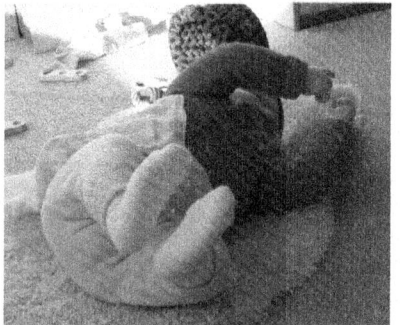

In this photo, the flexors are the prime movers to initiate the roll.

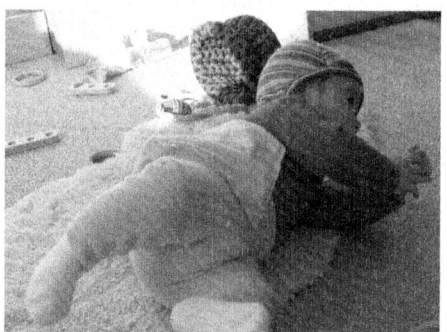

Midway through the roll, the baby is using both the flexors and the extensors in a balanced fashion.

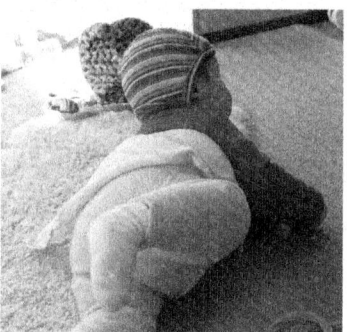

To complete the roll, the extensors are the predominant muscle group.

Experiences in the horizontal positions provide optimal opportunities for the development of a balanced, coordinated use of these two foundational muscle groups. Thus, when the child reaches the vertical positions of sitting and standing, they are well prepared and their posture reflects this. It is not surprising that the children reared at Lóczy were recognized for their beautiful, upright postures.

A Complex Coordination of Muscle Tension

Whenever we move, the tension in the various muscle groups of the body makes ever-changing adjustments. For example, when we bend our arm, the biceps contract and shorten, and in similar measure the opposing muscle group, the triceps, relax and lengthen. When the two groups work in a finely graded, complementary fashion, smooth, fluid movement follows. Szanto-Feder cites Julian de Ajuriaguerra[*] in describing this phenomenon as a "kinetic melody."[17] This happens at an unconscious level via

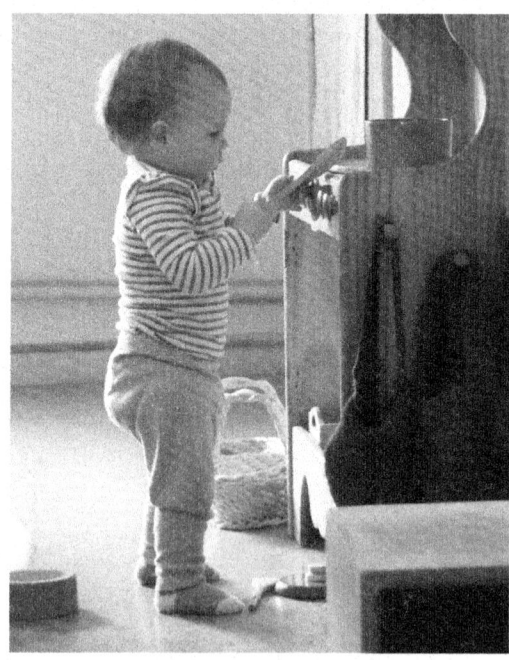

Note the beautiful, erect posture of this child, who has been raised according to the Pikler approach.

[*] Julian de Ajuriaguerra (1911–1993) was a Spanish-French neuropsychiatrist and psychoanalyst who wrote extensively on pediatric psychology.

a sensory feedback loop. Thus, the length and tension of the muscle fibers are constantly being adjusted for coordinated movement to manifest.

When babies are placed prematurely into positions that they cannot move into or out of by themselves, the positions are too difficult for them. This happens when we turn them onto their tummies, sit them up, or stand them up before they can get into these positions of their own accord. They can't move and play within the position, and they can't balance there. Instead, they tense up and "hold on for dear life." Consequently, coordinated interplay between the opposing muscle groups does not develop well. One muscle group becomes tight with overuse, while the opposing muscle group becomes overstretched. This interferes with the development of ease-filled, harmonious movement. From a physiological point of view, it is helpful to understand that muscles operate most effectively in a certain range of their length. If the muscle fibers get too lengthened or too shortened, their ability to generate effective force is compromised. Additionally, Ajuriaguerra proposes that "excessive muscle tension and spasmodic muscle contractions are *unpleasant* negative experiences for the child [emphasis in original]."[18] It seems reasonable that this would be the case, when we consider the neck and shoulder discomfort that we have all likely felt when we have had excessive muscle tension in the musculature of these areas. Hence, is it helpful to pick up, carry, lay down, and handle infants so their bodies have enough support for them to feel secure. It is also helpful to refrain from placing children into positions in which they don't have the motor control to feel secure. When babies feel secure, they don't tense up. When babies move out of their own initiative, they don't strain. Instead, they practice moving with ease—this becomes their normal, habitual way of moving, and they compose beautiful "kinetic melodies."

The Importance of the Supine Position for the Development of Healthy Movement

Szanto-Feder describes the initial time spent in supine as "vital" and foundational for later harmonious movement.[19] She notes that there are ramifications if the child is not afforded the full benefit of the supine position: "If we ignore the peculiarities of this earliest age—especially if we put children in a prone position from a neonatal age or we put them in a chair, thereby limiting movement—their motor development will progress differently."[20] She explains that Dr. Pikler placed newborns on their backs. This was the only position known by the child (except perhaps during brief instances during caregiving) until they turned—out of their own volition—to the side and then on to prone. In supine, newborns have more possibilities to move than in any other position. They can move in an unhindered manner here because they do not have to manage the weight of their head and their body—something they are not yet able to do without straining. The supine position offers the most possibility for the newborn to look around at their environment, and this includes looking at their primary caregiver. Here, the child can easily turn their head in every direction in order to orient visually and auditorily to what is going on in the room. They can locate the adult visually, and then try and draw the adult's attention to them when they want to. Placing an infant in back-lying also affords the optimal condition for the adult to see and communicate with the child.

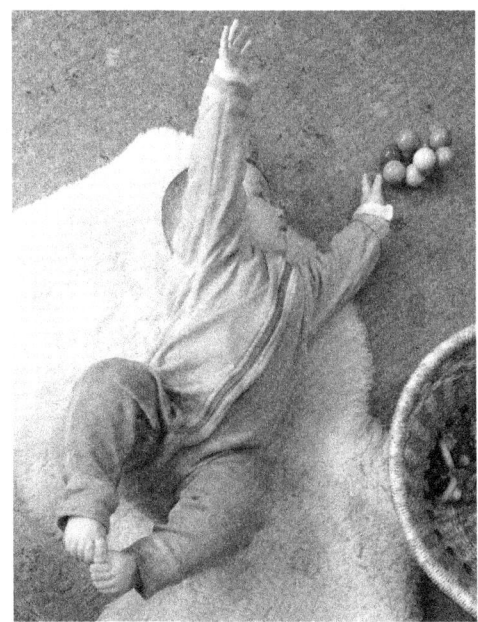

This baby is receiving significant proprioceptive input as they stretch to reach for a toy.

Additionally, the supine position sets the stage for optimal proprioceptive development. Proprioception is the sense that gives us information about what our muscles and joints are doing; because of this sense, we know the positions and

43

movements of our body segments (for example, we know that our fingers are bending or straightening without having to look at them).

The supine position affords the most possibilities for the young infant to move, and to *sense* their movements (at an unconscious level.) As described throughout this chapter, the sensing component of sensorimotor development is a critical factor for the development of healthy movement. Because the sense of proprioception is not fully developed at birth, the infant needs to see their arms and hands in order to help recognize what they are doing. The supine position affords more visual access to the arms and hands than does the prone position, because when a young infant is placed in prone, the arms are often tucked up underneath them. In supine the conditions are optimal for the child to move their arms and hands in all three dimensions of space and to see this movement. Hence, it is more possible for the infant to integrate visual and proprioceptive input, thus positively influencing brain development.

An Additional Attribute of the Supine Position

The supine position affords another valuable opportunity for the infant—the opportunity to even out mild asymmetries in the shape of the skull. Mild asymmetry is not uncommon with vaginal deliveries. The Mayo Clinic describes greater movement between the skull bones of the newborn than between those of the adult. The skull bones of the newborn are still growing. They are smaller than those of the adult, not only in literal size but also relative to the size of the infant's head; there are spaces between them (known as fontanels) that we don't see in the adult skull. This results in subtle movement of the skull bones, which then accommodates the rapid growth of the brain in the early months. It also helps the baby fit through the tight vaginal space during vaginal births. This can result in a head that is shaped "unevenly," but which usually rounds out over time.[21]

The infant's head can also change shape after birth if the infant spends time lying in one position for "too long." This can occur after the initial birth-induced skull asymmetry has resolved. This is known as positional molding or positional plagiocephaly.[22]

Certainly, when plagiocephaly is marked, consultation with a medical provider is warranted. Plagiocephaly is often accompanied by tight neck musculature on one side, known as torticollis or wry neck. Much can be done to prevent and avert mild conditions of positional plagiocephaly and wry neck from worsening—and, under the right conditions, mild conditions can resolve. The key factors appear to be the degree of mobility of the infant and the type of surface the infant is placed on. Additionally, one can carry an infant and strategically lay them down in positions whereby their interest will be drawn to one particular side, and then they will likely turn their head to that side. In this way the shape of the head and the tightness of the neck can be favorably impacted. For example, one can place a baby in a Pikler box, open side up, on top of the kitchen table, so the child's interest will be drawn to where the action is in the kitchen. They will volitionally turn to look to that side, thus actively stretching out the tight side. (The Pikler box is described in appendix 1.)

In response to a 2013 study on positional plagiocephaly by Dr. Ariane Cavalier, Szanto-Feder observes:

> As it turns out from their study, the back part of infants' heads will only flatten to a significant extent if they are limited to passivity and immobility for extended periods in their crib, baby carrier, or [car seat]. Alert and active children, raised on their back and in the spirit recommended by Pikler from the beginning, move a lot, especially move and turn their head a lot in all directions. Their head might indeed be a little flatter on one side, depending on which side they turn their head to while asleep; but this is reduced by the continuous "massaging effect" their head experiences when awake. The flatness of the skull will only be pronounced in the case of children restricted to being immobile.[23]

It is not uncommon for infants to have slightly misshapen heads, and many times these conditions resolve, especially when the child is reared according to the Pikler approach from the beginning of life. In the Pikler

Chapter 3: Qualitative Movement Findings from Pikler's Research

approach, infants are placed in supine on *horizontal, firm surfaces* and this allows the infant to independently move their head. Dr. Pikler did not hang mobiles above where the infant lies on their back. She did not want to set up an environment which would encourage an infant to look at a mobile for an extended period of time, thereby limiting movement of the head. Instead, after the child "finds their hand" the toys are placed to the sides of the baby, so that the baby will turn their head to both sides, further facilitating the "massaging effect" on the skull from the firm, horizontal surface. (For a detailed description of horizontal, firm surfaces, please see appendix 1; for more on how a child "finds their hand," please see chapter 7.)

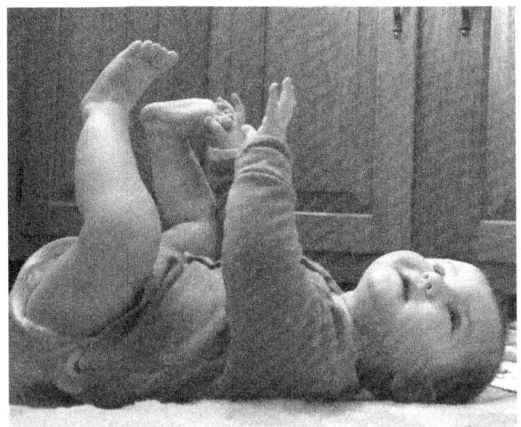 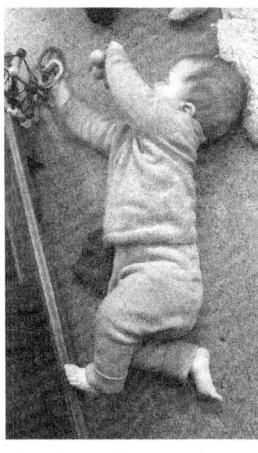

Above left: Here, the baby is looking at something of interest behind her, and this serves to massage the skull. Above right: Here, the baby is massaging the skull in side-lying as they look at the toy they are playing with.

When infants are afforded these conditions, they frequently move the head into all manner of positions in order to look around.

As noted above, this activity massages the skull and helps to even out plagiocephaly. The massaging effect is further enhanced when the child starts to roll from supine to side-lying and back again.

Tummy Time: How It Began

The "back to sleep" campaign began in 1994 in order to reduce the incidence of sudden infant death syndrome, or SIDS. In response to the back to sleep practice, the American Academy of Pediatrics recommended periodic placement of infants on their tummies, or in the prone position, when they are awake. Thus began the push for tummy time, where newborns and young infants are placed on their tummies before they can achieve the position on their own. Parents are instructed to place their newborns in prone two or three times per day for short periods initially, and then to gradually increase the length of the tummy time sessions. Parents are encouraged to get down on the floor, talk to the baby, and encourage the baby to lift up their heads and look at them, or to place toys in front of the baby, move the toys, and make sounds, so the baby is enticed to lift up their head and look at the toys.

It is helpful to understand the difference between self-initiated tummy time and prematurely placing the child on their tummies. Self-initiated tummy time is a very valuable phase of development for the child. The prone position is an especially good position for the development of eye tracking, for example. However, the timing of tummy time—dictated by whether the child achieves the position on their own or is placed there prematurely—has significant ramifications for the subsequent stages of the child's motor development. Agnes Szanto-Feder observes that placing a child onto their tummy from birth, into a position that they have not accomplished on their own, can forestall the child's natural course of development.[24]

Back-Lying versus Tummy Time:
The Initial Innate Imbalance between the Flexors and the Extensors

Newborns and young infants have not yet developed a synergistic relationship between the flexors and the extensors, as mentioned above. The extensors are not balanced by the flexors—there is a fundamental state of imbalance present. If young infants who have this imbalance are placed on their tummies, they overly tense the extensors, which can then become cramped—they must strain to move. With repetition of such strain, the extensor muscles become tight and shortened. Szanto-Feder observes, "When children feel without support or in a state of imbalance occasionally or for a longer period, *it is primarily this flexibility of the body that is jeopardized* [emphasis added]. If children are turned onto their tummies before they can turn over on their own, the above applies even more: as the underdevelopment of the synergistic system does not allow the shoulders and arms to support the head properly, children will only be able to lift their head by contracting the back musculature, which results in the spasmodic stiffness of the torso."[25]

When the spinal extensors overpower the neck flexors and the trunk flexors (or the abdominals), there is poor alignment of the spine, with characteristic neck and low back hyperextension. This poor spinal alignment, along with the mismatched muscular forces, then negatively influences the child's ability to balance.

Dr. Judit Falk explains that the imbalance between the spinal extensors and the abdominals can have other consequences. She cites research by R. Bernbeck as reporting that lumbar hyperlordosis (excessive arching in the lower back) and the weakness of the abdominal muscles, characteristic of children who have been placed in prone, "often go hand in hand with rectus-diastasis,"[26] a condition where there is an abnormal separation of the connective tissue between the rectus abdominal muscles—the two long vertical muscles in the front of the trunk. This condition results when there is significant weakness and lengthening of the abdominals, to such an extent that a split occurs. In a worst-case scenario, the separation can lead to a hernia. However, the condition often resolves by four years of age.[27]

Dr. Falk explains that "Infants raised on their tummy miss out on the 'exercise' aimed at strengthening the abdominal muscles in their first months, with which an infant kicking on [their] back develops [their] abdominal muscles to such an extent that, by the time [they turn] to the stomach and [start] working on [their] back muscles, there will be no risk of the abnormal lengthening of [their] abdominal muscles."[28] In other words, there are checks and balances inherent in free motor development which are protective to the physical body. The abdominal strengthening, which occurs in supine before the child turns to prone, precludes any overstretching of the rectus abdominal muscle when the child gets to prone. This protects it from separating.

Tummy Time: Other Consequences

Other orthopedic challenges in the legs can be associated with prematurely placing young infants in the prone position. When a child lies on the back, the joints of the legs can move without the resistance of the surface in three dimensions (up and down; right and left; and inwardly and outwardly). When the child is prematurely placed in prone, they miss out on all of these possibilities of movement, because the prone position precludes such extensive movement. In prone, the feet often remain in more static positions, whereby the feet either turn in or turn out, and this can sometimes lead to orthopedic issues. Dr. Falk notes that in back-lying, the movements of the legs are optimal for the continued proper forming of the hip sockets, which are not completely formed at birth.[29]

Dr. Falk describes how babies explore the prone position when they have assumed it through their own efforts. She explains that over time, these babies lift their "head without any cramped rigidity more and more easily and securely."[30] Since they have activated and strengthened their neck flexors and abdominal muscles, "there is no risk of the rear extensor muscles becoming overdominant."[31] She describes that, since they have gradually acquired prone through their own efforts, they are agile, at ease, and move with sureness as they raise their chests up off the surface. Falk gives a concrete example of this group of children's ease of movement: when they come to prone on extended (straight) arms, they typically bear weight through open hands rather than on fisted hands, as the babies who have been prematurely placed on their tummies do. Fisted hands indicate that the baby is moving with strain. Fisted hands also signal an active palmar grasp primitive reflex, which typically would be less pronounced by this time. (The palmar grasp reflex will be further discussed in volume 2.) Another concrete difference becomes apparent between "tummy time" babies and back-lying babies when they begin to belly-crawl. Often, the babies who have had tummy time predominantly use their arms and drag their legs passively behind them. The babies who were not prematurely placed on their tummies are more fully able to prepare themselves in supine and side-lying for prone locomotion, and these babies typically belly-crawl using all four limbs.[32] In other words, the quality of the child's movement is significantly affected according to whether they have been afforded the opportunity to turn to their tummy in their own time.

The Corrective Effects of Free Movement

Szanto-Feder explains that insofar as free motor development is provided for prematurely born children, and they are laid on their back from birth, their movement will end up being just as secure and harmonious as other children who are born at their "due" time. Prematurely born children's development, however, will be slower.[33]

4: Free Movement and Opportunities to Develop Self-Regulation

In the Pikler approach, besides sleeping, the infant engages in two qualitatively different activities throughout the day: caregiving activities and periods of free play. Free play includes playing with toys and objects, and it also includes free movement, as initially the infant *plays* with the movements of their body. Caregiving makes free play possible, and similarly, free play is a determining factor for the successful activity of respectful caregiving. During caregiving, the adult attends to the bodily care of the infant, including feeding, diapering, dressing and undressing, cutting fingernails, combing hair, bathing the infant, and so on. During caregiving, the adult builds a respectful, cooperative relationship with the child.

This chapter explores free movement during the two distinct activities of caregiving and free play, which occur rhythmically throughout the infant's day. The chapter also delves into the development of self-regulation. In both caregiving and in free play, the child is given opportunities to self-initiate their activity. Self-initiated activity and self-regulation are intimately related, and this relationship will be explored.

Free Movement during Free Play

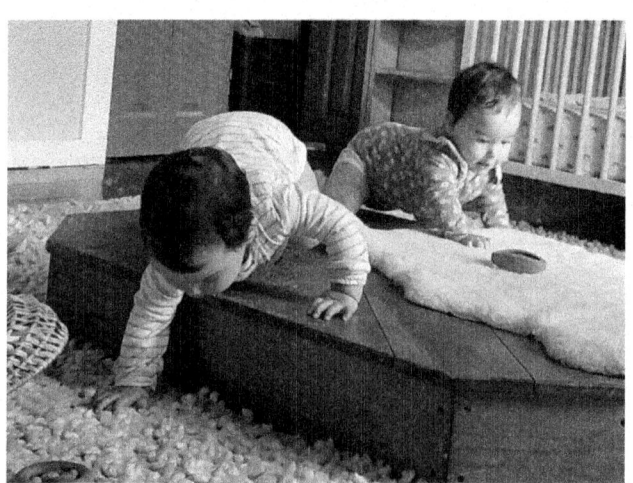

These two babies are playing freely in a movement space created for them in their home.

The adult chooses the appropriate toys and wooden climbing structures for the infant, older baby, and toddler, and then prepares the movement space for them. The adult's choices are based upon their observations of the child's movements and interests. Which toys and climbing structures are the child drawn to? The goal is to meet the child developmentally and also individually, so that the child has a fulfilling experience of moving. The child is placed into the movement space and then is free to move as they see fit—they are solely responsible for how, and how much, they move and play.

The children are not stimulated or encouraged to move in a particular way during free play; they are not placed into positions that they cannot get into or out of independently. No restrictive baby equipment is used. Babies are not prematurely placed on their tummies—rather, they turn to their tummies when they can do so on their own. Babies are not pulled to sit nor propped to sit, and their hands are not held in order that they are assisted to stand or walk. Sometimes, children want their hands held when they are first starting to walk. However, at the children's home in Budapest, the caregivers did not oblige the children in this situation. Rather, the caregivers held to their belief that when the child does what they are capable of independently doing, they are doing exactly the right thing. The caregivers focused on providing the child with opportunities for satisfying experiences in their current stages of development—crawling, climbing, and cruising. Each stage in the developmental sequence was considered valuable in and of itself, as well as preparatory for the subsequent stage. Simply put, when the child is ready to walk, they will. It is actually not helpful to assist a child in something that they cannot yet achieve entirely through their own forces. Offering a hand—or even a finger—to a child in order to help them walk, even when they ask for it, introduces an outside force to the child's system and actually interferes with the child's learning to balance.

Later, when the children are accomplished walkers, if the child offers their hand to the adult (during a walk, for example), the adult will take the child's hand and will hold it for as long as the child indicates. Here, the adult's hand is an emotional gesture of attachment, rather than a gesture of physical support. Walks in the neighborhood around Lóczy were introduced at sixteen to eighteen months to give the children an experience of the world outside the children's home. An adult accompanied a group of two or three children on the walk.[1] Myriam David and Genevíeve Appell explain, "At this age, the walks never have a specific destination. The distance covered is of little importance; what matters is discovering the surroundings. The initiative comes from the children themselves, who go from one thing to the next, exhausting their curiosity before moving on to another object of interest."[2]

During free movement time, the adult does not impinge upon the child with their expectations of how the child "should" be moving, nor have the attitude, for example, that the child "should be walking by now." They do not hold the child to an external timetable of motor milestones. The child is sensitive to the adult's inner state, and will readily perceive the adult's underlying attitude—the relationship will be negatively affected if the adult's expectations are beyond the child's ability and will to move. At the children's home, Dr. Pikler was dealing with children who had been orphaned, abandoned, or suffered other forms of trauma. It was important that the children felt accepted and affirmed for who they were in every way. Dr. Pikler also gave these recommendations to the parents in her private practice, which she had before she founded the children's home.

In the Pikler approach, the adult does not intervene frequently in the child's free play. Any intervention by the adult would be to "maintain the optimal conditions for self-initiated activity."[3] However, the caregiver is vigilant and is aware of the child's accomplishments. The caregiver will occasionally comment on a child's accomplishment, especially when the child looks to the adult, indicating a desire for recognition of what they have done. The adult acknowledges the child's achievement and shares in the child's joy without praising or encouraging them.[4] This is done to enhance the child's awareness of their body and of their Self.

Dr. Myriam David and Genevíeve Appell in their book, Lóczy, explain that there were three types of situations when the caregivers at the children's home in Budapest would directly intervene during the free play period: "if the child has a problem, if there is a conflict, or if [the child] shows signs of boredom or fatigue."[5] A "problem" would be the child's getting into a position that they cannot move out of, and their crying escalates, such as when they first turn over onto their tummies. Here, the adult may orient the child—letting

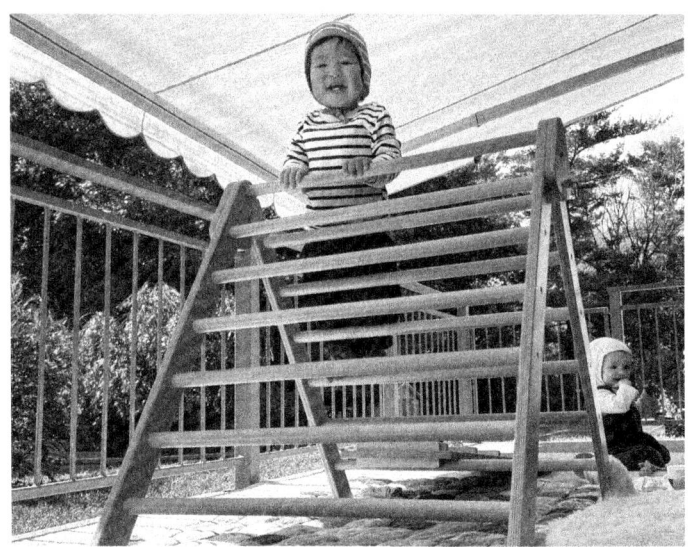

Here, the caregiver may acknowledge the child's achievement by saying something like, "I see you have made it to the top of the triangle."

them know what happened, for example, that they turned onto their tummies and are stuck. Next, they tell the child what will happen—that they will turn the child back over onto their backs—and then the adult does so.

Second, David and Appell relate that if there is a conflict between children at play that "continues and escalates, [the caregiver] tries to settle it by calling and talking to the children from a distance. [The caregiver's] voice never expresses anger, but tries to explain or reason. If this intervention proves insufficient, [the caregiver] approaches, separates and comforts them, then directs them to a new activity. If the aggressor starts again, [the caregiver] may end up putting [that child] to bed."[6] Please note that putting the child to bed at Lóczy was not

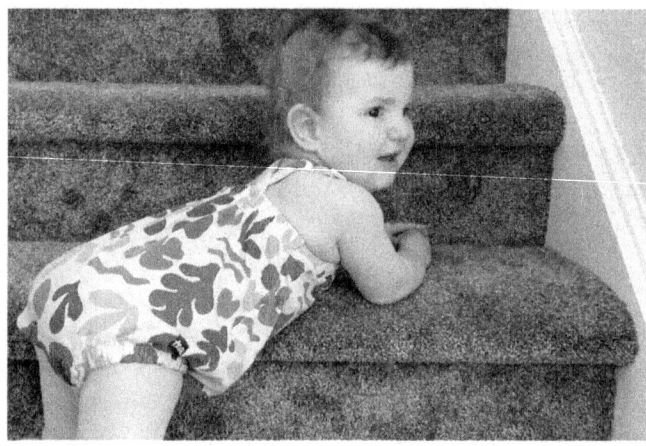

This baby has climbed up a couple of stairs and is unable to get down. This is another situation where the adult would intervene by orienting the baby to what has happened and what will happen, and then lifting them off the stairs, without teaching them how to come down.

punitive, but rather a support for the child in managing the strong feelings and impulses, and we can use the bed in the same way. In their bed, they are in a safe place, with a "transitional object," such as their cloth doll, and can rest from the intensity of the play situation and "gather" themselves. The caregiver always tells the child why they are going to bed. A play pen, cozy corner, or other delineated space (such as a blanket spread out on the grass) can also be used instead of a bed. (See, for example, "Sheltering Spaces for Self-Regulation," later in this chapter; it is often desirable for the child to associate the bed and bedroom exclusively with going to sleep.)

Third, David and Appell explain that if the caregiver interprets a child's behavior as the child being bored, the caregiver may introduce a new toy, rearrange the toys, move the child to another location in the play space, or open up a gated-off area to give the child more options. If the child appears to be tired, the caregiver may give the child some tea or put the child to bed, explaining what the caregiver is doing and why. If the child is old enough to express themself, the caregiver may even let the child contribute to the solution.[7]

Free Movement during Caregiving

It is easy to see that during free play, the child has wide open opportunities to move within the carefully prepared movement space. The child also has opportunities for free movement during caregiving times, and nothing is imposed upon the child during caregiving. For example, David and Appell report that at Lóczy, "Toilet training is not forced and babies are not systematically set on the potty."[8]

Let us consider dressing. Obviously, the free movement possibilities of the child are less, because the Pikler changing table is smaller than the play area. However, the child has free movement in that they can choose which position they want to be in, and they can change their position on the changing table. The various parts of dressing may be performed in supine, side-lying, prone, sitting, hands-and-knees, and standing while holding onto the railing.

Toys are not brought to the changing table, because toys would impede the child's ability to pay attention, participate in the dressing activity, and build a rapport with the adult. There can be other distractions on the changing table as well. Once, I had a sweater with two-inch-diameter polka dots on it that I liked to wear. I soon realized that my seven-month-old granddaughter was fascinated by the polka dots. She would reach for them and hang onto the sweater when I was changing her diaper. As this interfered with her engagement with me and with her ability to participate in the dressing, I stopped wearing the sweater.

Whereas in free movement, the child sets their own goals, in dressing the adult sets the goal and tries to elicit engagement and cooperation from the child in achieving the goal. The child has free movement in that they may choose to oblige the adult's request or not. The goal of the adult is quite precise. For example, the adult may ask a newborn, "Will you hold your arm out, so I can put on your sleeve?" This is a very specific movement. The adult needs to grade the level of difficulty of the request so it's achievable, and this changes over time—even from moment to moment, depending upon the state of the child.

I witnessed a one-week-old infant being dressed. The mother showed the infant the rolled-up pant leg, asked the infant to put her leg into it, and then waited. Eventually, when the infant did straighten her leg, the mother adeptly moved the pant leg over the leg and then thanked her daughter. The movement of the infant's leg may have been a random occurrence; however, it is noteworthy that the parent held the conviction that her daughter was capable of freely participating at her own level of development. The thoughts and feelings of the adult are a significant part of the environment from which the child forms their identity. Here, the infant was having a positive experience of herself.

The child generally wants to participate in the caregiving activity, and may freely chose to do so, because they enjoy being with the caregiver, and also because they learn that together with the caregiver, their distress goes away, be it hunger, fatigue, thirst, feeling cold or hot, or discomfort from a soiled or wet diaper. With regard to the above-mentioned newborn, it soon became apparent that this infant clearly did not like to be cold, and she would settle right away as soon as she was dressed in her woolies. At this early age, she was learning that she—in conjunction with her parent—had agency to relieve her discomfort of being chilly.

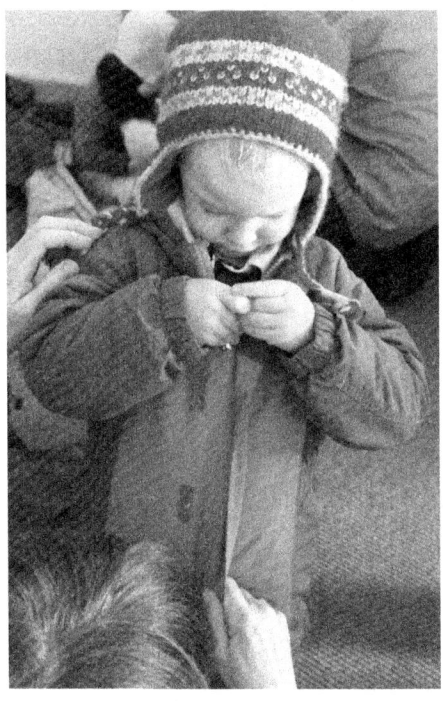

This child was invited to zip up their coat. The caregiver set the stage by stabilizing the bottom of the coat for them, and they readily joined in the activity.

Free Movement through Invitation during Caregiving

As mentioned above, during caregiving, the child is invited—but not required—to participate in the activity. Inherent in the concept of an invitation is the invitee's ability to say no. For example, if the one-week-old infant mentioned above had not extended her leg after a reasonable amount of time, the mother would have simply moved the pant leg up over the infant's flexed-up leg. The mother would not have taken the infant's foot and pulled it down through the pant leg. If she were to have done this, it likely would have triggered a primitive reflex, resulting in the infant pulling against the mother. Had the mother continued, this would have led to the unfortunate circumstance of the mother overpowering the infant in order to force her leg into the pants. In this situation, there would be no free movement for the infant. One can perceive that there would be a subtle element of violence to this, and Pikler considered this type of action to be a mini-aggression.

Mini-aggressions occur "when the adult doesn't realize [they are] being violent ... A baby or young child should never be treated with anything other than absolute reverence."[9] Elsa Chahin and Anna Tardos explain that in a group care setting, the adult may act aggressively because of an impersonal relationship and also "because of mechanical treatment of the children" during caregiving activities.[10] What mitigates mechanical treatment of children is that the adult learns to be aware of their own actions, and of the children's responses to them. Additionally, the adult must take charge of their own emotions. "When faced with a challenge, the adult must work very diligently to overcome [their] own reactivity and remain centered at all times when relating with children. ... Because children will test us, will cry to catch our attention, and will take a little longer to accomplish a task than what we had scheduled according to our expectations, this is not reason for us to become aggressive toward them. An adult must work with continuous patience and presence to maintain equanimity and emotional balance."[11] Mini-aggressions can be very subtle. Chahin and Tardos maintain that "Acting violently toward children doesn't necessarily have to do with physical or verbal force but could also be the result of not accepting the child or expecting [them] to be anything other than [they are.]"[12]

During caregiving activities, we are not forcing the child to perform a particular movement. However, we are consciously guiding a child into a formed activity through our consistency, our gestures, and our orienting language. The adult provides the framework for the activity, inviting the child into the formed activity, and the child self-initiates their own participation. The adult must remain flexible—the form of the activity changes over time as the child develops. In fact, each caregiving experience is created anew, and comes about through the child's and the adult's mutual cuing and responding to each other.

Here is a lovely example of a formed activity in which a baby participated out of her own free will—with a little ingenuity on the part of her parents. The baby was crawling and just beginning to pull to stand. Her father had just opened the oven door, and unfortunately, in the blink of an eye, the girl crawled over and started to pull to stand on the hot oven door. As a result, she burned three of her fingers. Her parents called the emergency room, and they were instructed to keep the baby's hand in ice water for twenty minutes. The parents filled a bowl with ice cubes and water; the child stuck her hand in it, and then promptly took it out. Her parents were faced with a choice. They could either force their daughter to keep her hand in the ice water, or they could try another way. Luckily, in their moment of need, they received an inspiration. They dropped a canning jar lid into the bowl. The baby put her hand in the cold water, picked it up, and put it on the table. The parents continued dropping canning jar lids, one after the other, into the ice water. Children this age are fascinated with dropping and picking up objects; so, this game occupied the baby for the full twenty minutes!

Exquisite Use of Gesture during Caregiving

It is helpful to consider the adult's use of gesture during caregiving activities. In a sort of spontaneously choreographed dance, the caregiver uses open-ended gestures and waits for the child to respond to them, which in turn impacts the adult's next action. In this way, a trusting relationship is woven. There are three characteristic gestures used by the caregivers, known as open hand gestures. Anna Tardos identifies them as "calling with gesticulation, offering something, and asking for something."[13]

Each of these three gestures is a half-finished movement of expectation. Each of them expresses an expectation on

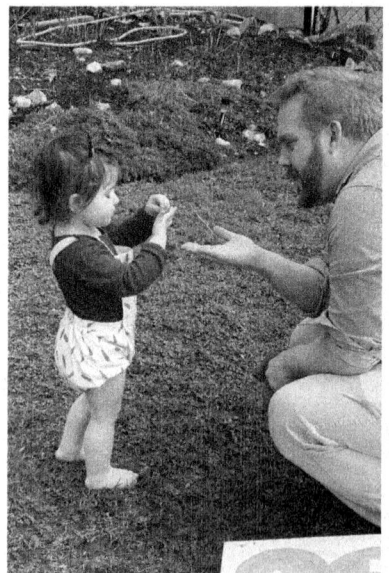
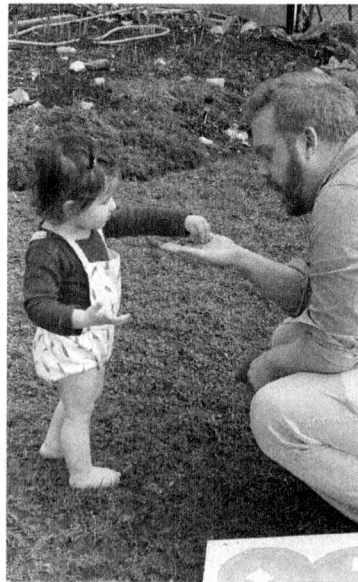

Here, the adult asked the child to give him the seeds they were holding. He gestured with his open hand, waited, and the child willingly responded.

the child's behalf, a possibility of choice. Such a half-finished movement allows the child [their] own activity.... The act of asking for something plays a particularly important part in the togetherness with an infant or a toddler. Just like calling and offering, the movement that asks for something is the expression of a peaceful approach to the child. It indicates that the person who is asking will not make use of violence in order to assert [their] wish. It is an expression of the fact that the adult doesn't intend to act alone, rather [they wait] for the child to act. [The adult anticipates] that [the child] will put something into the expecting, open hand for example—a piece of apple, with which [the child] has already begun to play, or [their] slipper, that [they have] just taken off.... The asking, expecting attitude of the adult offers the infant the possibility of decision, the possibility to meet out of [their] own free will the adult's expectations or not.[14]

Free Movement Does Not Prolong Caregiving Activities

Caregiving activities at Lóczy were never hurried. "Although the [caregivers are] constantly busy, [they never give] the impression of being in a hurry and [they seem] to give the child as much time as [the child] needs."[15] Additionally, barring something urgent and out of the ordinary, the care is not interrupted. Rather, the caregiver "finishes what [they have] started with a child and respects [their] individual rhythm.... These last two features might give the impression that the time allotted to each child is long, whereas, each care situation, is, in fact, fairly short."[16] Because the adult uses the aforementioned open-ended gestures and is an expert in reading the movement cues of the child, a sort of gentle harmony between the movements of the adult and those of the child comes into being. However, "the care is not prolonged in this way, for the [adult] avoids provoking any time-consuming resistance to [the adult's] actions."[17]

Medical examinations at the children's home were similarly conducted, and similarly, they did not last very long. "The doctor, verbalizing and explaining [their] actions, uses the child's movement and elicits [the child's] participation. [The doctor's] movements are gentle, nothing is forced or done with haste, and [the doctor] is in constant contact with the child."[18] As a result, the interactions with the doctors were pleasant for the children and they liked visiting the doctor, whether they were sick or for routine visits. The visits were opportunities for the child to become more aware of their body, and "for the older children, to learn the names of its different parts."[19]

Free Movement during Feeding

As in the other caregiving activities, the adult provides the frame for the feeding activity. Self-initiated activity of the child is the goal here also. At Sophia's Hearth we have used the principles of Ellyn Satter's work since our inception, and we have found them to be very effective and in line with Pikler's approach. Satter is a renowned feeding and eating specialist, family therapist, author, and speaker. She works with parents to support healthy eating practices in families. Her guidelines for parents create the conditions whereby children can self-initiate eating. Here are her guidelines, in a nutshell: "Successful feeding demands a division of responsibility. Parents are responsible for the *what*, *when*, and *where* of *feeding*; children are responsible for the *how much* and *whether* of *eating*. Put another way, parents are responsible for what food they serve to their children, and when and where they serve it; children are responsible for how much of that food they eat and whether they eat any of it at all [emphasis in original]."[20]

When parents ponder the idea of offering babies and young children nutritious foods at consistent times of the day, and letting them decide whether and how much they eat, some parents worry that their children will not get enough to eat. However, this has not been borne out in our experience at Sophia's Hearth, and also in my experience in working with families. The child may not eat much at one setting, yet, in the long run, it averages out.

A classic study performed by Dr. Clara Davis in 1928 also bears this out. At this time, in the United States, "pediatricians dictated precisely the amounts, types, and frequencies of food for children from 7 months to 3 years . . . it was assumed that infants lacked the ability to regulate their own food intake."[21] Three babies, aged eight, nine, and ten months took part in the study, which occurred over six to twelve months. Here are the fascinating results.

> At first babies chose foods and spit them out again, but after the first few meals they promptly recognized and chose what they wanted, no matter the location on the tray, and they stopped spitting out foods. It was impossible to predict what a child would eat at a given meal. An infant might eat from 1 to 7 eggs a day or 1 to 4 bananas. Milk consumption ranged from 11 to 48 ounces. . . . At the time he was enrolled in the study, one infant had rickets caused by vitamin D deficiency. He was offered cod liver oil in one of his little dishes—cod liver oil is a rich source of vitamin D. Over the first several months of the experiment he voluntarily consumed almost 9 ounces of the strong-tasting cod liver oil overall. Although he continued to be offered the cod liver oil after the rickets had healed and his diagnostic tests indicated his vitamin D status to be corrected, he stopped taking it.[22]

Ellyn Satter states that this study is sometimes construed to mean that it is okay to let youngsters "freely graze for food."[23] However, she maintains that this is a misinterpretation. The researchers chose and offered nutritious foods, and they selected regular times and places to serve them. In other words, the researchers created the eating environment, and the children were responsible for whether and how much they ate.

At Lóczy, similar feeding practices were and are still employed. "No child is forced to eat more than [they want]. At the first sign of refusal, [their caregiver] stops feeding [them] or lets [them] stop, and does not try to make [them] eat more. 'Not a single spoonful more' is the established rule."[24] Dr. Judit Falk, a long-time pediatrician at the children's home, sums up the caregivers' goals. "During the feeding [the caregivers] are not interested in whether the child eats all the food offered to [them] or leaves some of it, but the fact that [they eat] what [they] want with a hearty appetite and with pleasure, that [they explore] the pleasure of good tastes and the satisfaction of the feeling of fullness."[25] No cases of anorexia occurred at the children's home.[26]

Supporting the Development of Self-Regulation

Newborns don't have a mature capacity to self-regulate. Initially, the infant and adult engage in co-regulation. Here the infant relies on external cues and supports. Over time, the child matures and develops the ability to self-regulate. This is an internally organized capacity to manage situations with appropriate behavior. Co-regulation and self-regulation overlap throughout childhood, with self-regulation gradually increasing and co-regulation gradually lessening. However, co-regulation does not decrease linearly, and it is helpful for the adult to be sensitive to the child's changing needs. During periods of schedule changes, illness, or other stressors in the child's life, the adult may need to step in to offer more support with co-regulation during activities that the child was previously able to manage. Indeed, there are times that—even as adults—we need help to regulate. It is the general belief in the scientific community that the need for instances of co-regulation continues throughout life. Co-regulation is considered a "biological imperative; a need that must be met to sustain life."[27] I remember a time when my husband helped me co-regulate. We were at the ocean. I had gotten into the water, was getting too cold, and the rocks—moved by the waves—were hurting my ankles. I was having trouble keeping my footing and was starting to shut down. My husband saw that I was dysregulated. He came close to me and spoke calmly, clearly, and simply. His manner, in and of itself, helped me regulate. He said, "Do you want to go back to shore?" I answered, "Yes." He continued, "Turn around." Then he waited for the moment when the waves were opportune and said, "Go now." I'm not sure I would have made it back to shore without him.

What Is Self-Regulation?

Regulatory capacities refer to a person's ability to modulate their response to sensory input. In the above example at the ocean, I was not managing my response well to the sensations of the cold, the wind, the rocks, and the waves. As I write this chapter, my eighteen-month-old granddaughter is sick, and she is having meltdowns when it is time to change her diaper. Previously, diaper changes went well. However, since becoming ill, we have ascertained that she is not able to modulate her response to the sensation of the cold wipe on her skin, and her parents are starting to use a warmer for the wipes. So far, this appears to be resolving the issue. Inherent in self-regulation is the ability to discern and filter out relevant from non-relevant input and to use self-soothing strategies. For example, some people have trouble going to sleep in a room with a ticking clock or paying attention in a conversation when a fan is running. They are unable to filter out the errant sounds.

A landmark therapeutic treatment program for children with challenges in self-regulation was created in 1996 by two occupational therapists, Mary Sue Williams and Sherry Shellenberger. It is called the Alert Program, also referred to as "How Does Your Engine Run?" Williams and Shellenberger offer a very practical description of self-regulation: "the ability to attain, maintain, and change arousal appropriately for a task or situation."[28] Arousal refers to a state of the nervous system. For example, we would likely have a very high level of arousal if we were at the Super Bowl and our team made a touchdown in the final seconds to win the game. We would likely jump up and down and cheer loudly. This behavior would be appropriate for the setting. Williams and Shellenberger substitute the term "alert level" as a more user-friendly version of the medical term "arousal level"; different situations call for different levels of arousal or alertness. Other examples of when it is appropriate to have a high level of alertness include times when we are in a dangerous situation and must be highly aware of our surroundings; or when we are running a race and giving it our all. When we want to listen attentively to someone and develop a rapport with them, it would not be appropriate to have this level of alertness. Instead, we would want to keep ourselves calm and steady, without overreacting if something is said that pushes our buttons—here we would be modulating our emotions and our behavior. We would be operating out of a mid-level of alertness. If we were tired and started to become drowsy during the conversation, we would try to increase our alert level so that we could continue to be attentive. Later, at bedtime, we need to unwind and settle ourselves for bed—shifting to a low level of alertness is necessary to get to sleep. Indeed, the ability to "shift gears"—to modulate our behavior so as to act in an appropriate, functional manner in relationship to the specific situation—is a very complex skill. This develops with maturation of the nervous system. Additionally, it is helpful for the development of self-regulation that the child be given opportunities in which they can learn to self-regulate.

A concerning trend today is the increasing use of electronic devices to calm young children. Although giving a young child a smart phone to watch a video may serve to quiet them in the moment, in the long run it does not help them learn to self-regulate. Instead, when we give a young child a phone or a tablet or turn on the television, we create a vicious cycle. In order to better understand this phenomenon, it is helpful to look at the activity of dopamine during device use. Dopamine is a powerful neurotransmitter and is commonly known as the "feel-good" hormone. It is released with pleasurable experiences and also with arousing experiences. It is released in the brain when a child (or person of any age) views engaging content on a screen. When the screen is taken away, the dopamine is no longer released, and this causes irritability. The child seeks out the screen again and again. Dopamine "helps sustain people's interest and attention, which is why it can [be] hard for people to tear themselves away from a situation or behavior. It's also self-reinforcing. The more times people experience the behavior, the more dopamine is released, and the more driven they are to return to the behavior."[29]

Co-regulation

As described above, the adult sets the emotional tone for the infant. Ideally, the adult develops the capacity to stay calm when the infant is crying and upset. This can be a daunting task for a new, sleep-deprived parent, and they need support! When parental leave from work, breastfeeding support, and medical care are available, it can make a big difference. Other supports for new parents include tried-and-true customs such as bringing food and offering to take older siblings on outings.

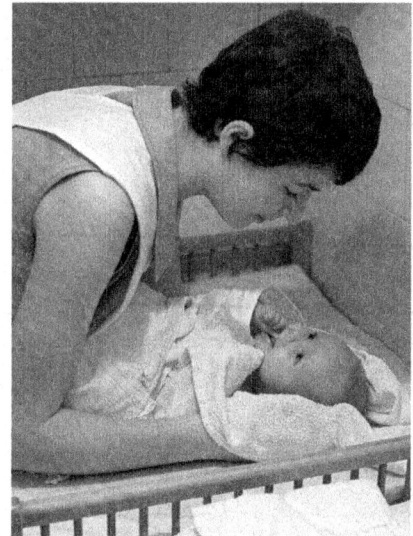 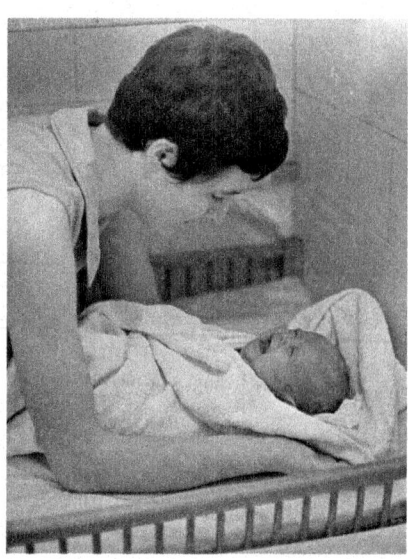

Here are two photos that were taken at the children's home in Budapest, in which a caregiver is dressing a baby. The two photos were taken on two different occasions. However, it is the same caregiver. In the first photo, the baby is smiling at the caregiver. In the second photo, the baby is crying.

What is striking about these two photos is that the caregiver has the same countenance—the same expression of calm and serenity. The caregiver has not allowed the state of the child, nor anything from their personal life, to negatively impact their own regulation. As Rudolf Steiner says, in the presence of the children, "we must train ourselves to lay aside [our] moods."[30] He says that when we can "strip off our narrower, personal self like a snake skin," the children will benefit.[31] When we have control of our emotions, we function as an anchor for the child. The adult, serving as a model for imitation, guides the child back into a more regulated state. This is an essential feature of co-regulation.

The adult also helps the infant regulate by taking care of their physiological needs and by providing them with appropriately graded sensory input—such as moving them slowly, predictably, and tactfully. Dr. Pikler instructed her caregivers to move the infants in such a way they that did not lose their balance. In this way the child is not made to startle unnecessarily, which takes the child out of a regulated state. Additionally, Dr. Pikler taught her caregivers to orient the child to what will happen *before* the action takes place, so that the child may respond rather than react. For example, when the adult approaches the infant, waits for eye contact, and says, "I'm going to pick you up," the child may "set their muscles" in anticipation of being picked up. The adult waits for this subtle response from the child, and then picks them up.

Anticipating and responding to a known event—as opposed to reacting to a sudden, unexpected occurrence—involve different parts of the nervous system. When anticipating and responding, the child is less likely to go into a state of fight or flight, and they can learn to meet the world in an optimal state of regulation. When a sudden, unexpected event occurs, they are more prone to go into a fight-or-flight response. The younger the child, the more this is likely, because of the immature condition of the nervous system at birth and the prevalence of the Moro reflex. If the child goes into fight or flight repeatedly over time, this state can come to be what the child recognizes as their "normal" state, and then it can become challenging for them to downgrade their regulation and settle down. (The Moro reflex, which triggers a fight-or-flight reaction, will be discussed in further detail in volume 2.)

Another practice that helps the child anticipate is to administer care in a fixed order—for example, diapering or bathing the children in the same order every day. This is described in detail in David and Appell's book *Lóczy: An Unusual Approach to Mothering*.

> When the [caregiver] takes one child, she goes to the next child and tells [them] that [their] turn is coming soon, showing [them] the child she will bathe first. In the same way, when she lays down the child she has just taken care of, she again tells the next one that it will be [their] turn as soon as she has put the other one to bed or attended to something else.... This order is strictly observed: even if a child cries, [they] have to wait [their] turn. Yet the child is not left alone to cry. The [caregiver] looks for a way to restore [their] feeling of well-being; for the babies, a change of place in the play area or being put back to bed; for the older children, a new toy. All this is accompanied by spoken encouragement.[32]

Here, the adults are helping the children co-regulate. Over time, the children understand the order, and can be comforted by the knowledge that they will receive the adult's full attention when it is their turn. Predictable order facilitates self-regulation. This is a good example of how co-regulation gradually declines and how the child becomes more able to regulate on their own.

The child has very particular opportunities to develop self-regulation during the periods of free movement and also during the caregiving activities. Let us begin with self-regulation during the self-directed movement time.

Self-Regulation at Lóczy during Free Play

During my two weeks of study and observing the children at Lóczy, I witnessed a remarkable degree of self-regulation. The children were very active, although not in a hyperactive way, and I did not observe signs of sensory processing disorders in the infants and toddlers. Instead, I observed an extraordinary degree of focused engagement. I did not expect this, considering the children's histories—the majority of them had experienced some form of trauma, and some were born to birthing parents with drug addictions. However, these children were exploring their world with joy and interest.

When I inquired about this remarkable degree of focused attention, I was told that the children were modulating their attention levels through unrestricted self-initiated movement. This concept is in alignment with basic principles of sensory integration therapy, but I have never seen it carried out with such understanding. Therapists were not needed to prescribe sensory diets of specially designed, scheduled activities meant to provide adequate sensory input for the child's nervous system to come into a more regulated state. Rather, at Lóczy, the infants created and carried out their own sensory diets, in the moment. This was possible through carefully sculpted play environments and through the generous time allowed for unhindered motor exploration. The play space was designed such that fine motor (emphasizing the hands and arms; reaching, grasping, etc.) and gross motor activities (emphasizing the legs and the whole body; running and jumping) were not dictated by an adult. Gross and fine motor activities were possible in the same space, and the children were free to choose when and how long they engaged in each type of activity. This practice has a remarkable effect upon the child's ability to self-regulate and attend.

At Lóczy, the development of attention has been observed, studied, and documented in depth. The research found that in approximately the first three years of life, periods of focused attention happen very frequently, although the periods themselves are short. The child will quiet their body and engage in fine motor exploration (via playing with a toy or object) for up to two minutes, and then they will need to move. During the motor stages between side-sitting on extended arm and walking, the children engaged in fine motor play for slightly shorter periods of time—for less than ninety seconds. The study concluded that the refined attention of the fine motor play and the active large motor explorations are recuperative for each other. They reinforce each other.[33]

Younger infants and babies will engage in a fine motor activity for a period of time, and then stop and perform a gross motor activity. The fine motor and gross motor are separate, unrelated activities. However, older toddlers will engage in a fine motor activity for a period of time, and then—within the context of the fine motor activity—perform a gross motor activity. The gross motor and fine motor activities are integrated into a whole. For example, a child may be sitting at a table and coloring for a period of time, and then get up and walk around to the other side of the table to retrieve another crayon, even though a crayon of the very same color is next to them. Or a child may be building with blocks for a period of time, and then get up and run across the room for another block, even though a block of the same shape is nearby. The child is extending their ability to continue the fine motor activity by performing a gross motor activity. The sensations from the gross motor activities exert a regulating influence. Only the child knows when they need a large motor movement. These are lovely examples of the relationship between self-initiated activity and self-regulation.

Sheltering Spaces for Self-Regulation

At the children's home in Budapest, the play spaces were separate from where the children slept. However, Dr. Pikler would place one or two toddler beds in the children's play spaces. These beds were not designated for "time out" or for napping, but as places for a child to retreat, be alone, and rest for a few moments—perhaps with a book or a stuffed animal. The caregiver saw to it that the other children did not come onto the bed when it was being used. The caregivers would say something like, "Johanna wants to be alone right now," if other children tried to join the child on the bed.

Additionally, there can be other quieting places in the play space such as little "houses" made of silks and play stands, or several fleeces arranged in a corner. These can be places where a child may go to rest for a while, but where other children may also join them. Thus, they do not afford the same degree of sequestering as the beds do, where the child is left alone. These two different types of spaces are designed to give the children opportunities for varying levels of self-regulation. In order to develop skills of nuanced self-regulation, children need nuanced environmental support. Children raised in institutional settings (and this includes childcare settings) need to be able to retreat and have some privacy from time to time. These sheltering spaces are particularly helpful for them, especially if they are there for long periods of their day. However, they are also appropriate for home settings, especially when there is more than one child.

Adult Discernment in Timing
Co-regulation and Self-Regulation

In the Pikler approach, when the child inevitably struggles at learning a new motor skill, the adult learns to view this struggle in a positive light. In letting the child experience a degree of struggle, we widen the child's tolerance for frustration. Importantly, we also learn to discern when the child's struggling turns into suffering, and therefore, when our intervention is needed. We don't want the baby's mood to escalate to the point of not being able to return to a calmer state. Hence, we may need to employ co-regulation—we may come close to the child and speak to them in a calm manner. This may be enough, or we may need to pick them up and comfort them—yet without solving the problem. The timing of our interventions is a delicate matter, and we can cultivate a sense of knowing when to intervene. We want to give the child the opportunity to self-regulate and to solve their own problem. For example, if a self-initiated play activity is not working out for a child and they become frustrated or bored, they may choose to stop and rest and then move on to something else. Sometimes, we subject the child to our misinterpretations of their actions. We may think that the child is frustrated, that they are experiencing a problem, and that it is our duty to jump in and "help" the child. Unfortunately, the child may not identify that what is happening is a problem! They may simply be observing how the world works.

Henri Wallon, a French psychologist, gives us insight here: "An observer should be cautious not to attribute such complex meaning to a child's actions that those same actions would mean in the case of adults. Regardless of how identical they may seem, the only meaning that should be attributed to them is that justified by the current behavior of the child. . . . Paying attention to such diversity of the meanings of behavior is probably the most significant difficulty, and at the same time an indispensable condition, of observation."[34]

"A Bit of Help"

Dr. Pikler describes the effect on the child when an adult "helps" them to move:

> The independence, the feeling of competence of the child is often checked by the way the adults are trying to help [the child's] development. The attitude by which the child is deprived from initiative under the pretext of "helping" and "teaching," from attempting things, and from completing an action "they" had started, should be revised. The so-called "a bit of help," i.e., "I'll only just give [them] a hand to help [them] complete what [they have] begun" deprives the child from the joy of self-dependent achievement, from the feeling of efficacy, just like the traditional modes of helping, when the child is dealt with like an object."[35]

What is lacking here is the adult's recognition of the baby's deeply rooted motivation to determine their own activities.

Here is a lovely example of what can happen when we refrain from helping our children. This incident was relayed to me by Ute Strub, a movement pedagogue, physiotherapist, and champion for free movement for children and adults, who worked closely with Dr. Pikler in the 1970s at the children's home. A toddler was out of sorts and couldn't be comforted. He went with his mother and Strub to an outside area containing sand. The boy filled the mother's hand with sand. The mother started to intervene by patting the sand. However, Strub asked the mother to wait and see what the boy would do by himself. The boy kept filling the mother's hand until the sand started to fall off her hand, and then he turned her hand to dump the sand. The boy repeated this filling and dumping thirteen times. Then he found a small board that he used as a tool to scoop up sand into the mother's hand, and again he dumped the sand out when it started to fall out. This happened another five times. The boy had noticeably settled by the end of this activity and remained well regulated for the rest of the day. Here, we see the intimate connection between self-initiated activity and self-regulation.[36]

Self-Regulation during Caregiving

As mentioned above, during the caregiving activity of getting dressed, the child moves freely into their position of choice, be it back-lying, tummy-lying, hands-and-knees, sitting, or standing while hanging onto the railing of the changing table. Additionally, they can change their position in the middle of the dressing activity. During dressing, the child is allowed to freely move, within the more limited confines of the changing table. Some of the child's movements may not appear to be related to the activity of dressing. For example, when they are asked to lift their foot in order to put on their pants, the child may side-step around the railing of the changing table. We could possibly interpret this behavior as the child misbehaving, or being distracted, or not wanting to engage in the dressing.

It is worth pondering the question: why would a child side-step around the railing of the changing table, when the goal is to be putting on their pants? Why would the adult allow this side-stepping, expect it, and even want this? The answer is that the child has to move in order to pay attention to the dressing task, which is a complicated task and which requires a lot of attention. The child is modulating their attention through the modality of self-initiated movement; they are self-regulating! If the adult understands this, and recognizes that the child's seemingly extra movement is actually an important part of their effort to participate, the dressing may have a breathing quality between the child and the adult.

Common Cultural Practices that Promote Dysregulation in Children

It is not uncommon in the wider culture for adults to regularly treat young children as if they were little adults. Our expectations are often not in line with the child's stage of development. For example, we prematurely expect the young child to operate in an intellectual mode. Hence, we speak to them in ways that are "over their heads." On the other hand, we "talk down" to them—even speak "baby talk" to them. These types of activities can be confusing, disorienting, and dysregulating to children. There are other common interactions with children that can be dysregulating to them. We pat their heads and entice them do "cute" things in order to "show them off" to our friends. We "egg them on," which sometimes leads to their having a meltdown, and then we wonder why they don't behave better. We cause them to laugh in order that we may be amused—all the while failing to recognize that the baby's laugh is not a gentle, spontaneous laugh, but rather a forced, tense laugh. We shake rattles in their faces, unaware of how we would not like it if someone did this to us. We toss older babies up in the air and catch them. In these examples, we are interfering with the child's ability to self-initiate their own activity—and hence, also, with their ability to self-regulate.

Similarly, we tickle young children. Magda Gerber,[*] a student of Pikler, expresses her thoughts regarding tickling: "I don't believe in tickling children. Tickling is invasive, almost an assault. It changes the way a child feels by making [them] 'laugh.' Laughter should come from the soul and be a sign of happiness, contentment, and joy. When a child is tickled, [they laugh] hysterically, and behind the laugher, there may be fear. I believe that this laughter is a nervous reaction on the child's part."[37]

What is missing in these examples is an interaction between adult and child in which the baby can act out of their own volition. Instead, something is imposed upon the child—and there is little freedom for them when this happens. Dr. Pikler sums up what was the state of affairs decades ago. She said that it was not uncommon for "the child [to be] seen as a toy or as a 'doll,' rather than a human being."[38]

The optimal situation is for the adult to see the infant as a unique, capable individual in their own right, no matter their level of development. According to Rudolf Steiner, we are able to perceive the infant in this light because of our sense of the ego of the other. The sense of the ego of the other is one of the twelve senses he defined. With this sense, we perceive the spiritual—or cosmic—essence of the other person. If we are able to perceive this aspect of a child, or of any person, regardless of their outer trappings, we won't treat them as an object, or as a "doll." Thankfully, we have the possibility to continue to develop this sense over the entire course of our lives.

---

[*] Magda Gerber (1910–2007) built a legacy of her own. She fled Hungary during World War II and came to the United States. She settled in Los Angeles and founded RIE, Resources for Infant Educarers.

5: Aspects of Self-Initiated Movement

Emmi Pikler and Rudolf Steiner didn't know each other, and they came from very different vantage points, yet they were remarkably similar in their fundamental belief that the infant is capable of achieving verticality and walking without the help or instruction of an adult. In this chapter, we will explore some of the commonly held beliefs of Pikler and Steiner, as well as some of their differences.

Teaching Babies and the Very Young: Embedded into Our Culture

Dr. Pikler was acutely aware of the widespread cultural practice of teaching babies to move. At that time, adults typically did not consider how this may affect the child, and this is still true today. For example, we commonly teach a baby to play peek-a-boo. Actually, there is no need to teach a child to play peek-a-boo. Babies will come to this game in their own good time, and then they will have the joy of discovering it themselves. When you teach a child something, you take away forever their chance of discovering it on their own.[1] It takes consciousness and restraint for an adult to hold back, though.

What Happens If We Don't Teach Infants to Move?

The questions of whether we need to teach infants to move, and what happens if we don't, had never been scientifically researched when Dr. Pikler began her private practice as a pediatrician in Budapest in the 1930s. However, numerous studies had been done identifying the motor milestones of babies who had been "taught" to move. These studies identified, for example, the average age when babies maintained the sitting position after having been placed there by an adult, rather than when a baby assumed the sitting position entirely through their own efforts. Dr. Pikler set out to explore the nuances of self-taught motor development versus adult-taught motor development in babies.

Dr. Pikler's research began in 1931 with the birth of her own child, who was reared according to the Pikler approach.[2] She observed her child's development, and the results were very favorable. After this, she established her private medical practice in Budapest, developing and perfecting the Pikler approach with the families in her care. She worked with over a hundred families during a ten-year period from 1936–1946 and observed the results of the Pikler approach upon these children and their families. Upon completion of these preliminary studies, she concluded, "Not only did the children learn to sit, stand, and walk by themselves, but they were apparently more independent, more sure in their movements, and, in general, more content and quiet in their behavior than were other children of the same age, reared in the customary way."[3]

When Dr. Pikler founded and directed the children's home in Budapest, she expanded her research, conducting an extensive study of self-initiated movement with the children who lived there "for varying periods between 1947 and 1964."[4] In the conclusion of one of her research papers from this extensive study, she states, "On the basis of systematic observation it was established that . . . 'teaching' by adults—is not a necessary condition for infants achieving gross motor skills if they are of normal mental level and are kept under appropriate conditions for self-movement. Untaught gross motor activities, such as turning to prone positions, sitting up, standing up, etc., appear regularly."[5]

Dr. Pikler continues, "Long years of experience have led the author to the conviction that children who have reached the stages of sitting and walking on their initiative, through their own independent efforts, move more steadily, less spasmodically, with more adroitness and harmony than do other children. Though children uninstructed in motor skills are very courageous in practicing movements, they are less prone to accidents under normal circumstances."[6]

With these groundbreaking and remarkable findings in mind, let us continue our exploration of self-initiated motor development.

Why Don't We Need to Teach an Infant to Move? Steiner's View of the Higher Self

According to Pikler, during the first two years of life the child learns the basic elements of movement. She clarifies, "The question is not how we can 'teach' an infant to move well and correctly, using cleverly thought up, artificially constructed, complicated measures, using exercises and gymnastics. It is simply a matter of offering an infant the opportunity—or, more precisely, not to deprive [them] of this opportunity—to move according to [their] inherent ability."[7] In other words, we don't need to teach the infant because they have an inherent ability to learn to move.

A. Jean Ayres, founder of the sensory integration therapy movement, speaks about the child's inner drive. She says, "Within every child, there is a great inner drive to develop sensory integration. We do not have to tell [them] to crawl or stand up or climb; nature directs the child from within. Watch how a child searches [their] environment for opportunities to develop and how [they try] over and over again until [they succeed]. Without this inner drive toward sensory integration, none of us could have developed."[8] During a therapy session, the goal of the sensory integration therapist is to tap into the child's inner drive.

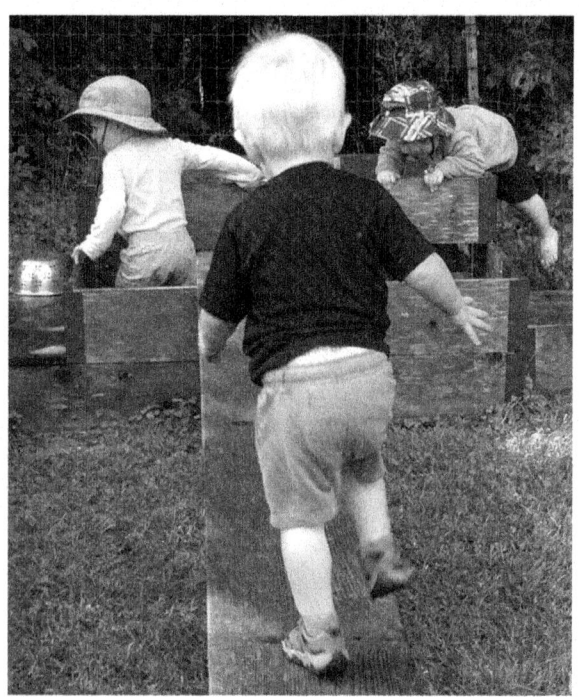

These two-year-olds self-initiated their play on the incline and climbing structure. They are fully vested in their activities—they have tapped into their inner drive.

Neither Pikler nor Ayres address how it comes to be that the child possesses an inner drive to develop sensory integration or has an inherent ability to move. Where do these come from? Rudolf Steiner exerts considerable effort to address their origin. In a 1921 lecture he states, "What children learn during this first two-and-a-half-year period is extremely important for their whole life. They do so through an incoming activity and from what they have brought with them from prenatal existence."[9] During this very early time of life, the child's higher self is active in directing their development, including their motor, speech, and cognitive development. Through its direct connection to the spiritual world, the higher self receives "incoming activity," or guidance from the spiritual world.[10] (The higher self will be discussed in greater detail in volume 2.) In other words, this incoming activity from the spiritual world, along with what the child brings with them from their pre-birth experience, combine to guide the learning of the infant and very young child. Where do we find this activity of the higher self during the period of early childhood—where do we see the infant and young child learning?

Chapter 5: Aspects of Self-Initiated Movement

The Deeper Meaning of Children's Play

In a 1912 lecture, Rudolf Steiner explains:

> Where do we find what works on the child as a higher Self, and which belongs to the child, but doesn't enter [their] consciousness? Astonishing but true: it is *children's play,* the meaningful, well carried out play of all children, that the higher self works on. . . . What is accomplished in play happens basically through the self-activity of the child, through everything that cannot be confined to strict rules. Indeed, the essential, educational aspect of play is based on the fact that we call a halt to our rules and to all our arts of education and leave the child to [their] own impulses. For what does the child do when we leave [them] to [their] own impulses? When playing with external objects the child can try out whether this or that will work through [their] own activity. [They bring their] own will into activity, into movement. Because of the way in which the external objects behave under the influence of the will, it then happens that the child educates [themself] for life, simply through play, in a completely different way than through the influence of an older person or of someone's pedagogical principles. *For this reason it is so very important that we mix as little of the rational or intellectual as possible into children's play. The more that play has to do with what cannot be comprehended but is simply beheld in its living character, the better it is* [emphasis added].[11]

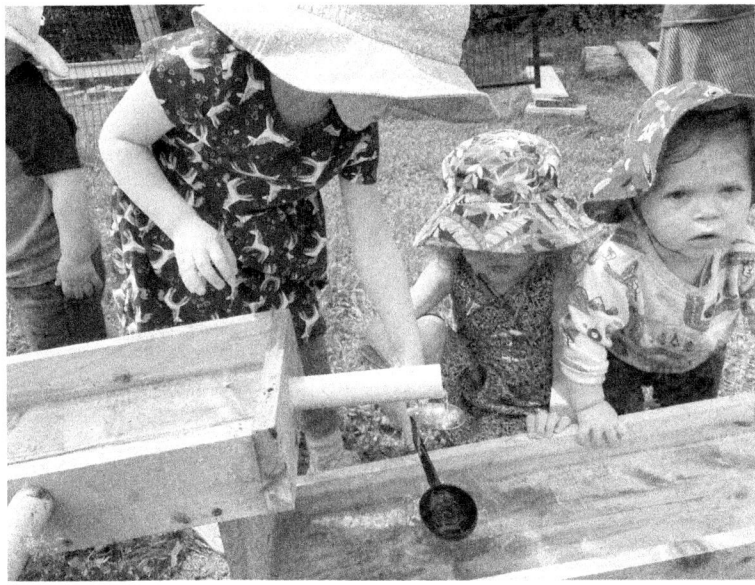
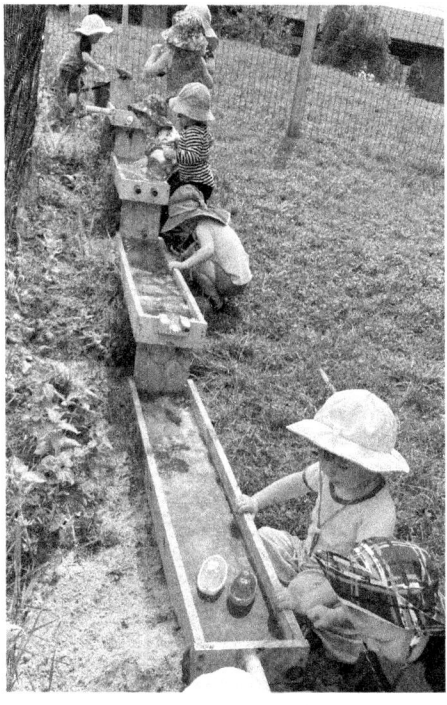

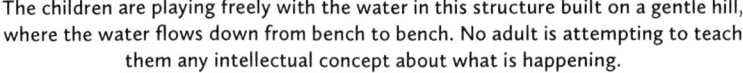
The children are playing freely with the water in this structure built on a gentle hill, where the water flows down from bench to bench. No adult is attempting to teach them any intellectual concept about what is happening.

Interestingly, Emmi Pikler says something remarkably similar. "What is essential is that the child discover as much as possible for [themselves.] If we help [them] to perform all of the tasks [they meet], we deprive [them] of just this, which is of greatest importance for [their] intellectual development. [They gain] a very different kind of knowledge through experimenting independently, than from knowledge presented to [them] ready-made, complete. . . . Therefore, we allow a child to experience [their] environment in [their] individual way, and according to [their] individual development."[12]

Earlier in the same article, Pikler says,

> What is most important, however, is not the result, but the way to it. This learning process will play a major role in the whole later life of the human being. Through this kind of development, the infant [develops their] ability to do something independently through patient and persistent effort. . . . While learning during motor development to turn on the belly, to roll, [crawl], sit, stand and walk, [they are] not only learning those movements, but also how to learn. [They learn] to do something on [their] own, to be interested, to try out, to experiment. [They learn] to overcome difficulties. [They come] to know the joy and satisfaction which is derived from this success, the result of [their] patience and persistence.[13]

In other words, the child is developing their will. Both Steiner and Pikler note the positive ramifications of childhood play for the entirety of the person's life.

During the initial period of life, play and movement are indistinguishable. Pikler explains: "During the first two years, [the child] is busy—or better, [they are] 'playing' with each movement for days, weeks, sometimes months."[14] Pikler goes on to speak about the child's joy of moving and of learning:

> The joy of learning, by the way, does not always depend on the result. Trying something out without arriving at the goal can be as joyful an experience as a successful experiment. The moment itself brings joy and it would be difficult to decide in which instance the child learns the most[,] "successful" or "not successful." These playful experiments are necessary parts, and form the basis of future development. There will be a loss, perhaps an irretrievable one, if the child stops experimenting too early, or never gets to experience this attentive, patient, concentrated occupation with [themselves].[15]

Now let us continue our exploration of the unrestrained play of babies and very young children.

Nuanced Variations of the Young Child's Movements

In free, unhindered movement and play, the activities are child-led, rather than adult-taught. This is the optimal situation for the infant and young child, and it changes over the course of one's life. A teenager or an adult may want to perfect a particular movement, and they may seek out a coach, whereby they receive external input and undergo instruction and training. Teenagers work to get their tennis stroke or their free throw just right, repeating these very singular, particular movements again and again. This is in contrast to what infants and young children do. If we saw a youngster repeating the exact same movement in a series of repetitions, we likely would be concerned that the child was perseverating. Babies and very young children do repeat movements in order to learn them. However, their movement have a different quality to them than those of the teenagers mentioned above. The movements of babies and very young children are embedded into play scenarios, and there is much subtle variation in them. The little ones' movements are within the context of the physical and social environment. They move to explore their surroundings with nuanced variations.

Here is a lovely example: A baby is playing with toys in back-lying and in side-lying. She lies on her back with both legs extended up in the air. She reaches up with her hands to her feet, and after a time she manages to pull off both socks. She holds onto her toes with her hands—right hand on the right foot and left hand on the left foot. She shifts her weight slightly to one side and then shifts back to the middle. She brings her feet together—sole touching sole—at the middle of her body. She moves them apart and back together again, as if she were playing patty-cake. She lets go of one foot and continues to keep it extended in the air. She brings the freed foot to touch the other foot, which she is still holding onto. She pats the airborne foot against the held foot. She slides the soles of her feet together—toes to heels and heels to toes.

Next, she lets go of the other foot, lowers both feet to the floor, picks up a nearby toy, and holds it with both arms extended. She brings her feet back up into the air. Her feet are separated and she moves them asymmetrically in the air. She brings her feet together—this time side by side, rather than sole to sole. She bends and straightens her legs rhythmically, still keeping her feet together. She separates her feet, extends both legs, and places her feet slowly on the floor. As she lowers her feet down to the floor, she rhythmically waves the toy in the air with her two hands. She stops moving for a moment, and looks across the room. She raises her feet back up into the air and bats the toy against both of her feet. She holds the toy in one hand and simultaneously holds the backside of the toy with the toes of the same-side foot. She holds her other foot with her other hand. In this fashion she rolls to the side. She releases both feet and extends them out farther to the side. She leaves her feet in the side-lying position and rotates her upper body ninety degrees to the supine position, and then she rotates her upper body back to side-lying. She hasn't finished at this point and continues to play. There seems to be no end to the nuanced variations of her movements.

I observed this same baby five days earlier. In this short time, there has been a noticeable increase in her motor control and stamina—she can hold her legs up in the air for longer periods, and she can shift her weight through longer excursions without losing her balance. If one were taking a Pilates class and doing what this baby is doing, it would be an advanced level class!

During this exploration, the baby is well-regulated. She paces herself. She does not rush. There is no strain in her movements. She moves with control and ease. She is fully engaged and interested in what she is doing. Pikler comments that the baby "is following [their] own movements with extraordinary interest and amazing patience. [The baby] attentively studies one movement innumerable times. [The baby] enjoys and becomes absorbed in each little detail, each nuance of a movement, quietly taking [their] time in an experimenting mode."[16] Pikler's comments are very applicable to this baby in this situation. Dr. Michaela Glöckler and Dr. Wolfgang Goebel regard the capacity for interest as one of the vital parts of health. They describe that health includes "the ability to be open to and interested in the phenomena of the world around; furthermore, to be in a position to share in the world's problems and to do all in one's human power to set them right".[17]

Note that no one interrupts the baby in the above scenario. No one interferes with her full engagement. I once observed an older two-year-old happily playing, singing as she was playing. She was singing bits and pieces of a song. She was not singing the song "correctly"—words were mispronounced or replaced, and she kept changing the words as she repeated the song. An adult relative heard her and started singing the same song, only with the correct lyrics. Perhaps the adult wanted to teach the child the correct words. Perhaps she wanted to engage with the child and have a shared singing experience. Whatever the relative's motivation was, unfortunately, the result was that the child stopped singing, and stopped playing. My interpretation was that the adult's singing was an abrupt intrusion into the child's play—even resulting in a little jolt to the child's dreamy consciousness.

A Deeper Look at the Movement Scenario

Let us consider what the baby is working on in the scenario illustrated above. In chapter 3, the development of a balanced relationship between the flexor muscles (which act to bend or curl the arms, legs, and trunk) and the extensor muscles (which arch the back and straighten the limbs and digits) was discussed in depth. Recall that all babies start out with an extensor bias—it is easier for them to extend their bodies than to flex them. In order for harmonious movement to ensue, the baby must balance out the two muscle groups. In self-initiated movement, the baby starts out in supine (back-lying), which is the optimal position for the flexors to begin to develop and "catch up" to the extensors. If we don't interfere by holding the baby to an externally imposed time frame of motor milestones, they will naturally stay in the supine position until the flexors have had enough time to "catch up," and the timing for this is unique to each individual child. When one considers the history of this child, one can see that there are good reasons for what she is doing. Earlier in her life, she displayed a slightly exaggerated amount of extension—she had a prominent tongue thrust, which is an extensor pattern. She has wisely penetrated the supine position more fully. In the above scenario she is demonstrating mastery over quite sophisticated, refined flexion. As a result, the tongue thrust has largely abated at this stage of her development. Now, she is starting to explore other positions more—she is spending more and more time in side-lying and has started to roll onto her tummy.

This baby was nine months old when this movement exploration occurred. Many babies would have been farther along in their gross motor development at nine months. These same babies would likely not have mastered flexion activities to the degree that this child has. Fortunately, no one in this child's life tried to hurry her up and teach her to do something that she was not yet ready to do. If this had happened, she would have missed out on a valuable part of her development, and she would likely have retained the extensor thrust of her tongue. Her parents then would likely have needed to take her to physical therapy, where the therapist would have worked on improving her flexion control. Instead, the child developed flexion control entirely out of her own initiative, and she did so at the most opportune time for her, in the course of her development—before the tongue thrust had become firmly established in her habit body,

Earlier in the chapter, we explored Rudolf Steiner's insights regarding the unique condition of children under three. This period of life is distinctive in that the higher Self has a direct connection to the spiritual world, and therefore, the profound wisdom of the spiritual world acts to guide the child's development. This case study offers us an opportunity to witness divine intelligence at work during a child's movement journey.

What else is this wise baby learning in this movement scenario? When she reaches for her toes with her hands, she is integrating the top of her body with the bottom. When she rotates her upper body away from her lower body in side-lying, she is developing counter-rotation in her trunk—a crucial and complex movement needed for later reciprocal crawling. (Counter-rotation is discussed in detail in chapter 2.) When she transitions between supine and side-lying, she is developing her balance. When she looks at her hands, her feet, and her toy, she is developing the convergence of her eyes. When she looks away at something in the room, and then looks back at her hands again, she is developing the ability to focus between far and near. When she stops and rests, she is learning to pace herself. She is also learning the limits of her abilities, and each day they expand a little bit more. Yesterday, she could shift her weight from supine into partial side-lying and hold the position without falling, and today she can go a little farther into the partial side-lying position and still maintain control.

In the above scenario, the baby is self-directed. It is she alone who decides what to do and how to change what she is doing. She is fully engaged and interested in what she is doing. It is all about doing at this stage of life. Rudolf Steiner describes this type of activity as an example of the child developing their will. He explains that the first seven-year period is a time for developing the will, the second seven-year period for developing the feeling life, and the third seven-year period for developing the thinking life. Let us consider the development of the will in more detail.

Education of the Child's Will

Renate Long-Breipohl explains that, according to Rudolf Steiner, "in the early years, thinking develops best by itself within an environment where there is enough opportunity for sensory exploration and for imitation. Will, on the other hand *does* need education because at the beginning of life it lacks conscious purpose and direction. The task of early education is to provide this direction through work with example and imitation."[18] (Cognitive development, including the development of thinking, will be discussed in greater detail in volume 2.) In other words, educating the will unfolds through the indirect process of imitation. The ultimate goal of educating the will is that the child develops into a person capable of meeting what comes toward them in life, while at the same time exerting self-determination in their life. A famous quote, often attributed to Rudolf Steiner but actually written by his wife, Marie Steiner, sums up the "highest endeavor" of Waldorf education: "Our highest endeavor must be to develop free human beings who are able of themselves to impart purpose and direction to their lives."[19]

Renate Long-Breipohl continues that there is much controversy and confusion over how to best educate the child's developing will. Often, "children's expressions of will are misinterpreted." [20] It is not uncommon for the young child to be seen as self-centered, and for the adult to assume the job of teaching them otherwise. Unfortunately, a battle of wills sometimes ensues, whereby the adult's will is imposed upon the child. The adult may employ admonitions, reasoning, arguing, fear tactics, and reward programs. All of these means may serve to "suppress the child's will. *But we cannot refine the child's will this way* [emphasis added]."[21] We intuitively know that it is not a sound practice to try and break a child's will—that this can have a lasting negative impact on the child. Rudolf Steiner wisely states, "as long as you impose your wish upon anything at all, without this wish of yours being born from the thing itself, you injure it."[22] Instead, he says to "allow the heartbeats of the other to resound within you and do not disturb them by the pulse of your own heart."[23] He also advises us, "we must recognize the Will-element, and everything in another person's subconscious, as something which should on no account be intruded upon; it must be regarded as [their] innermost sanctuary."[24]

It is helpful for us to understand that "Education of the will means to *facilitate the child's learning to master [their] own will.*"[25] For the infant and young child, free play time serves as a wonderful time for the child to master their own will. In free play, babies and young children set themselves tasks and then exert their wills in order to carry out those tasks. This often requires perseverance, patience, creativity, and tenacity. It is very healthy for the child to engage their will. This is what we want them to do! We purposely set up the child's play spaces so that they may become fully engaged and exercise their will.

Only the child can develop their will. We cannot do it for them. However, we can support the child by serving as a model worthy of imitation. According to Renate Long-Breipohl, "Steiner states that the education of the will of children under three should consist first and foremost of the self-education of the adult. He asks that adults apply themselves wholeheartedly to all tasks that may come their way and approach life with an open heart and mind. In dealing with the young child the [adult] should develop sympathy with the child and lovingly embrace the child's will. Lovingly accompanying the child's steps into life will create warmth around the child and in so doing create the optimum conditions for the will to become active."[26]

Children under three spend an incredible amount of time moving! Self-initiated movement calls forth the Self—it engages the will. In order to "lovingly embrace the child's will" and "accompany the child's steps into life," then, it is helpful to understand some basic aspects of how a child learns—and remembers—patterns of movement.

A Different Type of Memory in the Young Child

As adults, we are (hopefully) easily able to remember things. We are able to create inner pictures, re-create them, manipulate them, and learn. However, the child is not able to do this until approximately age seven. In the young child, the development of memory occurs in a predicable sequence. (The development of memory will be discussed more fully in volume 2.)

Rudolf Steiner describes the first type of memory that starts to develop in the baby: "In the little child, the capacity for recollection and memory has not yet assumed the character of mental images; rather, it is a bodily or 'implicit' memory associated with 'habitual' soul behaviors."[27] In a 1921 lecture, Steiner elaborates:

> When we observe a very young child, we find that the capacity to remember has the quality of a soul habit. When a child recalls something during that first period of life until the change of teeth,

such remembering is a kind of habit or skill. We might say that when, as a child, I acquire a certain accomplishment—let us say, writing—it arises largely from a certain suppleness of my physical constitution, a suppleness that I have gradually acquired. When you watch a small child taking hold [of] something, you have found a good illustration of the concept of habit. A child gradually discovers how to move the limbs this way or that way, and this becomes habit and skill. Out of a child's imitative actions, the soul develops skillfulness, which permeates the child's finer and more delicate organizations. A child will imitate something one day, then do the same thing again the next day and the next; this activity is performed outwardly, but also—and importantly—within the innermost parts of the physical body. This forms the basis for memory in the early years.[28]

In this passage, Steiner points to how, at the start of life, memory begins with incorporating impressions into the etheric body. The etheric body is also referred to as the learning body, as well as the habit body. This habitual memory is our basis for learning, particularly for learning skills. We want the baby to incorporate lots of healthy impressions into their etheric body, as this sets the stage for the later development of more sophisticated types of memory; these will be covered in volume 2.

We commonly refer to the bodily, habitual type of memory as muscle memory or kinesthetic memory. In the scientific literature it is also known as procedural memory, a type of implicit memory where the repetition of an activity leads to it becoming automatic. This type of memory is involved in learning to tie our shoes, ride a bike, and drive a car. We continue to create and employ muscle memories throughout adulthood. These muscle memories serve to anchor us as we navigate our environments. They make life easier and more predictable for us.

Recently, the spring mechanism in the door of our dishwasher broke, and it took several weeks before the repair person came to fix it. My husband and I are both right-handed. When we bought the dishwasher, the muscles and joints in our right arms registered the weight of the door, as well as the arc and dynamic of the door's acceleration and deceleration as we lowered it to the horizontal position. Thus, the muscles in our arms learned to generate the appropriate forces with which to open the door. We soon developed a muscle memory—a bodily habit—of opening the dishwasher door. After the spring mechanism broke, when we opened the door, it would quickly fall—with a thud—down to a horizontal position, instead of moving more dynamically in an arc, as it did before. Initially, this startled us a bit. We had lost the orientation that our muscle memories had given us when we opened the door. After a couple days, we adjusted to the new "feel" of the door—we had mastered a new muscle memory. After the spring mechanism was fixed, we again experienced a slight feeling of unease from the change in the "feel" of the door, and we had to readjust our movement pattern again back to the original one.

My husband and I are mature adults with well-developed coordination, and though it wasn't a terribly big deal, we both commented on the perturbation that this experience with the door gave us. Our bodily memories provide us with an unconscious, foundational feeling of security as our bodies interact in routine ways with the world. Imagine how unsettling and confusing life could potentially be for a newborn, who has not yet mastered control of their body, nor developed bodily memories. This is why it is so helpful for the adult to use orienting language with infants—we tell the child what we are going to do with them *before* we do it. Even before the child is able to understand our words, they respond to our tone of voice and our manner. For example, "It's time to eat. I have the food all ready. I am going to pick you up now and take you to the kitchen table." As the child grows older and clearly has learned the routines, they no longer need such detailed orienting language. However, even as adults, whenever we are in an unknown situation, such as when we have a medical procedure performed, we still benefit from orienting language. With orienting language, we are not teaching abstract concepts to the child. We are not prematurely appealing to their intellect. Rather, we are anchoring the child in the here and now, giving them concrete orientation for what is about to happen, so that they are better prepared to meet the situation at hand.

Developing Skills and Habits in Free Play

We can support the child to establish movement skills and habits by giving them long periods of uninterrupted free play. For example, the baby learns to transition between positions and to roll, to belly-crawl, to crawl on hands and knees, and so on. The baby practices these movements over and over, with many nuanced variations, and it takes their full attention to do so. Imagine back to when you were learning to write. It takes attention and repetition to learn to write—ideally, without unnecessary interruptions. Once you have learned to write well, the task of writing can be accomplished without as much attention. For example, you can likely take notes while listening to a lecture, and even while reaching into your backpack for a tissue with your other hand. The baby and young child are still at the stage of learning basic foundational bodily skills. It is very helpful to refrain from interrupting the child during their learning, instead giving them the time and space to allow these processes of mastering movement skills to unfold naturally. Only the child knows when they have mastered the habit, and the baby is in various stages of learning several habits at once. In the above example, the baby is in the final stages of learning to reach for her toes, in the midst of learning to stabilize herself in side-lying, and just beginning to learn to roll to her tummy.

The child's establishment and mastery of healthy movement habits is supported by the adult's creating and supporting the daily rhythm of caregiving and opportunities for free movement, as described in earlier chapters. The ebb and flow of this rhythm gives a healthy, breathing quality to the relationship. There is an alternating "going out into the wide world" and then a "coming back home" gesture to this set up.[29] During the free movement periods, the adult "holds" the space with their warm, receptive presence, giving the child a chance to learn new motor skills on their own and find out what they can independently do in the world. Let us now consider how the adult can support the child in mastering new movements during the caregiving times, when they "come back home" to the security of a nurturing relationship.

Developing Skills and Habits in Caregiving Activities

We can support the child's learning movement habits and skills during caregiving activities by providing regularity when we ask the child to participate in a particular movement. Imagine that a baby is standing on a Pikler changing table, hanging on to the rail (see the description of the Pikler changing table in appendix 3). The caregiver indicates to the baby that the pant leg is ready, and they would like the baby to insert their leg into it. The caregiver speaks to the child and perhaps also touches the child's leg with the pants in order to cue the child. The caregiver waits for the child to process the request. The child responds by shifting their weight onto their other leg, and then picking up and inserting the airborne leg into the pant leg. This is a very complicated movement, requiring spatial orientation, body scheme, balance, and coordination. Over time, this movement becomes more fluid, and it gradually becomes established as a bodily habit, or muscle memory. We can consciously present the pant leg in the same fashion every time to the child, i.e., at the same height, at the same angle to the body, and on the same side of the body. This consistency helps the child as they develop the skill of donning their pants.

Here is another example. I witnessed a mother changing a six-month-old baby's diaper in the presence of a friend of the family, who was visiting. Instead of holding the baby's feet and lifting up her bottom by pulling the feet, as is the common cultural practice, the mother asked the baby to lift up her bottom so the mother could position a fresh diaper underneath her. The child easily and readily complied. This degree of motor skill in such a young baby is not typically expected in the broader Western culture. Indeed, the friend, who had raised three children of her own and who also had several grandchildren, was surprised at the baby's motor control and cooperation. This motor capacity did not happen overnight. The mother had been consistently engaging the baby in the diapering activity since birth, and the baby had developed this movement habit.

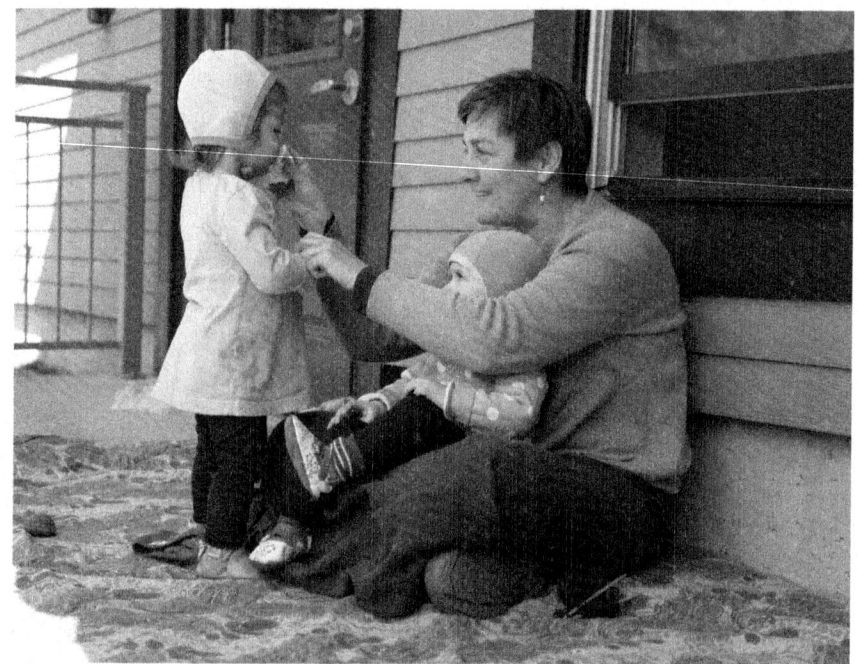

This caregiver is wiping the child's nose. She has elicited the child's participation, and it is a positive encounter for both parties.

Participating in wiping the nose is another habit that the young child can acquire. What sometimes happens is that the adult tries to wipe the child's nose, the child pulls away or runs away, and the adult "wipes the child's nose on the run." Or sometimes the adult approaches from behind and hurriedly wipes the nose before the child knows what is happening. In either case, the child is not engaged and is not developing a habit or a skill of participation. Rather, the child is developing the habit of avoiding cooperative activity with the adult, and unknowingly, the adult is setting the stage for this. In contrast, the adult can calmly approach the child from the front and orient the child, saying something like, "Your nose has some drips, and I'd like to wipe it." The adult then waits for the child's response—it can be the slightest movement forward of the face—and then the adult gently wipes the nose.

There are endless opportunities for cooperative engagement between adult and child. In another example, the child can develop a habit of joining in when their face and hands are wiped after a meal. Sometimes children go through phases where they object to having their faces wiped, or the child may have a sensitivity due to a skin rash on their face. Here, the adult can experiment with different approaches so the child can still have a pleasant encounter with the adult. Perhaps the adult simply needs to wait a moment until the child is ready. The child's attention may wander. The adult may choose to follow the child's attention and then lead the child's attention back to the matter at hand. Perhaps the child will better engage in the face cleaning if the cloth is wetted with warm water instead of cold water, if the adult dabs the face more firmly—or more lightly—instead of wiping it, or if the child wipes their own face first and then the adult finishes. Sometimes a different type of cloth is more acceptable to a particular child.

I witnessed an early childhood teacher readying a one-year-old for naptime in our childcare at Sophia's Hearth. The little boy and the adult were working together to don his sleep sack. The caregiver held the bottom of the zipper so that the boy could successfully zip it up. Upon completion of the task, he looked at the caregiver and beamed! The adult could have just "gotten the job done," and dressed the boy herself, but by eliciting the engagement of the boy, the boy was learning the skill of zipping. In addition, the relationship was nourished.

In another instance, at our childcare at Sophia's Hearth, three toddlers were sitting at a Pikler feeding bench with the teacher next to them. (See the description of the Pikler feeding bench in appendix 3.) One boy touched a girl's leg with his foot. The girl voiced her discomfort about this. The teacher oriented the boy, saying, "She is telling you that she doesn't like it when you touch her leg, and that it is time for you to stop doing that." The boy persisted, the girl again voiced her discomfort, and the teacher again oriented the boy. It is noteworthy that the teacher spoke very matter-of-factly and maintained her equanimity. After the fourth repetition, the boy stopped. Here, the boy self-initiated the quieting of his legs. He was beginning to learn the habit of keeping his legs still while eating at the table with the other children. The teacher wisely perceived that in order to learn the habit of sitting quietly at the feeding bench, the boy had to perform the deed himself. She did not force the boy to stop touching the girl's leg, but repeatedly invited and guided his engagement.

In all of these cooperative caregiving activities, the adult is supporting the child to learn a skill or a habit through their own self-initiated activity. There is a nuanced dance going on between adult and child in each encounter. The adult is confident that the task will be completed. However, the caregiver is open-minded, knowing that the roads to Rome are many. Based upon the momentary responses of the child, the adult may need to repeat or reform the activity so that the child can enter in out of their own will forces. The goal is to give up using power over young children and, rather, to support the child to come to the deed themselves.[30]

Here is an example of two young children who did not learn a new movement habit, and I was one of them! When I was a child, we frequently visited my grandmother. The front door of her house had a wooden screen door which was used all summer. Anxious to get outside and play, my sister and I would run out the door, letting it bang behind us. My mother would call after us, "Don't bang the door," after it had already banged. This literally happened for years, during which time the door banged merrily along. What was going on here? My mother was appealing to us verbally, but we didn't readily register verbal input at that stage of development. Rather, the child in the first seven years is better able to perceive gesture, or nonverbal communication. Additionally, in order to remember to close the door quietly, we needed to actually practice closing the door quietly so that it could become a kinesthetic memory—so that we could remember to do it with our limbs. My mother was asking us to remember something via our heads, in a way that we were not developmentally ready to do. It would have been more productive for all concerned if she could have met us at the door as we were going out of it and modeled closing the door quietly so it didn't slam. She wouldn't have had to say much—or anything at all. Her actions would have said it all. However, she would have had to repeat this over time, and have us do the correct movement after the first couple of times. If she would have met us at the door, it would have slowed us down and essentially served to head us off at the pass. In this way the conditions would have been ripe for us to learn the new movement skill of closing the screen door quietly.

6: The Complexity of Baby Equipment

Long ago and far away (in the Midwest), I began my physical therapy career. Conventional baby equipment was only moderately used. Its influence was tempered, because free play and time outside in nature for children were fairly common. There were no screens, except for movies and TV, which was generally not broadcast on a twenty-four-hour basis. Grade schools still had recess. The grandparents of the day remembered using playpens and putting infants down on the floor to play. Parents cooked supper holding the baby on their hip, where the baby actively engaged with maintaining their posture. When the parent fatigued, they moved the baby to their other hip, so the baby wasn't in one position for too long.

The baby equipment of the day primarily included doorframe jumpers, bouncer seats, wind-up swings, slings, and baby walkers. (These will be described below.) A physical therapy colleague of mine compared the trend toward baby equipment to the movement toward junk food. Junk food is not really good for us, but for most people, an occasional bit won't hurt. Some people can eat a lot of junk food, and it doesn't seem to bother them. However, for others, just a little bit of red food dye gives them the jitters for days, and for some it can be addictive. Similarly, although baby equipment does not provide conditions for the development of healthy movement, for most infants, a little bit won't significantly harm them. However, it can have a strong negative impact on babies who have certain conditions, such as cerebral palsy, developmental delays, or musculoskeletal issues.

Today, baby equipment is a big industry. It is common practice to use baby equipment in homes and childcare settings, however, pediatricians and physical and occupational therapists routinely speak out against *excessive* use of it. Unfortunately, sometimes a little leads to a lot. It may be so convenient for the adult to place the child into a piece of baby equipment that it can inadvertently become a habit, and before you know it, the child has spent hours during the day in various devices. There may be another, perhaps less understood, phenomenon occurring. Inherent in the horizontal position is the propensity for a decrease in consciousness. Parents who have been on bedrest for an extended period during a pregnancy often attest to this. It can go the other way too. When we're trying to get to sleep, if an interruption causes us to sit or stand up—even briefly—we may then have to start our bedtime routine all over again, because verticality calls forth increased consciousness.

Similarly, when babies come into sitting and standing, we often notice an increase in their awareness. During free motor exploration, the attainment of verticality is gradual, and with it, there is a gradual changing of consciousness. However, if we place an infant into a vertical position for extended periods of time before they attain verticality on their own, they don't fully experience the earlier, dreamy stage of consciousness, and their awakening may be more abrupt. If we then place that same child back down into a horizontal position, they may resist, perhaps because they have grown used to the consciousness of the upright.

Baby equipment has routinely been advertised as supporting motor development, however, significant research disputes this claim. In one study, infants were divided into two groups, one with significant baby equipment use and one without it. Developmental motor assessments were then performed at eight months. It was found that "infants who have high equipment use tend to score lower on infant development . . . and infants who have lower equipment use tend to score higher on infant development."[1]

In addition, baby equipment has become increasingly high tech, and with this, the baby's experiences when placed in the equipment have become more intense. Now, there are computerized baby cribs with sensors to sense when the baby is stirring, and then rock the baby back to sleep. Where infant seats used to be simple sling seats on a wire frame that bounced the baby when they kicked, today many infant seats are computerized. Some resemble an amusement park spaceship ride, with vibrators, flashing lights, whirring sounds, and spiraling, rocking, and ascending and descending movements. It seems there is no end to what can be done with baby equipment, and unfortunately, with the growing capacities of technology, this will surely continue.

The culture of forty years ago, which used to mitigate the effects of baby equipment, does not exist today. Today, most children spend less time outside in nature. They have less downtime and fewer opportunities for free play, more screen time, and more structured instruction—such as baby exercise classes and sports programs for youngsters. (That said, forest kindergartens and forest preschool programs are gaining traction as well.) These two factors—the cultural conditions and the increased intensity of the baby's experiences when placed into baby equipment—potentize the effects of the use of baby equipment.

Parents ultimately must make the decisions for their children, and there are many decisions to make. The issue of whether to use baby equipment is a complex one. This chapter offers several lenses through which to explore the baby's experiences when they are placed into a piece of baby equipment, in the hope that parents—as well as early childhood teachers and administrative staff at childcare facilities—can make informed choices about the use of baby equipment for the children in their care. If one is working with parents, it is helpful to remember that there is no useful purpose in making a parent feel guilty for having used baby equipment. Use of baby equipment is not necessarily a good indicator of a child's later abilities, as life is multifaceted.

A Look at Some of the Devices

Baby bouncers, car seats that can be removed and used outside of the car, infant seats, and infant swings are commonly used for newborns and younger infants. (Of course, a car seat should be used when the baby is in the car!) These pieces of equipment all have two defining features in common—they all put a baby into a semi-reclining position, and they generally have soft surfaces into which the baby's body sinks. As such, they severely restrict the baby's movement and limit the baby's position to one where the hips and knees are flexed up, and the back and neck are rounded. This is the common position of newborns. However, after birth, the entire musculoskeletal system gradually undergoes a complete transformation. For example, the long, rounded spine of the newborn eventually becomes the three gentle undulating curves of the neck, thoracic, and lumbar spine. Firm horizontal surfaces support the baby's ability to move, and the movements serve to lengthen, strengthen, and balance the muscles and ligaments around the entire spine, whereas the soft, semi-reclined seats thwart the child's ability to move, effectively stunting the transformation of the musculoskeletal system.

Full-term newborns are nearly always born with very slight asymmetries, because of the tight quarters inside the womb and the fact that they have not been able to move freely during the last few months of pregnancy. In order to balance out the newborn's subtle asymmetries, then, they need to be able to move and stretch out! As adults, we get stiff if we sit too long in one position, and this is very apparent on long plane trips. (I have flown to China and Australia from the United States, and after several hours, there are always people—including me—who pull out their stretchy exercise bands to quietly "work out" in their seats or find a place in the plane to do standing yoga postures and stretching.) In many cases, when the young infant has opportunities to move and stretch on a firm, horizontal surface, the asymmetries will resolve. If they are placed into semi-reclining, soft types of seats for extended periods, their asymmetries may continue and even progress. It is particularly problematic when infants sleep in these types of seating devices, not only because of the potential to exacerbate asymmetry, but also because it places them at higher risk for SIDS. According to the American Academy of Pediatrics: "Babies should not routinely sleep in car seats, strollers, swings, infant carriers, and infant slings. Some of these products keep the baby in a position where their breathing could be compromised while sleeping."[2]

Occupational therapist Rachel Coley writes about another common consequence of extended time spent in "container devices," or "baby buckets," as they are often referred to by pediatric occupational and physical therapists. "One of the most obvious negative impacts of lots of time spent in infant positioners is flattening of the head. It's common to blame Back to Sleep recommendations for increased head flattening in infants. But the plethora of baby gear our newborns lounge in during the day is a huge contributing factor to head flattening that we CAN safely change."[3] (See Chapter 3 for more on this topic.)

There are other options besides soft, semi-reclined seats for newborns and younger infants, such as a Moses basket, in which the infant is horizontal. A Pikler box placed open side up on the kitchen table provides a firm horizontal surface up off the floor, and the child won't be able to roll off the table.

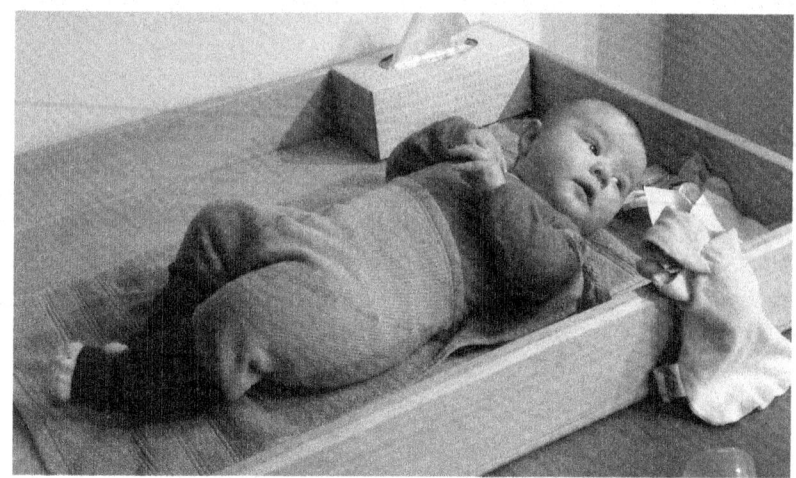

Pikler box on a kitchen table.

Baby walkers are wheeled devices with suspended seats in which the child is positioned in an upright position before they can assume it on their own. The device allows them to propel themselves in all directions, using the balls of the feet. Baby walkers are not as popular as they used to be. Perhaps this is because babies have been seriously injured while using them, especially when the baby walker fell down stairs or was tipped over by siblings. However, they are still on the market, and advertised as helping a child learn to walk while the child has fun, because the devices also provide entertaining sounds, melodies, and lights. This is marketing claim does not survive critical thinking! The claim implies that the child needs help—that they aren't capable of learning to walk on their own. It implies that the motor sequence is boring, that it is without consequence to skip some of its early stages, and that the child needs to be entertained in order to learn a motor skill. These ideas are not true, and are antithetical to what both Steiner and Pikler espoused.

Baby saucers are similar to baby walkers except that they are considerably safer, in that they don't have wheels, and the child stays in one place in the room. There is a domed surface on the bottom, with the convex side down, which allows spinning and rocking. The advertising for these products implies that a baby needs one, or they won't get enough exercise. If you've ever gotten down on the floor and imitated a baby's movements even for a short period of time, you can realize how much exercise they are truly getting, without the aid of a saucer!

Doorframe jumpers are seats that are usually suspended with straps from a doorframe for the purpose of supporting a baby to bounce before they are developmentally ready to stand or jump. Of all the baby equipment on the market, these give me the most cause for concern, as numerous children have sustained ankle sprains from jumping and landing on ankles that are not developmentally ready to withstand such strong forces placed upon them, and infants have also received serious injuries from hitting the door frame, including head injuries. In addition, they (along with baby walkers and saucers) may position the baby in such a way that the child is up on their toes, and this can contribute to toe walking later on. In contrast, the baby on the floor gets a lot of input to their heels, thus preparing the healthy pattern for walking with the heels down. For example, babies play on their backs and kick their legs, sometimes sliding their heels along the surface as they kick, and often coming to rest with their heels in contact with the surface. In back-lying they also push down through their heels to lift their buttocks up off the surface into a bridge position, and they dig their heels into the surface to scoot backward across the floor.

Push-type baby walkers are also on the market. Their design is similar to walkers for the elderly, in that they have handles and wheels. These baby walkers are specifically made to assist babies who are not yet able to walk on their own, but who are pulling to stand and standing. However, it is not necessary to hurry a pre-walker to walk! They will walk when they are ready to. Additionally, if the child is given such a device before they are independently walking, the child typically assumes a poor posture with a forward head, a forwardly inclined trunk, and excessively flexed legs. This pattern is not one that is conducive to coordinated movement.

Harnesses have become increasing popular. Harnesses fit snugly around the baby's torso—over the shoulders, under the armpits, around the chest, and under the crotch. In many of the various brands, the crotch strap is removable. Harnesses also include a strap for the parent to hold.

Years ago, harnesses were used primarily for safety. When I was a toddler, my family visited San Francisco. I have two siblings very close in age, and so it is not surprising that my parents found it challenging to keep track of the three of us in such a busy environment. I wandered off, and they lost me. Luckily, a woman from the bar in our hotel found me and brought me back to my frantic parents. My parents quickly purchased a harness. In those days, the harnesses did not include the strap under the crotch. My parents used the harness for the rest of the trip whenever we were in crowded conditions, as they didn't want to lose me again. This was a reasonable way of using this piece of equipment under those conditions.

Today, harnesses are advertised as having an entirely different purpose. Many parents walk behind their child, holding their child's hands from above in order to help them learn to walk. This maneuver requires that the adult leans over. The harnesses are advertised as a means of "teaching your child to walk" without breaking your back. Thus, the child is walking with adult assistance for longer periods of time. Initially, the full harness is to be used. It fits around the upper body and also covers the crotch. Later, the crotch part is to be removed so that the harness fits only around the upper body. If the child stumbles, the adult pulls up on the harness so the child won't fall to the ground.

Harnesses are advertised as helping the child learn to balance, and as a way for the child to get over their fear of falling. Unfortunately, this is clearly not the case! Using a harness in this manner actually interferes with the child's learning to balance, because it short-changes the sensory feedback that is necessary for learning to balance. Using a harness puts a child in a contrived situation whereby the child is asked to perform a motor task that their body is not yet prepared for.

Harnesses are also advertised as a way to bolster a child's self-confidence and as a way to spend quality time with your child. Again, I beg to differ.

Decreased Free Movement in Baby Equipment

To state the obvious, when a baby is in any piece of equipment, they are not able to do the things that they would be doing if they were free to move on a firm, horizontal surface. Skipping the early stages of development before sitting and standing is really the crux of the baby equipment question. There is inherent wisdom in the self-initiated motor sequence. Each stage lays a firm foundation upon which the child can take their next step, and also, each stage—in and of itself—is valuable. For example, during free movement exploration, the baby typically goes through a stage in which they use their feet like hands, in that they manipulate toys and objects with their feet. This may happen when they are on their back, where they hold an object between their two feet. They often pass objects back and forth between their feet and their hands. Sometimes they have an object in their hands and simultaneously another object between their feet, and they bang the two objects together. In these activities the child is sensing the objects with their feet (as well as with their hands.) The child may also play with a toy with their feet while lying on their tummy. In this position, the baby can't see their feet or the toy, and so the need for the child to sense out beyond their feet in order to perceive the toy is even more pronounced.

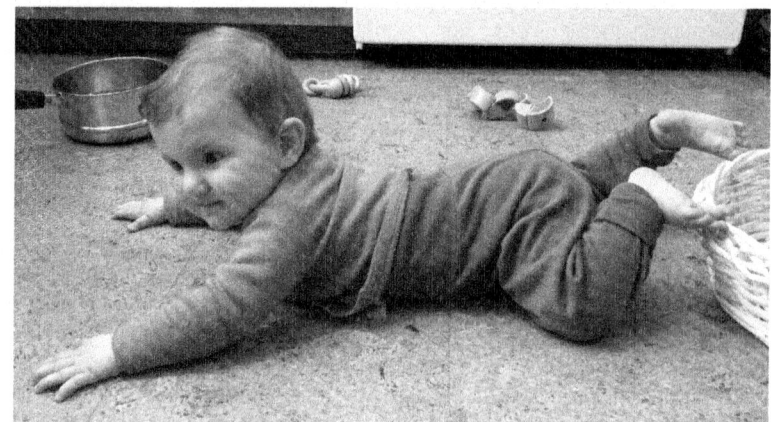

This baby is playing with a basket with their feet, tapping it and moving it. In order to do so, they must sense the basket with their feet.

If the child spends a substantial amount of time standing prematurely in baby equipment, they don't fully experience the early sensing phase of their feet in the horizontal positions. This is unfortunate, because sensing in the horizontal positions helps prepare the feet sensorily for balance while standing and walking. Walking toddlers and people of all ages need to be able to sense beyond their feet, into the surface beneath them, in order to perceive whether it is horizontal or inclined, firm or yielding, and whether there is an irregularity such as a clump of grass, a random toy, or a change of surface—from secure to slippery, for example. This is referred to as "orienting to the supporting surface." When babies can do this accurately, their bodies automatically make the necessary adjustments, thus preventing a fall. *The capacity to balance is built upon the capacity to sense.*

When the baby is born, the development of virtually all of their basic systems is not complete. We recognize that their digestive system is immature compared to that of an adult, and we take care to nourish the baby with breast milk or formula. We watch and wait until they are ready to try solid foods. Then we mix the cereal with formula or breast milk to make it just right. We don't feed them honey until they are one year old, when their systems have developed enough to safely handle it. Their other systems—such as the various sensory systems, the musculoskeletal system, and the neurological system—are also immature and need this same degree of care and attention. For example, the infant's tactile system (or sense of touch) is not fully developed. When the baby plays in supine, side-lying, and prone, and also when they roll and belly-crawl, they are receiving a significant amount of tactile input from the floor to all the various sides of their body. This serves to nourish and support the developing sense of touch. The opportunity for nourishing tactile input is diminished in baby equipment. In the tactile system, sensory information comes from the skin, which informs us about the boundary of our body. (See chapter 12, discussing the sense of touch.)

What all baby equipment has in common is that it restricts the child's movements, and with it, the child's sensory experiences and opportunities to choose their own sensory experiences. The baby is not free to move into and out of the devices, and there are limited opportunities for movement within the devices. In contrast, children engaged in free movement (outside of devices) are able to move a greater amount and with greater variations to their movements. The gesture of baby equipment is to distract and pacify the child rather than to provide them an environment in which their will forces can develop, i.e., in which they can find and create unique activities that interest them. In free motor exploration, the activity of interest may be a large motor movement, such as rolling or belly-scooting, or it may be a small motor activity such as playing with a toy or object. The child frequently switches back and forth from large motor to fine motor play. It is the child who chooses when to switch activities and when to continue what they are doing. In this way, the child is learning to modulate their engagement. This is not possible in baby equipment.

In baby equipment, the child may experience movement, as in the mechanized seat described above, however, they don't move by employing their own will forces. Instead, they are passively moved. The sounds, melodies, and lights of baby equipment are also experienced by the child, however, the child is not actively involved in creating them in the same way that a child can create visual and auditory experiences on the floor in free play. For example, a child playing on the floor may create sounds by banging two objects together, banging one on the floor, batting at an object, or dropping it. They may find a particular sound interesting, reproduce it, and also vary it. Or they may not like a sound and will stop making it. They may create changes in the light falling upon a metal bowl by batting at it and wiggling it. This may catch their eye, and they may do it again, or not. In free movement on the floor, the possibilities for sensorimotor experiences are endless, whereas they are much more limited in baby equipment.

A Specific Example: The Saucer

In free motor development, when the child first stands alone without holding on to a coffee table or other support, they typically have strikingly good spinal alignment. They may be remarkably upright with the head centered over the trunk, and the trunk centered over the feet. Their posture at this point is a result of all their previous experiences of strengthening, elongating, and balancing the muscles and ligaments of the spine that have occurred in the previous horizontal stages of the motor sequence. When they first stand without arm support, they bear full weight through the legs, the heels are down on the floor, and they use their muscles efficiently. All of these conditions provide good proprioceptive input and contribute to the development of this sensory system. (In the proprioceptive system, sensory information comes from the muscles and joints and informs us about the positions and movements of our body parts.) In addition, the infant is employing balance in order to stand, and their trunks are incredibly active, further developing their posture.

In contrast, the infant in a saucer is not bearing full weight through their legs and not using their muscles as extensively as the child who comes to standing on their own. Thus, in the saucer, they are not receiving the same degree of proprioceptive input. They are partially sitting on the sling seat, and they often lean forward on the tray in front, i.e., the trunk is inclined forward, with the head out in front of the body. Often, the baby will then arch their head backward in order to compensate for the forward-leaning trunk. Thus, the posture of the child is negatively affected. The child may also lean back to sink into the backside of the saucer, with a slumping posture. Here, the child is not using their trunk. This is especially pronounced in very young babies who are placed into the saucer.

In addition, when very young babies are placed upright before they have the ability to hold their heads up—which requires a degree of maturation of the deep tonic muscles of the spine—there is the possibility of inadvertent compression of the vertebrae.[4]

Saucers have a rounded base. With this design, the child can spin around, and rock forward and backward, side to side, and diagonally. Because a child doesn't have access to a horizontal surface with their feet when they are in the saucer, they are not getting "true" feedback from gravity. Typically, when we push down into a flat surface, our body is displaced in a predictable way, according to the laws of physics. There is a clean feedback loop which gives us a means to learn to manage the weight and mass of our body in space. Because of the convex bottom surface of the saucer, sometimes, when the baby pushes down into it with their foot, they tip forward, sometimes they tip sideways, sometimes they spin clockwise, sometimes they spin counterclockwise, and so on. The laws of physics are still working here, but the convex surface complicates the situation, and for a young infant who has very little experience with balance and spatial orientation, it is much harder to come into relationship with these force vectors. In other words, it is harder for the child to develop an orientation to one of the most pervasive and important features of the earth—gravity. When we have a healthy relationship with gravity, this can give us a basic sense of security in the order of the world and in our ability to cope with it. Indeed, the children who do not have this fundamental relationship with the supporting surface are said to have gravitational insecurity.

Babies are typically placed into saucers before they are able to stand on their own. It is nearly impossible for these infants to develop any significant degree of balance while in a saucer, because they are developmentally not prepared, and the biomechanics don't stack up! As described above, they literally can't align their bodies correctly. Instead, they typically posture in one of two ways. They either strain to pull up off the surface—literally tensing up all the way into their shoulders and necks, rising up onto their toes—or they sink down and collapse into the seat and bar. Neither of these responses is conducive to developing a heathy working relationship with the surface, which is perhaps the most important part of learning to balance. (The development of balance is covered more fully in chapter 15.)

When they tip in the saucer, they are practicing movement that is not coordinated, in that they are hurling their bodies. However, they don't experience the true consequence of their movement, because the rim of the saucer catches them. If the rim weren't there, they would fall to the ground. This setup gives them faulty feedback with which to learn to manage their bodies in space, and perhaps even more importantly, to develop judgement about their abilities. As a result, they may be less safe in future situations, when there isn't anything there to block a fall. The specific features of a saucer combine to actually work *against* a child's learning to walk!

The toys on the saucer are secured, so that the baby is not able to pick them up and manipulate them singly and in conjunction with the other toys. Toys that the child can pick up and manipulate are more open-ended, and the baby has free range for how they want to play with them. They can drop them, stack them, roll them, put one inside the other, and so on. In doing so, they may feel agency. They can better understand what they are doing and how they are impacting the world. Instead, the toys attached to a saucer have limited possibilities, thus limiting the child's ability to do and to learn by their doing. They are designed for the baby to push buttons and slide levers in order to turn on recorded music and light shows. One can ask, what is the child learning here? Perhaps they are learning that the world is a yes/no, on/off situation. This is very different than when the child plays on the floor and manipulates objects, where more nuanced learning can occur. For example, they can place one block on top of a second block, and if it is mostly centered on top of the second block, it will stay there. If their placement of the first block is off center, it may or may not fall off, depending upon how far off center they place it. If they place a large block on top of a smaller block, then it really has to be centered, or it will fall.

After a period of time, the lights and the music may stop in the saucer, but the child did nothing to stop them. The world seems random and arbitrary. When they push a button, and a light turns on and changes colors, they don't really have the ability to understand how that works—not in the same way that they can understand how the placement of a block affects whether it will fall or not. The mechanisms behind the lights and the melodies are hidden from the child, and they are complex. I have observed that infants often lose interest in these types of toys rather quickly, because they really can't do much with them besides turn them on and off. Infants are hungry to understand and meet the world, and it is helpful if we take steps—like providing simple toys—in order to make the world more digestible for them.

A Note about Screens

In chapter 4, we discussed screens in relation to self-regulation. Let us now also consider the huge sensory differences between a child's interacting with the real world versus receiving transmissions from a screen. In healthy perception in the "real world," a person experiences bidirectional movement—subtle incoming and outgoing movements. In *The Renewal of Education*, Rudolf Steiner explains that when we listen to another person or look at something, we "fall asleep"—that is, we put aside our own thoughts and feelings and enter into the outer world. Our comprehension of what has occurred in the outer world happens when we re-enter our own world, inside our bodies, experiencing a kind of "awakening." Steiner states: "While we are listening or looking at something, there is a continual awakening and falling asleep, even though we are awake. It is a continual undulation—waking, falling asleep, waking, falling asleep. In the final analysis, our entire relationship to the external world is based upon this capacity to move into the other world, which could be expressed paradoxically as 'being able to fall asleep.'"[5] In other words, healthy perception occurs on a two-way street. We go out into the world and have an experience, and the location of this experience is "out there" in the world. Then we come back to ourselves in our bodies and register what just happened. There is a reciprocal ebbing and flowing.

Jaimen McMillan explains that one of the things that is so tragic about young children and videos is that their perception is passive, a one-way street, with everything pouring in. There is not an outgoing streaming gesture from the child. The perception is deadpan and takes place inside the body of the child. In addition, there is no filter. Much like an embryo that must take into itself everything the pregnant person eats and drinks, the young child must helplessly ingest through their eyes all that is projected directly into them.

This is especially concerning when we consider Steiner's statement above, "In the final analysis, *our entire relationship to the external world* is based upon this capacity to move into the other world, which could be expressed paradoxically as 'being able to fall asleep [emphasis added].'"[6] Indeed, if we observe children who are using a screen or tablet to watch a movie, there is a certain hollow paleness that they may develop. Their pupils dilate and their bodies become immobile. We can sense a gesture of withdrawal—as if they are retreating into their bodily shield, trying to avoid the assault of the incoming images. Indeed, the child may appear as just a shell of themselves after being exposed to a video for an extended period. Children need to cultivate the back-and-forth, two-way gestures of perception in their interactions with other people and with the real world, and videos do not afford this spatial opportunity.[7]

Give Caregivers a Break

As we have explored in this chapter, baby equipment does not support motor development. The child's sensorimotor experiences, while they are in a piece of baby equipment, are far from optimal, and the time spent in baby equipment is time not spent exploring the important foundational stages of motor development. Yet, the use of baby equipment is still widely accepted as a normal part of child-rearing. Most medical professionals recommend limited use, but they seldom recommend avoiding it altogether. While car seats are an example of necessary safety equipment for infants, the ubiquitous use of other baby equipment seems to indicate underlying challenges inherent in the cultural practices and expectations surrounding infant care.

In the United States, typical interactions between adult and baby demonstrate the opposite of Dr. Pikler's recommendations. In the Pikler approach, the adult gives their full attention to the child and encourages engagement from the child during caregiving activities. Through the encounter, the child is "filled up," so to speak, so that when they are placed into the prepared play space, they are generally ready to explore their movements independently. The child is never left completely alone here. The adult is always ready and willing to support the child if needed; however, the child's movement period is generally a time when a healthy degree of separation occurs. After this time of relative apartness, both parties are ready to come back together again for another caregiving encounter.

In contrast, during typical caregiving activities in the United States, the adult often does not give their undivided attention to the child, nor do they try to draw the child into participation. The adult may be multitasking, and their actions may take on an automatic quality, such that the caregiving activity is done to the child, rather than with the child. The child may react to this, leading to a situation where the adult interprets the child's behavior as uncooperative. Unfortunately, neither party perceives the encounter as pleasant or rewarding.

Also, children are typically rushed through development in the United States. The vast majority of American adults are not familiar with Pikler's research on self-initiated motor milestones, and motor development is viewed through a narrow lens of timetables. Parents, grandparents, neighbors, medical professionals, and friends routinely compare an infant's development to that of another, and this can cause high levels of stress for a parent, especially if their child's development is not meeting the expectations. It is common practice for parents to "teach" and encourage their children to move, as we have discussed in previous chapters. Many times, too, parents feel they must entertain their children (which is not to be confused with simply enjoying the company of their children). These practices are often not sustainable, and so parents resort to screens and baby equipment in order to take a much-needed break.

Fortunately, Dr. Pikler gives parents and caregivers another option.

Dr. Pikler recognized that when parents don't have rhythmic periods of time where there is a healthy degree of separation from the child, they can become exhausted and depleted, and may even develop a festering resentment toward the child. Unfortunately, the child is well aware of the parent's emotional state, and this can affect the relationship. In this scenario, also, the child is not given time to explore their movements and the world on their own, which would otherwise allow them to develop a sense of self-confidence and agency. Dr. Pikler realized that, although the child must never be completely left alone—the adult must be nearby and available, should the need arise—it is beneficial for *both* the parent and the child to have breaks from each other. Inherent in Dr. Pikler's approach are rhythmic breaks from parent-child interactions throughout the day—without the use of any screens or baby equipment. The genius of the Pikler approach is that it creates a natural process of breathing in and breathing out between the primary adult caregiver and the infant. There is intimate time together during the caregiving times, and more independent time for both the child and the adult during the child's free movement exploration time. When parents and childcare professionals adopt the Pikler approach, the need for baby equipment goes away.

7: The Interplay Between Fine and Gross Motor Development

I write this chapter out of my observations, over many years, of babies' movements. My observations have been colored by my NDT[1] training (training in neurodevelopmental treatment). I am indebted to my NDT instructors, Judi Bierman PT and Laura Vogtle OTR, for much of the content of this chapter. I am also grateful to Jaimen McMillan, founder and director of the Spacial Dynamics Institute. Through my study of Spacial Dynamics, I have developed new capacities with which to observe. My observations have also been influenced by my study of the work of Dr. Emmi Pikler.

The development of the hand is also known as fine motor development, as the muscles in the hand are some of the smaller and finer muscles of the body. Gross motor development involves actions of the whole body, such as rolling, crawling, running, and jumping, which require the larger muscles of the body. This chapter will explore the interplay between fine and gross motor development.

One cannot really get a complete picture of fine motor development without considering that it is embedded in gross motor development. Please note that this is a daunting task, because motor development is complex, varies from child to child, and it is not linear! For example, in the Pikler approach, we recognize a general sequence in which a baby first lies on their back and looks at their hand, then looks at toys, and then manipulates the toys. However, in reality, there is much overlap among these three phases, and they can all occur simultaneously. Please take this into consideration when reading this chapter.

The pattern of acquiring new fine motor skills is the same as it is in acquiring new gross motor skills. "At first, the new form of activity is sporadic, then very frequent, and finally gradually declines, though it does not completely fade away, while in parallel, the next form of manipulation appears and develops following the same pattern."[2]

In the developing baby, cognitive development is more closely tied to fine motor development than to gross motor development.[3] (Cognitive development will be discussed more fully in volume 2.)

To a typical adult, it may look as if a young infant lying on their back is not doing anything, and that they are not engaged in a developmental process. As a result, a well-intentioned adult may feel compelled to step in and stimulate the child, in order to get the ball rolling. It has been my observation that when adults hone their observation skills and are able to discern some of the "less spectacular" and less recognized states of motor development, they realize that the infant *is* doing something—and then the adult is more likely to refrain from imposing their agenda upon the infant. One of my goals in writing this chapter is to help parents and caregivers see what their infants and babies *are* doing. In my mind, from the point of view of the baby, all the stages of motor development are equally spectacular!

A Deeper Purpose for Fine Motor Development

Before we delve into our topic, let us consider what we do with our hands. We work with our hands. We build and destroy with them. We offer comfort, fight, bless, and curse with our hands. We hold hands with a loved one in tender or critical moments. We give our hand in marriage. We give our word with a handshake. And we create with our hands. Michelangelo's famous painting, *The Creation of Adam*, on the ceiling of the Sistine Chapel, is an archetypal example of this. God reaches out with his *hand* to give Adam the spark of life.

There are drawings from ancient times depicting eyes on the palms of the hands. Perhaps the drawings indicate that the hands were considered organs of perception—organs with which we may *see* in a unique fashion. Interestingly, Frank Wilson, author of the groundbreaking book *The Hand*, says that the hands give us knowledge that can "be obtained *only* by acting on the object being held [in the hand]." He goes on to say that this knowledge is then registered in the brain, where it is "written in the tactile and kinesthetic language of manipulation."[4]

One could say that Waldorf education is a celebration of the hand! Steiner is a strong advocate for hands-on learning. In *Practical Advice to Teachers*, he recommends that on the first day of school, teachers talk to their first-grade students about their hands. He suggests that the teachers say something like, "Look at yourselves. You have two hands, a left one and a right one. These hands are for working; you can do all kinds of things with them."[5] Indeed, the children in Waldorf schools learn to do many things with their hands. In the kindergartens, this may include finger games, finger knitting, felting, and sewing. Handwork in the grade schools may include knitting, crocheting, and cross-stitch. The students also use their hands in playing the recorder, form drawing, woodworking, hand-clapping games, drawing, and painting. Penmanship includes printing, cursive writing, and calligraphy.

These are all wonderful ways to support an older child's fine motor development. In this chapter, I hope to show what adults can do to support fine motor development from the very start of life—specifically, through the medium of self-initiated movement. Let us start with the state of affairs in the newborn.

The Newborn

The newborn's body has been influenced by being in the fetal position in the womb. It's a tight fit during the last few months! The fetus is all tucked up into the fetal position, so that at birth, the full-term newborn's spine is in a long C-shaped curve. Gradually, the form of the spine changes, and the cervical, thoracic, and lumbar curves emerge. Indeed, a transformation of the entire musculoskeletal system transpires in the early months and years of life. The newborn is overstretched on the backside and contracted on the front side in the shoulders and hips—the newborn has considerably less range of motion at their hips and shoulders than the mature adult. The newborn's arms are generally flexed up and close to the body. Additionally, the shoulders are elevated toward the ears, so that it looks as if the newborn doesn't have much of a neck—but, of course, they have a neck! At rest, the hands are generally held in fists—initially, often with the thumb inside the fist. The head is rotated to one side, often with the neck extended. The newborn does not yet have midline orientation (orientation toward the central position in the body between right and left). The newborn is characteristically a little asymmetrical. "As a rule, the newborn always turns the head to the same side."[6]

A Lack of Head Control in the Newborn

The newborn does not have any significant degree of head or trunk control. When the baby is born, the muscles acting upon the spine are not developed adequately to support the baby's relatively large, heavy head in the vertical positions. Therefore, it is beneficial to support the young infant's head and neck when you are picking them up and carrying them. It is also advantageous to lie the newborn in the supine (back-lying) position and let them progress to side-lying and prone (tummy-lying) in their own time and through their own efforts. These positions are the optimal ones to strengthen, elongate, and coordinate the spinal muscles.

Agnes Szanto-Feder, Pikler pedagogue and author, recommends avoiding holding a baby in a vertical position until they move into verticality on their own during free play.[7] (This was also Dr. Pikler's recommendation.) Szanto-Feder explains that it takes time for the spinal musculature to develop in order to properly support and protect the integrity of the vertebral column in the vertical positions. Vertebral discs exist between all of the vertebrae, and each disc serves to provide nutrition to the vertebra above and below. In the horizontal positions, the proper spacing is maintained between the vertebrae so that the discs can provide nutrition to the vertebrae. However, in the vertical positions, gravity exerts compressive forces upon the spine, and so the musculature must be adequately developed in order to keep the correct spacing between the vertebrae. In self-initiated movement, the child comes up into verticality very gradually, and this is the optimal manner for the musculature to develop. In this way, the discs are continuously providing these young spines sufficient nutrition all throughout the motor journey into verticality.[8] Here, we see the tremendous wisdom at work in the self-initiated motor sequence.

Head control commences to develop in supine when the baby becomes interested in objects in their environment and wants to look at something. Here, young infants learn to hold their heads still in order to look at something, and they also master turning their heads volitionally, in order to track a moving object. Control of the head gives a stable basis off of which the eyes can work. In other words, looking at objects of interest contributes to head control, and head control is foundational for visual coordination. The role of interest is noteworthy here.

Early Movements of the Newborn

Just after my second grandchild was born, I spoke with the midwife. She told me that the baby came out of the birth canal in a spiral motion. This is not an uncommon way for babies to be born, she said. It is as if the baby catches a wave, as one does in surfing, and rides it out into the world—only the wave is in the form of a spiral. Indeed, I saw similar spirals in the first days of my grandchild's life as her fingers opened and closed, spiraling around a diagonal axis of her hand. I have seen these same spiral motions in older babies as they lie on their backs and look at their hands.

It is not uncommon for the newborn's arms to have tremors, as myelination is not yet complete. Myelin is a fatty substance which surrounds the long fibers of the nerve cells, and myelination is "a major contributor to processing speed."[9] Additionally, the newborn exhibits random movements of the arms and legs—qualitatively, these movements are abrupt, jerky, unsophisticated, and without voluntary control. These types of movements are characteristic of the primitive reflexes—stereotypical movements that emerge in the womb, which are important during birth and the period after birth. They continue over time, and gradually their impact lessens as the child develops motor control. (The primitive reflexes will be discussed in greater detail in volume 2). When the primitive reflexes recede into the background of the child's movement repertoire, they are said to become integrated. When a reflex is manifesting, there is no isolation of the movement of one body part from that of another; instead, the various body parts move as a unit, and in this situation, the child's movements are not free. For example, in the Babkin reflex, there is an involuntary mirroring between the hands and the mouth. The Babkin reflex commonly manifests when the baby nurses or bottle feeds: when the mouth sucks, the hands also perform a kneading or sucking pattern, as if the entire body is sucking. This can also happen in reverse—a kneading motion of the hands can stimulate sucking of the mouth.

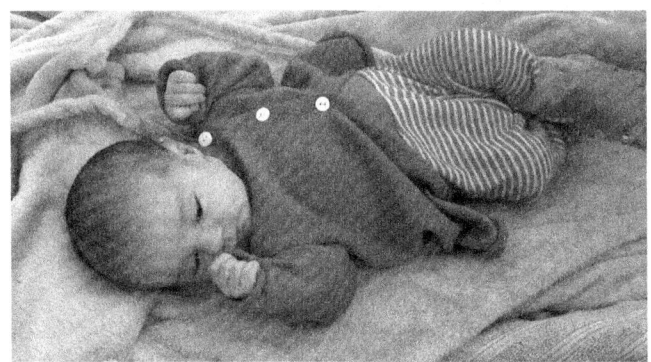

Here is a newborn manifesting a palmar grasp reflex. Often, the thumbs are positioned inside the fingers at this early stage of life. Note also that the infant's head is to the side.

Another one of the primitive reflexes, the palmar grasp reflex, is in full force in the early weeks of life.

In the palmar grasp reflex, if an adult places their finger into the palm of the newborn's hand, the newborn's fingers will flex into a fist. If the newborn's fingers are then drawn gently upwards, the newborn's grip increases with the traction, "and it would appear that the baby could support [their] own weight if so suspended."[10] Needless to say, this would be a very disrespectful action to subject a baby to, and I don't recommend it, but it shows the tremendous strength of the grasp reflex. This reflex is often described as helping a newborn cling to their birth parent for safety during our evolutionary history. The Moro reflex is also strong. In its full-blown manifestation, the Moro reflex has two stages. The first part involves total extension; the head and trunk extend backward, the baby inhales, the arms and wrists extend, and the fingers open. In the second part of the reflex, a mass flexion pattern manifests; the head and trunk flex forward, the baby exhales and cries, and the arms, wrists, and fingers flex inward.

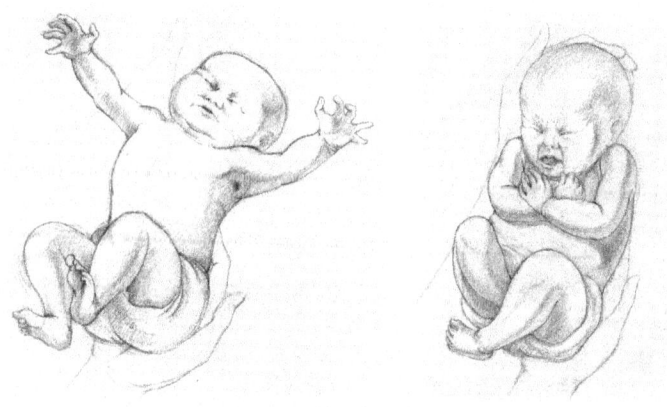

With a fully manifesting palmar grasp reflex, the fingers flex into tight fists. With the Moro reflex, the fingers first open completely and then they fully flex. Thus, the baby experiences strong muscle contractions when the fingers are at the end ranges of motion—when the fingers are completely extended and completely flexed. These strong contractions at end-range positions help the baby feel their fingers. Dear reader, please stop for a moment, make a tight fist, and hold this for about ten seconds. Then completely extend your fingers and hold this for about ten seconds. Take notice of how your fingers feel. Chances are that through the muscle activity, you feel your fingers more. At the beginning of life, the newborn does not have good awareness of their fingers—nor, indeed, of their whole body. The end-range movements of the primitive reflexes serve to help them establish perception of the various parts of their body.

In all three of these reflexes—the palmar grasp, the Babkin, and the Moro—the fingers do not move in isolation of each other. They all flex, or they all extend. If these reflexes were to continue to act in later life, the person would be challenged in activities such as playing the piano, typing, or performing sign language, for example. Additionally, there are other primitive reflexes whose patterns are such that all of the fingers move as a unit. The asymmetrical tonic neck reflex is one such reflex, and it is described below.

The Asymmetrical, Sprawling Stage

Several weeks go by, and the baby is not so flexed up anymore. The newborn has been out of the confining space of the womb for a while. As a result, the baby sprawls out somewhat—at rest, the arms and legs are a little farther away from the body, and the elbows are straighter.

The arms are moving more, out to the sides of the body and in large circular patterns—somewhat like a windmill moves. The hands are more open at rest, although the palmar grasp reflex still manifests strongly if something is placed in the palm of the hand. At this stage,

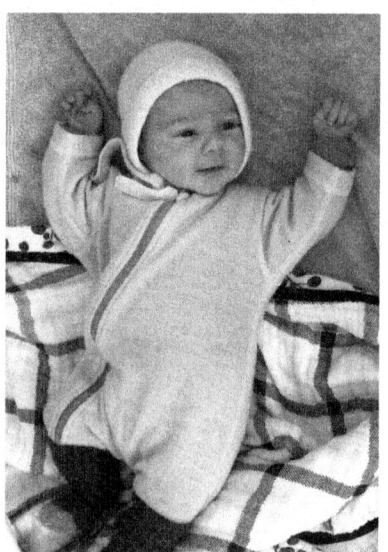

This photo captures the infant's posture during the "sprawling stage" of development.

the baby still can't keep the head in the midline position, and the neck is still extended. In fact, the baby is even more asymmetrical than at birth, due to the increased influence of the asymmetric tonic neck reflex (ATNR). In this reflex, if the head is turned to one side, the face-side arm and fingers extend, and the skull-side arm and fingers flex.

The Importance of Vision in Fine Motor Development

As one hand moves across the baby's visual field, they may notice it. However, initially, the baby does not perceive their hand to be part of them, and only gradually do they come to recognize it as theirs. This happens as the baby looks at their hand and as they move it while watching it. They move it closer and farther away from their face, they turn it around, and they open and close their fingers, for example. Gradually, vision and movement of the hand become integrated. This is a significant milestone for the development of hand-eye coordination. Dr. Pikler's wisdom is apparent in her consideration of when to give the baby their first toy. She did not give infants toys until they had "found their hand." At this stage, it is noteworthy that the baby can look only at one hand at a time and can only pay attention to one hand at a time. They initially look at their hand at the side (rather than at the middle of their body) because of the influence of the ATNR.

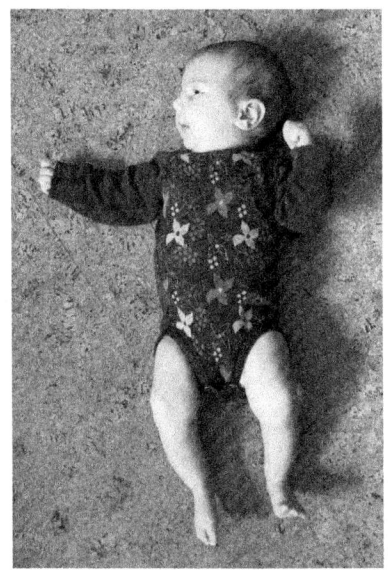

Here is an eight-week-old baby displaying a classic posture of the arms when the asymmetrical tonic neck reflex (ATNR) manifests.

The child's visual interest in their hands tames the chaotic movements of the arms and hands. "[The child] observes [their] hands; we could even say [they take] possession of them with [their] eyes. [They discover] that these are [their] own hands. Under the constant guidance of [their] eyes [they learn] to move [their] hands with coordination and purpose."[11] Because of an immature proprioceptive system—a mature proprioceptive system allows us to sense the positions of our body parts relative to each other, independent of vision—the child must look at their hands in order to know what their hands are doing and to gain mastery over their hands' movements.

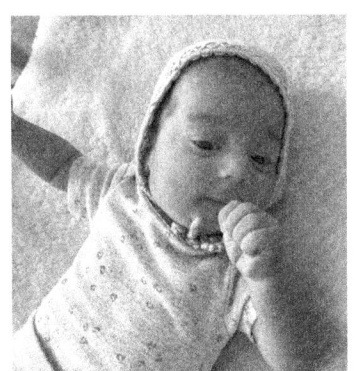 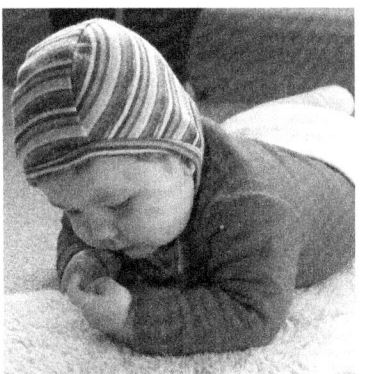 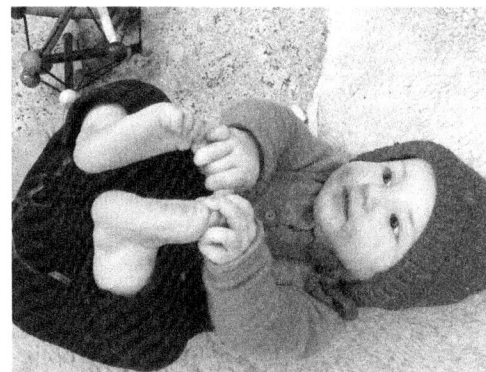

Above, left: In this photo, we see the influence of the ATNR, as the baby looks at one hand at the side of their body rather than at the midline. We also see the influence of the palmar grasp, as the hand is fisted. Above, center: The discovery of the hands continues for months. This baby has discovered their index finger. Above, right: This baby is exploring their toes.

Here, again, the vital role of "interest" in the acquisition of motor control is noteworthy, and the child's interest in their hands is very great! Dr. Pikler states, "As a rule, an infant's interest in all the possibilities of moving the hands and fingers is *inexhaustible* [emphasis added]. Later [they] will play in a similar way with feet and toes, but never as long and as persistently as with hands and fingers."[12]

The Sprawling Stage Eases and the Symmetrical Stage Emerges

The early stages of head control continue to emerge when the baby is lying on their back. They learn to tuck their chin, instead of holding it in an extended position, as in the early newborn stages. They also learn to bring the head to the middle of the body and keep it there for short periods. The new midline position of the head is liberating. The eyes converge and better eye tracking is possible.

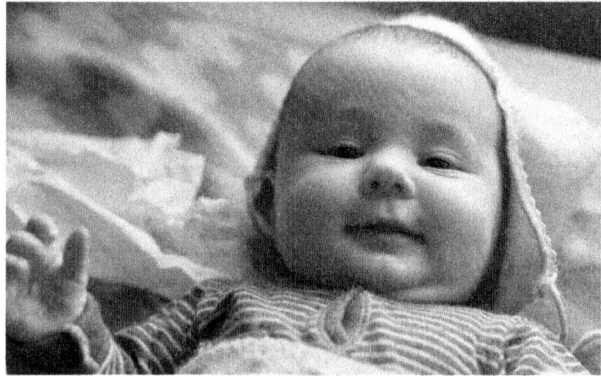
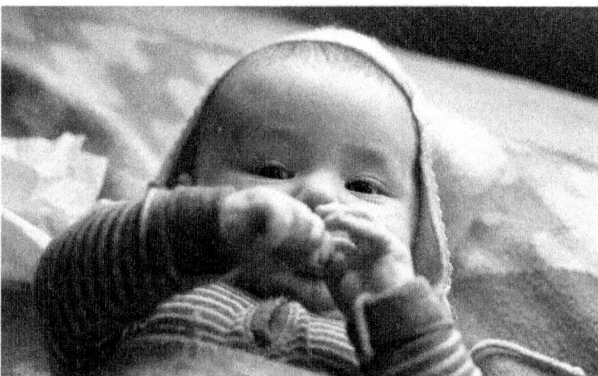

This baby has mastered a midline position of the head. Note the convergence of the eyes.

They also learn to bring the hands together at midline.

Over time, the grasp reflex exerts less and less influence over the baby's movements. Therefore, the hands are predominantly open at rest, and the very early stage of a volitional grasp begins. In this very early stage, the baby can't yet combine reaching out with grasping. Grasping is a flexion pattern, and reaching is an extension pattern. Combining the two patterns at the same time is too complicated. However, the baby begins to grasp their clothes at their chest in an immature manner, because here the fingers and arms are both flexing.

Symmetry and Midline Orientation Bloom in Full Glory

Time continues to march on, and the baby comes more fully into the stage of symmetry and midline orientation, a noteworthy accomplishment. Previously, under the influence of the asymmetrical tonic neck reflex, asymmetrical movement was the norm—the head was turned to the side and the arms were in asymmetrical positions. Now, the head easily comes to the midline position and stays there for long periods of time.

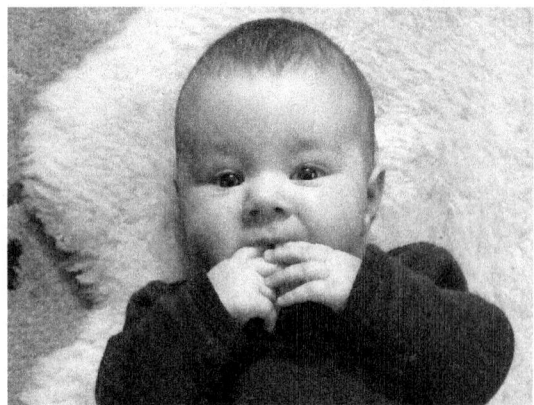
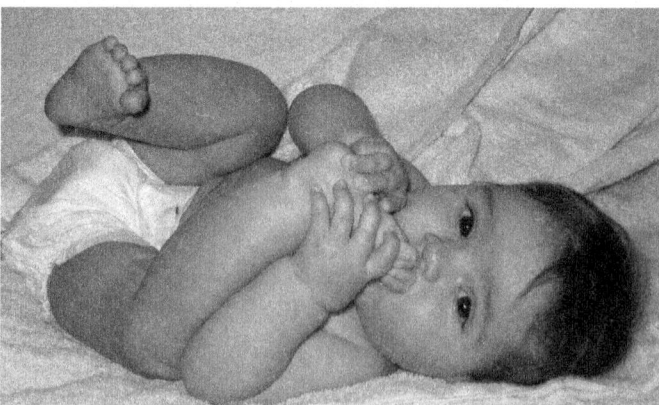

The hands also come to the mouth, a very popular midline location!

This baby frequently put a foot into their mouth during the supine stage of development.

Chapter 7: The Interplay Between Fine and Gross Motor Development

This is a remarkable transformation of the child's spatial orientation, when one considers that previously, the baby could only look at one hand at a time, and that hand was off to the side. Now the arms easily assume symmetrical positions at midline and around the midline—with the arms equidistant from the midline, such as when the infant bats their arms (and legs) in the air symmetrically.

The baby progresses to play in supine with their elbows extended. In this position especially, the shoulders come down lower, and the neck starts to be revealed. Playing in this position is very conducive to building strength in the arms and upper body. If you have ever lain on your back and worked with your arms up like this, you may relate to how much strength the position requires.

Soon, the hands find the knees and then, in another few weeks, the feet—which then also go in the mouth!

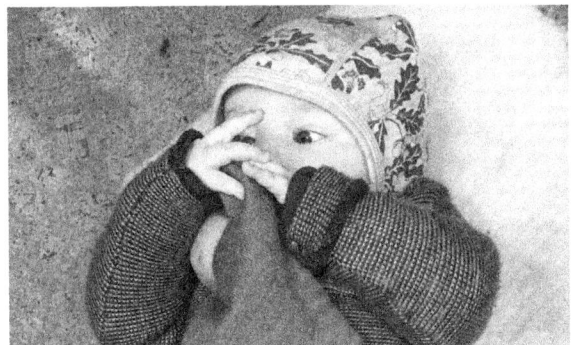
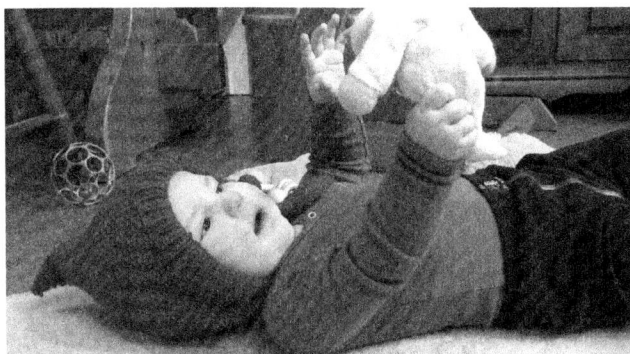

Above left: The baby is playing at midline. Initially, the baby plays with toys in supine with the elbows bent.
Above right: This baby is playing at midline with arms extended, which takes more strength.

Please note that limb-to-trunk proportions of babies are different from those of an adult. This allows the baby to put a foot in their mouth, whereas it would be unlikely for an adult to accomplish this. The baby can also lift their feet up off the surface and reach them with their hands; they hold onto their feet; they bat at them. This raises their center of gravity, making them top heavy. They may turn to look to the side, which shifts their weight just enough so that they plop over to lie fully on the side. This characteristically happens at first by accident, and then the baby learns to do it intentionally.

Also, at about this time, when the baby is lying on their back and looking at a toy to the side, they will reach for it with the same side arm. Over time, they will roll to one side and reach with the top arm.

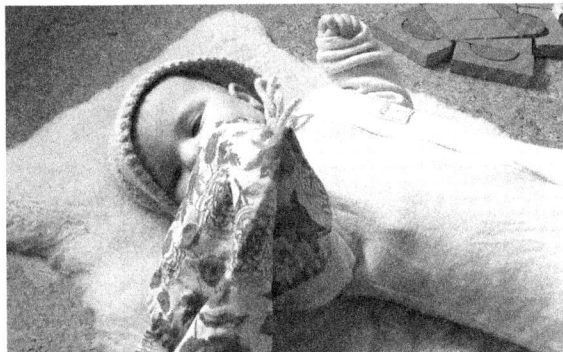
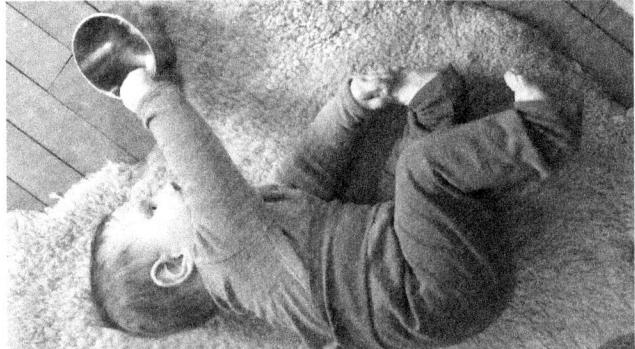

Above, left: Here, the baby is looking to the right and reaching with the right hand. This activity does not involve reaching across the body.
Above, right: This baby has rolled to their left side. They are reaching across with their right hand to bang the toy on the floor on their left side. Simultaneously, they are grasping their toes with their other hand. In this scene, the baby rolled repeatedly from supine—where they waved the toy in the air—to side-lying—where they banged the toy on the floor.

During this type of maneuver, the baby is learning to use the supporting surface to initiate the roll—they push into the floor with a particular part of their backside in order to begin the movement. For example, if they reach across their body with their right arm, they typically push down into the floor with their left shoulder blade. If they reach across the body with their right leg, they typically push down into the floor with back of their left pelvis. Dear reader, please lie on your back and try this. It is very helpful to understand that pushing down into the supporting surface is a vital part of coordinated movement; this is often overlooked by adults.

The baby will roll to one side, and then back to the middle, and then roll to the other side and back to the middle. Here, they are more fully establishing midline orientation, always coming home to midline. This is a noteworthy milestone in the integration of the asymmetrical tonic neck reflex. The baby continues to refine the control of their hands at the midline, and they start to explore volitional release via the mouth. Transferring a toy, such as a napkin or soft cloth toy, directly from one hand to the other is a very complex task. In one hand, the fingers must open to release the toy, and in the other hand, the fingers must close to receive the toy. This requires a significant degree of bilateral integration (where both sides of the body work together), and is too difficult, initially. The baby may come up with an ingenious solution. They hold the napkin in one hand, put it in their mouth, and let go with the first hand. Then they grasp the napkin with their other hand and pull it out of their mouth. Here, they are using the mouth as a third hand. Over time and with practice, they learn to transfer an object directly from one hand to the other.

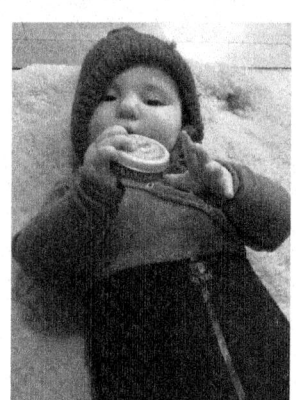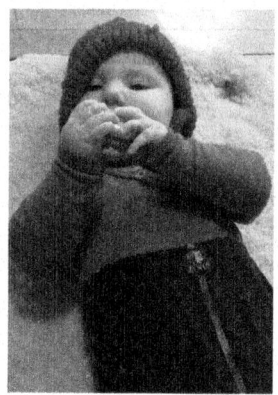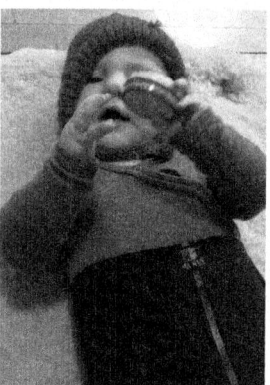

This baby is mastering the skill of transferring a toy directly from one hand to the other.

Reaching and grasping

Let us look more carefully at the developmental stages of volitional reach and grasp. The palmar grasp reflex is strong, initially. As it gradually fades, the baby starts to reach for toys. The early volitional grasp is an immature grasp, called the *ulnar palmar grasp*. The ulna bone is one of the two long bones in the forearm, and it attaches to the bones of the wrist on the pinkie side of the hand. Hence, in the ulnar palmar grasp, the baby uses the pinkie and ring fingers to grasp a toy and press it against the palm of the hand, without involvement of the index finger, long finger, and thumb. The cotton napkin is a wonderful first toy when the baby is employing the ulnar palmar grasp, because the pinkie and ring fingers are able to easily grasp the flexible cloth and hold it against the palm.

At this stage the baby reaches with poor aim, and frequently overshoots the toy. They will later correct the reach in midstream and thus fine-tune the aim. The reach is visually directed—the baby must see their hand as well as the toy. They need vision because their sense of where their body parts are and what those body parts are doing (proprioception) is far from fully developed. Additionally, the baby bangs objects with a strong downward motion, i.e., they use more force than is necessary. Again, this is because their proprioceptive system is still immature, and so they can't yet perceive, and thus control, how hard the muscles are contracting.

Chapter 7: The Interplay Between Fine and Gross Motor Development

With all this activity of the hand, the baby begins to purposely reproduce an interesting result that occurred initially by chance. In other words, they capitalize on eureka moments. Here we see the intimate relationship between fine motor development and cognitive development. As I write this chapter, I am observing my third granddaughter, who is just starting to roll over onto her tummy. However, she still predominantly plays on her back or her side. A couple of days ago, she was playing on her back with a small skillet. She played carefully and didn't let the skillet fall on her face. She initially lay on her back, holding the skillet with two hands by its pan. Then she moved one hand to the handle, but she seemed to immediately sense that this was too risky. She couldn't control it adequately by the handle and switched back to holding the pan with two hands so that it wouldn't fall onto her face. Here, she is learning about the properties of a skillet and developing judgment regarding her capacities. Next, she turned to her side, held onto the skillet by its handle, and slid it on the floor, away from her and toward her. This is a classic stage of fine motor development, defined as "sliding" by Dr. Pikler. This movement made a sound. She slid the skillet a couple times, stopped, and then repeated this. She would slide it with different numbers of excursions and in slightly different directions. She explored in this way for an extended period. It was as if she was realizing that the skillet made a sound while she was sliding it, and perhaps she also realized that it was *she* who was sliding the skillet in order to make the sound. Then my granddaughter returned to her back and kicked her legs vigorously while vocalizing. Shortly thereafter, she returned to playing with the skillet. This is a good example of the complementary nature of gross and fine motor activities. She engaged in a focused, fine-motor activity with the skillet for an extended period, and then she switched to the vigorous gross motor activity of kicking. The kicking provided her with substantial proprioceptive input, which served to prepare her again to be able to attend to the skillet. In a similar fashion, adults will work at their desks for a period of time, and then they get up and walk around the building. Here, the walking provides them with the proprioceptive input that they need in order to come back to their desks and attend to their task again. In both cases, the baby and the adult are modulating their attention with movement.

Exploration in the Prone Position Influences the Hand

The baby rolls in and out of side-lying and plays in side-lying, gaining balance and control in this position. Then, one day, they roll all the way over to prone (tummy-lying). They usually get their arm stuck under them, but not always. My third granddaughter recently rolled over for the first time, and she was able to get her arm out from under her trunk. However, she cried soon thereafter, even though she had just previously been very content to be playing on the floor. She wasn't able to settle back down, and her mother picked her up. Perhaps the new prone position was too much of a surprise for her. "What has happened? Where am I now?"

A couple of days later my granddaughter rolled to prone again, and this time she was not able to get her arm out from underneath her trunk. Her father gave her time to try and figure out how to navigate the situation, but it became apparent that she was not going to manage. Her father approached her saying, "You rolled over and I see you are stuck there. I am going to turn you back over now." He turned her to her back,

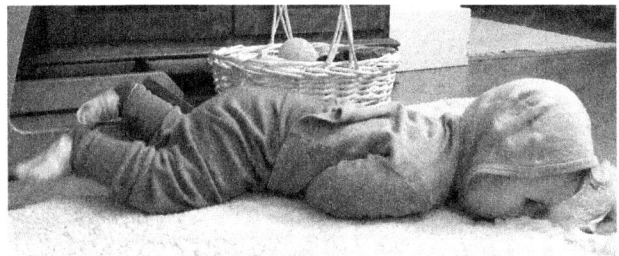 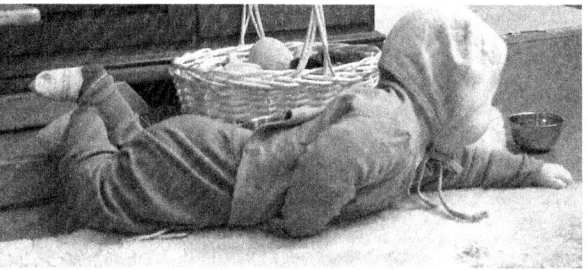

This baby rolled to their belly, landing with one arm underneath their trunk. They lay still for a while with head down. Then, they repeatedly kicked their feet. Soon, they started to lift the upper body. After several attempts, they started to fuss, but stuck with it, and eventually shifted to the side enough to pull the arm out from under them.

and soon, she rolled right back over onto her tummy again, only to get stuck again. Over time, she figured out how to free her arm on her own.

The child progresses to turn from prone to supine. At this point they roll from supine to prone and from prone to supine, in both directions. The baby gradually becomes more familiar and capable in the prone position—they become more active in prone and they start to scoot. (They also scoot in supine.) Almost imperceptibly, one realizes that the baby is ninety degrees from where they just were, or they have scooted off their sheepskin and are now in the corner of the kitchen. Dr. Pikler describes this stage: "A child bends, stretches [themself], makes minimal movement like a caterpillar. This slow and gradual stretching and reaching is one of the most important stages in the motor development of the infant. It goes on for months. During this time the asymmetry of the trunk with which the child is born disappears. Through these natural movements [in supine and in prone] the spine becomes straight; the trunk becomes elastic, flexible and muscular. *I cannot emphasize how important this stage of development is* [emphasis added]."[13]

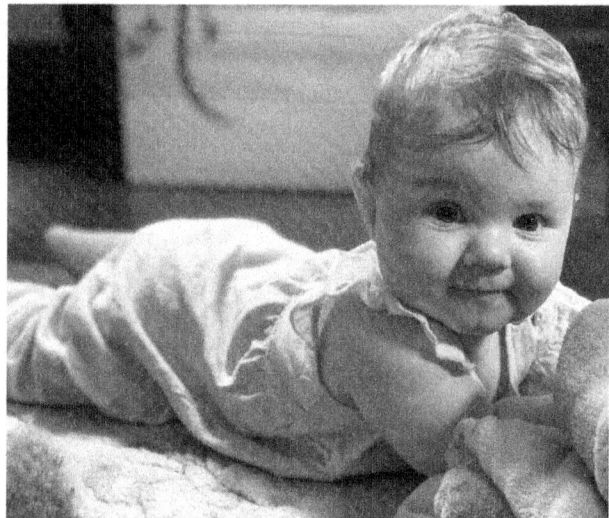 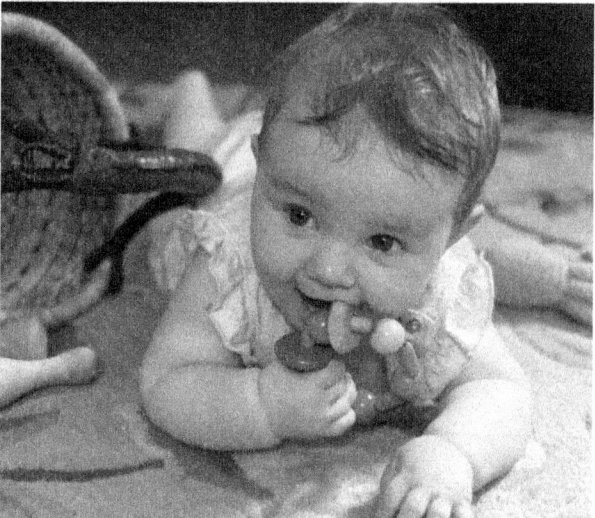

Above, left: This baby has assumed prone on their elbows. Note how free their head is as they look around. Note also that their elbows are in front of their shoulders. Above, right: A few weeks later, the baby's elbows are farther back, and they are bearing more weight in the shoulder joint. Thus, their hands are freer to manipulate toys than when the elbows are in front of the shoulders.

The baby continues to explore the prone position. They push down into the supporting surface through their forearms and, as a result, their head and their upper body are displaced up off the surface, and they assume the prone-on-elbows position.

With time, they shift their weight onto one forearm in order to reach for a toy with the other arm. Initially, they may collapse with this maneuver, however, over time the muscles learn to stabilize the shoulder blade on the trunk, and they gain more control of their reaching. In prone, they also spin around on their tummies in both directions—the palms of the hands push into the floor in order to accomplish this. They transition from prone-on-elbows to side-lying on elbow, and back again to each side. They are building strength in their upper bodies. Additionally, with all of these experiences in prone, the baby is receiving deep pressure from the floor into the various front parts of their bodies, including their forearms and their hands. This serves to increase the baby's awareness of these different body parts.

When they push down into the floor and come up onto extended arms in prone, more weight is borne through the hands than when they are on their elbows.

Chapter 7: The Interplay Between Fine and Gross Motor Development

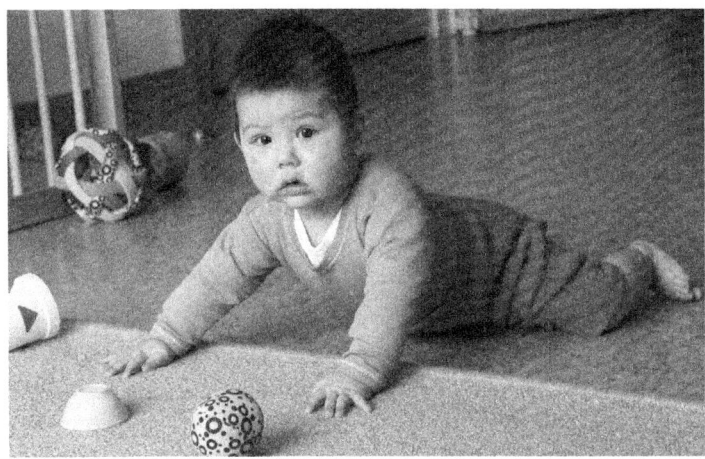

This baby is new to being prone on extended arms. Note how they are receiving deep pressure into the heels and palms of the hands.

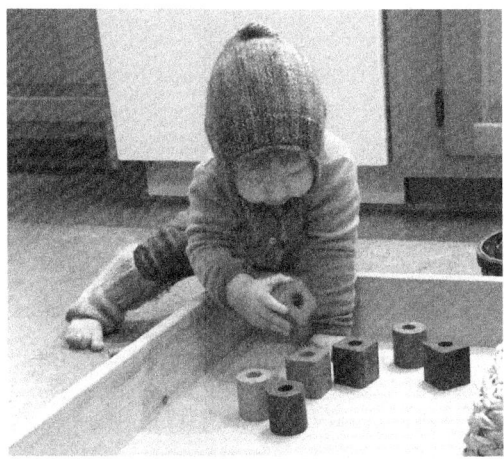

This baby is employing a radial palmar grasp. They are using the thumb along with the index and long fingers, and the block is in contact with the palm of the hand.

Here, they start to work on wrist control. Again, they shift their weight onto one side and reach for a toy. Initially, they may wobble with this maneuver as they are higher up off the surface—it takes more balance and more stability. Their stamina in the position increases so they can shift their weight onto one side, then onto the other, to reach for a toy. During these weight shifts, the weight is borne by the heel of the hand, through the pinkie side, and also through the thumb side. Thus, these parts of the hand receive more deep pressure input. When the thumb side of the hand receives more deep pressure input, this promotes more proprioceptive awareness and subsequent coordinated use of the thumb side of the hand. This contributes to a change in the grasp pattern. It changes from its initial use of just the pinkie and ring fingers pressing an object against the palm of the hand (*ulnar palmar grasp*) to the use of the thumb, long, and pointer fingers pressing an object against the palm of the hand (*radial palmar grasp*). The radius is one of the two long bones of the forearm. It attaches to the wrist bones on the thumb side of the wrist. Hence, the type of grasp using the thumb, long and pointer fingers is called the radial palmar grasp.

The baby also rolls to each side and pushes down through their arms to achieve side-lying on one extended arm, also known as high side-lying. As they gain more stability, they play in this position. Because the baby is bearing more weight through their hands in the prone positions and in high side-lying, thus gaining more awareness of their hands, there is less need for visually directed reaching. At this stage, the baby also employs a *raking grasp*, where all the fingers are partially flexed and perform a raking motion to move small objects. However, there is still no mature opposition of the thumb; thus, refined manipulation of objects is still challenging.

The baby is grasping many objects now, but they have no concept of pressure when they grasp. They will grasp objects very tightly. This is still a manifestation of the primitive grasp reflex. It sometimes remains in older school-aged children and can be observed when they hold their pencils with excessive pressure. At this point, the baby has mastered the extremes of grasping and reaching, i.e., they grasp too tightly (at the end range of flexion) and they release a toy with a fling of the entire arm (at the end range of extension). Soon, they will scratch with their fingers on the floor, and this characteristically happens when the baby turns to prone. Scratching serves to activate the midranges of grasp and release. This is another example of the incredible intelligence at work in the developmental sequence.

The baby employs their new, more sophisticated hand skills by exploring toys and objects in more complex ways, and their learning about the quality of these items expands. Cognitive development does indeed go "hand in hand" with fine motor development.

Far-Reaching Effects of the Horizontal Movements

All this exploration in the horizontal positions of supine, side-lying, and prone lengthens and strengthens the muscles that stabilize the shoulder blades on the rib cage, and the shoulder blades are stabilized in many different positions on the rib cage. This paves the way for coordinated reaching and use of the hands in many different positions later, when the child achieves sitting and standing. The increased stability of the shoulder girdle also makes possible the beginnings of reaching with the palm of the hand turned up (in a *supinated* position) rather than with the palm turned down (in a *pronated* position.) Supination and pronation involve a complex rotation of the forearm. It is only later, when the child has a degree of mastery in walking, that they will be able to open a jar or turn a doorknob—both of which require coordinated supination.

The baby more fully masters rolling. As noted earlier in the chapter, initially the baby rolls from supine to one side and back to the middle. They do this to both sides. Next, they roll all the way over onto their bellies—from supine to prone, and then later from prone to supine. Gradually, the baby progresses to roll from supine to prone to supine in one continuous motion. They do this to both sides. Recall that in the asymmetrical tonic neck reflex (ATNR), the face-side arm extends. Initially, the extension of the face-side arm blocks the motion of rolling from supine to prone. With successful rolling, then, the ATNR becomes integrated.

Additionally, in rolling, the rotation around the central axis of the spine is refined, and the abdominal muscles are further activated. The activation of the abdominals is significant, in that these muscles are important stabilizers of the ribcage. Developing the abdominals leads to increased lung capacity, which enhances the baby's vocalizations and contributes to their oral motor development. Rolling—as, indeed, do all of the baby's explorations thus far in the gross motor sequences—contributes to a flexible and dynamically stable trunk from which to control the head. Good head control is foundational for coordinated eye movements, which in turn enhance hand-eye coordination. Here, we can see the interrelatedness of gross motor development with oral motor development and also with fine motor development.

The possible explorations in the prone position are vast! The baby also assumes the "airplane" position with arms and legs up off the floor. They "swim" in this position and also rock forward and back on their bellies—both of which are an incredible workout for the core! They progress to belly-crawling and move longer distances through space.

Gradually Rising Up off the Surface

As described above, in prone, the baby pushes down through the hands and comes up onto both extended arms. From there, the arms push down and slightly forward into the floor, and the baby's body slides backward. During this motion, the shoulder blades glide downward on the ribcage, and the muscles and tissues are further elongated. Dear reader, please stop for a moment, try this movement, and see if you can feel your shoulder blades sliding down your back. This is an incredible transformation of the form of the body, when one remembers how, initially, the newborn's shoulders were elevated toward the ears, and it appeared that they didn't have much of a neck! In addition, when the baby pushes through extended arms, they are pushing through open palms and through the heels of the hands, which further increases their awareness of the hand and integrates the grasp reflex. In fact, all of the weight bearing through an open hand, noted above, has been integrating the palmar grasp reflex.

Gradually, the belly comes up off the surface; the child achieves the hands-and-knees position, and rocks forwards and backward. This rocking elongates the tendons at the wrist, developing more wrist control, and further helps to integrate the palmar grasp reflex. With self-initiated motor development, only now (after they have achieved hands-and-knees) does the child typically achieve the sitting position—Dr. Pikler defines sitting as the position of sitting on both sitz bones with hands free. The baby transitions from hands-and-knees to sitting and back again, to each side. Because they are higher up off the surface, more balance is required to negotiate these transitions, and there is even more weight shifting across the hand. They play freely in side-sitting on extended arms.

Crawling

The baby starts to crawl. They may crawl with the same-side arm and leg moving together, in what is called a homolateral pattern, or they may achieve the mature pattern of reciprocal crawling right away. Reciprocal crawling involves a complex counterrotation in the trunk, whereby on each side of the body, the upper trunk rotates in one direction and the lower trunk rotates in the opposite direction. Reciprocal crawling serves to integrate the various body parts into a unified whole—weaving together the upper body with the lower, the right side of the body with the left, and the front of the body with the back.

Crawling offers an additional opportunity to enhance coordination of the eyes. When they crawl, the baby will look from one hand to the other and back to the first hand—this is the same pattern that the eyes will use later, for reading. The baby also looks down at their hands, across the room, and back down again at their hands—this is the same pattern that the eyes will use later for copying from the blackboard to a paper on the desk and for catching a ball.

At this time, the baby picks up objects of different weights. The arm initially falls, and then readjusts according to the weight of each particular object. Gradually, as the baby has more and more experience lifting objects of varying weights, the proprioceptive system continues to develop. As a result, the arm will no longer need to readjust midstream but will achieve the right amount of muscle contraction right away.

Shifting the Body's Weight Over the Hand: Diagonal Movements

When spinning around in prone, transitioning between sitting and hands and knees, and crawling reciprocally, the weight of the body is transferred through the hand in a diagonal pattern. Dear reader, please get down on the floor and try these movements so you may feel the diagonal weight shift of the body over the hand. This weight transfer serves to develop the arches of the hand, as these are not present at birth. Additionally, these sophisticated diagonal weight shifts pass through the thumb, thus further increasing the proprioceptive and deep pressure input to the thumb and "enlivening" the thumb. As noted throughout this book, the various diagonal movements of the baby are very healthy movements!

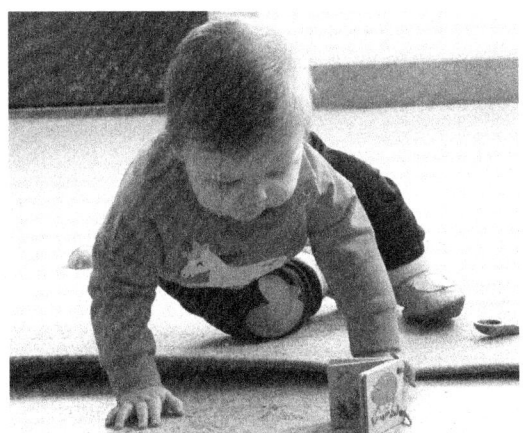

Note the open palm. The baby's body weight is passing over the palm in a diagonal pattern as they transition from sitting to hands and knees.

With these diagonal weight shifts of the body over the hand, the baby begins to use more mature patterns of thumb opposition, which occur in a variety of ways. In one pattern, the thumb pad opposes the side of the index finger (*lateral pincer grasp*). In another pattern, the thumb pad opposes the pad of the index finger (*inferior pincer grasp*). In yet another pattern, the thumb pad opposes the pads of the index and long fingers (*three-jaw chuck grasp*). The baby now becomes a human vacuum cleaner! They will pick up every piece of fuzz that they can find. The fingers of the radial and ulnar sides of the hand are now being used in differentiated patterns, with the thumb, pointer, and long fingers active and the ring and pinkie fingers resting. This evolved pattern is seen in writing with a mature pencil grip, sewing, cutting with scissors, putting on an earring, and using fine tools.

Gradually, the child will master a more sophisticated form of opposition, where the tip of the thumb opposes the tip of the index finger (*superior pincer grasp*) rather than using the pads of the fingers. This is a tremendous accomplishment, when one remembers that the newborn had little volitional control of the hand. The hand essentially could only open or close in reflexive patterns, with all fingers doing the same thing.

Also, in reciprocal crawling, there is a diagonal weight shift from the heel of the hand across to the tip of the pointer finger. This specifically serves to elongate and enliven the index finger tendon. Soon, the baby points and pokes with the index finger. Here, the baby is isolating one finger from the others, rather than using the total patterns of the hand, as in the newborn period. The baby frequently crawls with a toy in their hand, which further stretches out the tendons of the wrist, readying them for more sophisticated patterns of releasing objects.

The Progression of Releasing an Object

During this initial time of exploration in crawling, the baby may release an object into a container if the wrist is stabilized on the container's edge. Previously, in order to release an object, they needed to use the mouth as a third hand, as described above, fling the entire arm, or shake the entire hand. Gradually, over time, they learn to release an object in the air without needing to support the wrist. In order to achieve an airborne release, the entire body must coordinate and stabilize the hand. This can be a challenging motion to achieve until it is practiced. It is an incredible achievement—a culmination of all the motor activity that the child has accomplished thus far.

The trunk is key for this refined airborne release. All throughout the gross motor sequence, in all the many different positions, the trunk provides a stable position from which the shoulder blade can work—the shoulder blade would not work well if it did not have a stable base of support from the core. In turn, the shoulder blade fine-tunes its ability to move into various positions on the rib cage and to hold its position there, so as to provide a stable base of support for the next lower segment of the arm, the humerus (upper arm). Likewise, the humerus fine-tunes its ability to move and to hold itself in varying positions so as to provide a stable base for the next lower segment, the forearm. The forearms then serves to stabilize the wrist, and the wrist serves to stabilize the fingers. The foundation stone for this cascading stabilization of the fingers is the mighty trunk!

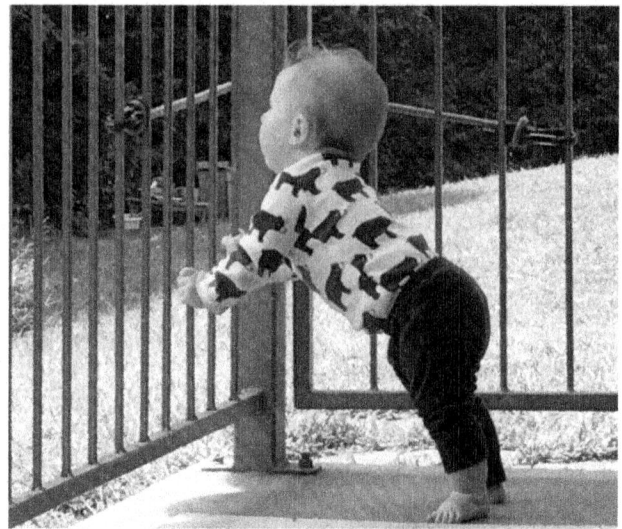

This is one of the first times this baby pulled to stand at the bars. Note the relatively large distance between their hands and feet. More weight is borne through the hands than through the feet.

The degree of fine-tuning and coordination between the various segments is truly miraculous. Coordinated use of the arm requires a significant amount of time to practice such delicate maneuvering, and indeed, babies seem to never tire of reaching, grasping, and releasing from so many positions throughout the motor journey.

Standing and Walking

Babies eventually progress to the pulling-to-stand stage of development. They don't actually pull themselves up. Rather, they push down on a stool or other surface, or push down on vertical bars, and their bodies are displaced up into standing. Initially, they push primarily through their hands—they bear the majority of their weight through their hands, rather than through their feet.

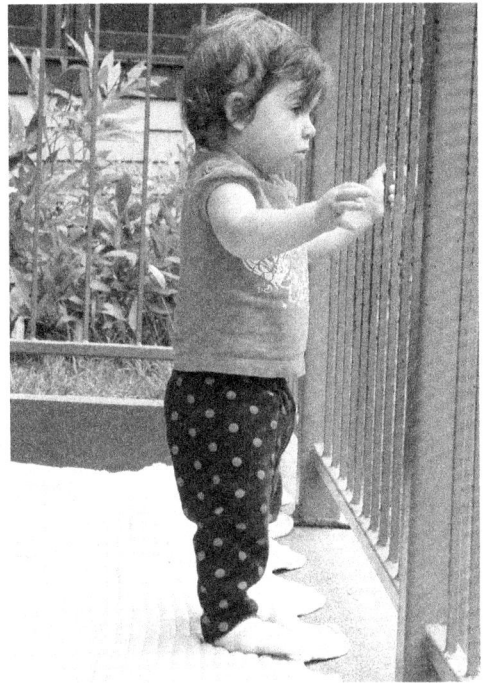 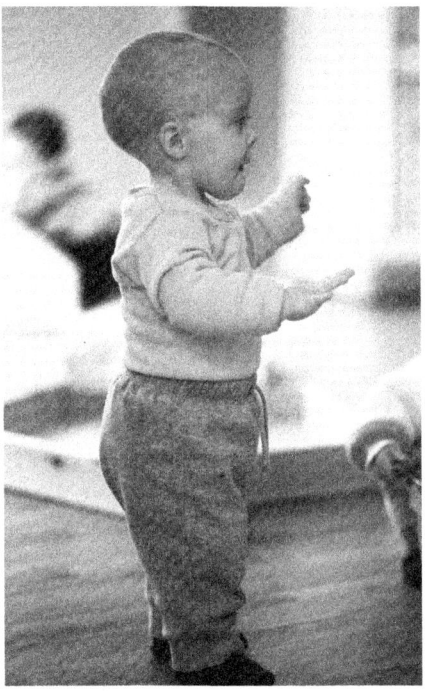

| This child is more experienced at pulling to stand and standing. Their feet are taking the full weight of the body, and one hand has let go of the bar. Note the beautifully aligned posture of this child, who has had free movement from the very start of life. | This photo was taken as this baby took their first steps. The arms are not yet free in walking, as they are being used to balance. Here we also see a beautifully aligned spine in a child raised according to the Pikler approach from the very start. |

Gradually, the child gets their feet underneath them, pushes down through the feet with greater force, and takes more weight through the feet. This begins the process of freeing the hands in standing.

Babies typically cruise sideways along a coffee table, a Pikler labyrinth, vertical bars, or a wall before walking forward.

When babies initially stand alone, and also when they first walk freely, the shoulder blades are often pulled back with the arms out to the sides and the hands up in the air. In this posture, the arms are not free. Instead, the arms and shoulder blades are serving to stabilize the child in this new, precarious position.

The Freeing of the Hands

As the child achieves more stability and balance in the upright, the hands come down, the walking and standing become more fluid, and only then are the hands free for activity in the standing position. This is an incredible musculoskeletal, physiological, neurological, and truly human accomplishment! Rudolf Steiner speaks about the freeing of the hands specifically. He says that the limbs of animals are not free—they must support and carry the animal's body from place to place. Similarly, during human motor development, the arms and hands assume a weight-bearing function during belly-crawling, hands-and-knees crawling, and pulling to stand. However, because the human being progresses into a balanced upright posture, the hands are freed for higher tasks, and this is one of the things that makes us truly human.

The freeing of the hands is a culminating moment in fine motor development, and the child celebrates by playing a favorite game: giving an object to another person and then asking for it back.

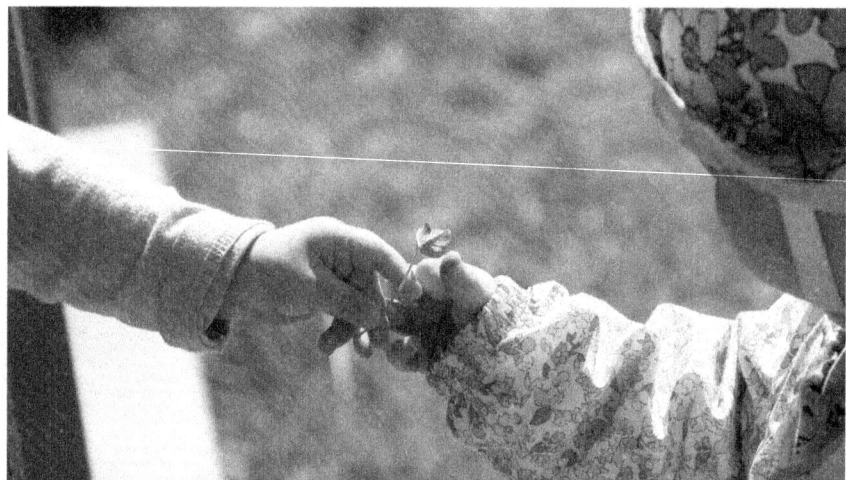

This photo was taken on our patio at Sophia's Hearth. The children like to pass flowers, leaves, and other treasures back and forth to each other through the bars.

This simple game of giving and taking, grasping and releasing, asking and receiving involves the archetypal gesture of reciprocal connection with others. This can also be a challenging motion to accomplish, until it is practiced. Fine motor development continues as the child grows older and, indeed, can continue throughout all of life, but in these early months and years, the child has achieved an incredible amount, and has laid a solid foundation for all that is yet to come.

Steiner typically refers to the arms and hands as part of the metabolic limb system. However, in the following passage from *Anthroposophy and Science*, he says they also can be seen as part of the rhythmical system. (The metabolic limb and rhythmical systems will be discussed further in volume 2.) He explains that after the hands complete their weight-bearing function, they are freed for the higher purpose of expression.

> The arms and hands, because of their specific location on the human body and through their life functions, can be seen as belonging to the rhythmic system. The most obvious demonstration of this connection is the way they are used freely in gestures to express feelings. When they are used in this way, they are lifted to a higher function than serving merely the body. In the case of animals, the corresponding members, the legs, are used only to serve the body, but in human beings the arms are freed for a higher function. Through the fact that they are used for gestures in connection with speech, they have the higher function of making the invisible aspects of speech visible.[14]

In a 1919 lecture series entitled *Practical Course for Teachers*, Rudolf Steiner describes the arms and hands as "externally the most beautiful symbol of the human being's freedom. There is no more wonderful symbol of human freedom than these arms and hands."[15] Ingun Schneider summarizes Steiner's thoughts from lectures four and seven of this same lecture series. She says, "The hands are the human being's most creative and selfless organs, in that our hands are free to offer service to others and to nourish and care for ourselves."[16]

8: An Introduction to the Twelve Senses

In order to be comfortable and successful in negotiating encounters with the world, one must first have a degree of comfort and competence in one's body. Here is a simple example of when this is *not* the case: If we have an inner ear infection, and as a result, we feel dizzy, it can be difficult to manage our daily affairs and even to walk across the room. In this case, our balance is disturbed and we are not comfortable in our body nor in the world. Here is another not so uncommon example: Some children bruise their shins because they run into objects and furniture. The child does not have sufficient sensory awareness of their own body to be able to safely maneuver it in relationship to the various objects in the environment. Safe maneuvering involves the ability to perceive the space of the body and its distance from the object, to control the body while moving through space, and to slow down and stop before hitting the object. *Healthy movement is based on healthy sensing.* Even more complex sensing is required when there are other moving beings in the child's environment, such as other children and pets. It follows, then, that a book about the development of movement in babies and young children would not be complete without a look at the child's sensory development, as the two go hand in hand.

The Twelve Senses, a Cosmic Whole

Rudolf Steiner distinguishes *twelve* senses. Interestingly, twelve is an archetypal number. There are twelve months of the year, twelve Jungian archetypes, and twelve signs of the zodiac. The major religions of the world recognize twelve as a significant number: twelve disciples of Christ, twelve sons and tribes of Israel, and twelve "jewels," or principles, of Islam. Musing on the number twelve, Steiner discusses the twelve knights of the Round Table during his visit to the ruins of King Arthur's castle in Cornwall, England:

> These knights of King Arthur could number only twelve. This came to me because one can still perceive today what it was that formed the basis for that number twelve. There are just twelve nuances of perception when you are concerned with this kind of cosmic perception that comes into being with the help of elemental beings; twelve modes of perception. If you want to embrace all twelve as a single human being, you find that one of them always makes another indistinct. So the knights of Arthur's Round Table shared the tasks among themselves in such a way that each could be regarded as one of these twelve nuances. . . . There could not have been a thirteenth knight, for he would have had to resemble one of the twelve.[1]

Steiner relates the twelve signs of the zodiac with the twelve senses: "As far as our senses are concerned, what is spread out over our nerve substance is organized according to the number twelve because the human being is in this most profound sense a microcosm and mirrors the macrocosm. . . . In the macrocosm the sun moves through twelve signs of the zodiac in the course of a year, and the human I lives here on the physical plane in the twelve senses."[2]

Karl König relates that Rudolf Steiner was the first person in history to describe the three highest senses—the sense of word, the sense of thought, and the sense of the ego of the other (the "I"-sense).[3] Additionally, König explains that "It took Rudolf Steiner many years to come to the idea of the twelve senses."[4] In 1909, Steiner gave four lectures on the senses, describing ten of them. In 1916, he spoke again about the senses and added the sense of touch and the sense of the ego of the other. Between 1916 and 1924, Steiner divided the twelve into three groups of four senses and differentiated each group.[5] The three groups are listed below.

The foundational, or lower, senses:

   (1) the sense of touch

   (2) the sense of life or well-being

   (3) the sense of self-movement

   (4) the sense of balance

The middle senses:

   (5) the sense of smell

   (6) the sense of taste

   (7) the sense of vision

   (8) the sense of temperature

The higher senses:

   (9) the sense of hearing or tone

   (10) the sense of word

   (11) the sense of thought

   (12) the sense of the ego of the other ("I"-sense)

Each of the twelve senses will be described later in the chapter. Each of the four foundational senses will be covered in more detail in chapters 12 through 15. (The middle and higher senses will also be discussed further in volume 2.)

The twelve senses can be thought of as doorways through which the ego may pass into three different worlds. The doors of the four lower senses can be pictured as opening in, toward the body; those of the four middle senses as opening out, into the social world; and those of the four higher senses as opening beyond the physical world, into the spiritual world. The twelve senses are also a means by which the higher ego or "I," is active and engaged; as Steiner expressed it, "The *I* is intimately related to the sphere of the senses."[6] It is very healthy for the child's higher self to be engaged. One area where we can recognize the activity of the child's higher self is in the child's sensing—specifically when the child can meet the sensations that come toward them from the world. We support this activity of the child's higher self by adjusting their sensory environment so they can meet the incoming sensations. This is discussed in detail in the subsequent chapters.

Waldorf education recognizes that "The early childhood domain is the lower senses, the body, the will."[7] The early childhood teacher is tasked with supporting the young child as they develop their physical body, and this includes supporting them as they develop their sense organs. The middle senses are more central to the experiences in the Waldorf grade schools, and the higher senses come to the foreground in the Waldorf high school.

The Foundational Senses Give Us the Spatial Features of Our Bodies

The four foundational senses include the sense of touch or the tactile sense, the sense of well-being or life or interoception, the sense of self-movement or proprioception, and the sense of balance. Through these four senses we come to know our bodies, and the different *spatial* aspects of our bodies. (The spatial aspects of foundational sensory development are further discussed in volume 2.) Through the *tactile sense* we perceive the boundary or border of our physical body. The organ for the sense of touch is the skin. By means of the *sense of life*, we feel that we take up the space inside our border. In other words, we perceive our inner volume, as Jaimen McMillan describes it. The organ for the sense of life is the autonomic nervous system. By means of the *proprioceptive sense*, we perceive where the different segments of our body are and what they are doing in relationship to each other, i.e., whether our elbow is bent or bending, or straight or straightening. The sense organs for the sense of proprioception are embedded in the muscles and joints throughout the body. The sense of *balance* tells us about the position of our head, whether it is stable, and whether it is speeding up or slowing down. Through the sense of balance, we can perceive whether we are falling or not.

Rudolf Steiner considers each of the foundational senses to be inner senses. They give us perceptions about what is going on inside our bodies. The foundational senses are also known as the basal or lower senses. However, lower does not imply lesser. Each sense has its unique place within the totality of the twelve.

The Foundational Senses Are Usually Sleepy

Rudolf Steiner explains that "all that has to do with the senses of balance, movement, life and even with the sense of touch . . . is connected with the will."[8] It follows, then, that since the foundational senses are will senses, "and the will sleeps, people sleep through these senses,"[9] we are largely unaware of our experiences of the foundational senses—unless there is something out of the ordinary going on. For example, the sense of touch gives us the perception of the edge or border of our body. Normally, the border of our body is not something we pay much attention to. However, we can be acutely aware of the border of our body if we have a painful skin condition, such as poison ivy, and we are boarding an airplane. In this situation, we may make every attempt not to bump into the airplane seats as we pass by them, because our skin is so sensitive to touch.

Rudolf Steiner describes the sense of life as the sense "for perceiving the condition of our body in the broadest sense. . . . Many people are very dependent upon this sense of life. They perceive whether they have eaten too much or too little, or whether they are tired or not, or whether they feel comfortable or uncomfortable. In short, the states of our own bodies are reflected in the sense of life."[10] Other people have less sensitivity in this sense and may not notice that they have missed a meal and are hungry and thirsty. Steiner also explains that "the harmonious collaboration of all the bodily organs expresses itself through the life sense, through the state of life in us. We usually pay no attention to it because we expect it as our natural right. We expect to be filled with a certain feeling of well-being, with the feeling of being alive."[11]

Our feeling of well-being is characteristically under the radar of our consciousness. We typically only notice the life sense when it is disturbed—when we feel ill or in pain, for example.

The sense of self-movement gives us the perception of the positions of our body parts. We aren't usually aware of the positions of our arms—how far bent or straight our elbows are, for instance. However, if we are learning a choreographed dance with a group of people for a performance, then we need to pay attention to the position of our arms.

Regarding our sense of balance, we typically take this sense for granted also—unless we are in a precarious position and are at risk of falling, or we are challenging our balance.

The Middle Senses

The four middle senses include the senses of smell, taste, sight, and temperature. Rudolf Steiner relates that everything that has to do with the middle senses, "with the senses of warmth, sight, taste and smell has to do with feeling."[12]

While the four foundational senses allow us to perceive our own bodies, through the middle senses, we venture out of ourselves to perceive the world. Steiner says that "The first sense to take you outside yourself is the *sense of smell* [emphasis added]."[13] However, he relates that with the sense of smell we don't go very far outside of ourselves. Interestingly, he says that we aren't much interested in interaction with the world through our sense of smell! "Furthermore, people do not want to have anything to do with the intimate connection with the world that a developed sense of smell can give. Dogs are much more interested. People are willing to use the sense of smell to perceive the world, but they do not want the world to come very close. It is not a sense through which people want to get very involved with the outer world."[14]

As a rule, we are more interested in our interactions with the *sense of taste*. "With the sense of taste we get more deeply involved with the world. . . . What is external is taken inward."[15] Here, we take into our bodies something from the outside world, break it down, mix it with our saliva, and taste it. With taste we distinguish sweet, sour, salty, and bitter tastes.

As we proceed through the middle senses, we become more adept at going out of ourselves into the external world. Specifically, with the *sense of sight*, we perceive the lightness or darkness of an object's surface as well as its color. We perceive just the exterior and nothing of its interior with the sense of vision. Steiner clarifies, "The sense of sight transmits to us the surface of external corporeality which confronts us in color, brightness or darkness."[16] In a passage from his diary, Karl König gives us a very nuanced insight regarding the sense of vision. He relates a particular visual experience of his, which he had upon waking and opening the curtain. He describes that "the eye is not for seeing things and objects but to prepare the space in which the things and objects 'can let themselves become visible.' . . . Through this space created by the eye—like a candle which is lit in the darkness—the objects in this space appeared and compelled me to perceive them."[17] It is interesting that babies sometimes appear compelled to look at something.

With the *sense of temperature*, we can perceive further into the external world than with the sense of vision. The interior of an object also has warmth or cold, and so with the sense of temperature, we perceive something of the inner condition of the object, not just its exterior surface, as with the sense of vision.[18]

The sense of temperature does not tell us whether we ourselves are hot or cold—that information comes to us from the sense of life. Rudolf Steiner gives a very specific explanation for the way that the sense of temperature operates: "Seventh among the senses is that of temperature, and again there is something in [human beings] that transmits it. It is the sentient body itself, which is of an astral nature. It transmits the sense of temperature by sending its astral substance outward. An experience of warmth or cold occurs only when the human being is really able to ray his astral substance outward, that is, when nothing prevents this."[19] The sentient body, also referred to as the astral body, plays a role in sensation.[20] Steiner says that our astral substance doesn't ray out when we take a bath in body-temperature water, because there is an equilibrium between our body and the water. "We only experience temperature when warmth or cold can flow out of or into us."[21] In other words, there needs to be a flow of warmth in order for us to perceive warmth or cold. If warmth flows from the environment into us, then we perceive the environment as warm. If there is a flow of warmth from us into the environment, then we perceive the environment as cold.[22]

The Higher Senses

The four higher senses include the sense of hearing, the sense of word (also known as the sense of language or speech), the sense of thought, and the "I"-sense, or the sense of the ego of the other. Rudolf Steiner says that through these senses, we "receive what is predominantly associated with the *idea*."[23] In another place, he refers to them as "cognitive senses."[24] Whereas we relate to the lower senses with our will and our middle senses with our feeling, we relate to the higher senses with our thinking.

With the *sense of hearing* we perceive sound and tones. As Rudolf Steiner describes this sense, "When we strike an object, its inner nature is revealed to us in tone, and we can distinguish among objects according to their inner nature, according to their inner vibration, when we open our inner ear to their tone. It is the soul of objects that speaks to our own soul in tones."[25]

When I was a child, my great aunt taught me how to tell the difference between lead crystal and pressed glass. When you flick your finger on the lip of a lead crystal goblet, it has a bright tone, but when you flick the lip of a pressed glass goblet of nearly the same size and shape, the tone falls flat. The lead crystal "rings true." The crystal's sound reveals its inner nature. One day the babies explored their sense of hearing in this manner while they were playing outside on our patio at Sophia's Hearth. One child spontaneously took a toy and started banging it on the bars which surround the patio. Soon the other three babies joined in the fun, each with a different object—one had a little wooden bowl, another a metal cup, and so on. Each object expressed its inner nature by making a different sound, and all together the babies created a little orchestra!

Similarly, when we hear the sound of a cat, we can perceive something of the inner soul condition of the cat. One sound can signal to us that the cat is just about to get into a fight with another animal. Another sound tells us the cat is hungry. Yet another sound (purring) tells us that all is well. Parents and caregivers employ the sense of hearing when they discern the meaning of an infant's different cries. Thus, with the sense of hearing, we can perceive something of the inner nature of another being or of an object, and we penetrate farther out into the world than we do with the sense of temperature. Recall that with the foundational senses we perceive conditions inside the body. With the middle senses we begin to venture into the outer world, and with the higher senses this continues. In fact, Steiner relates that with each subsequent higher sense, we journey more deeply and more intimately into the world.

With the *sense of word*, we listen *behind* the tones and sounds of the person speaking, and we perceive whether the sound they are making is a word or a random combination of sounds. I remember the first time I heard a language other than English. When I was a child, my family went on vacation to the Rocky Mountains, and went to an evening presentation at the lodge where people from all over the globe had gathered. I could tell that these people were speaking languages—that they were not just making odd sounds. I could identify their sounds as words through the sense of word.

Rudolf Steiner stresses that the sense of word is not identical to the sense of hearing. "To be sure, sounds open the inner world of objects to our perception, but these sounds must become much more inward before they can become meaningful words. Therefore it is a step into a deeper intimacy with the world when we proceed from perceiving sounds through the sense of hearing to perceiving meaning through the sense of the word."[26] We enter more deeply into the world when we perceive the meaning of the words through the sense of word. We perceive the meaning of words—not by thinking—but by *sensing* their meaning.

Next, we come to the *sense of thought*. This sense "has nothing to do with the formation of our own thoughts. . . . Our sense of thought is what gives us the ability to understand and perceive the thoughts of others."[27] The other person's thoughts are communicated by means of words or gestures. Sometimes, the person with whom we are communicating isn't able to express themselves adequately—perhaps they can't find the right words—yet we know what they mean. We listen *behind* their words and their gestures to grasp their intended meaning. We do this frequently with little ones who haven't fully developed language, with someone who has aphasia, and with someone for whom we don't speak the same language. We also use the sense of thought when we play charades!

Rudolf Steiner explains that the sense of thought allows us to go out more deeply into the world than does the sense of word. In the following passage, he compares the sense of thought with the sense of word:

And yet, when I perceive a mere word I am still not so intimately connected with the object, with the external thing, as I am connected with it when I perceive the thoughts behind the words. At this stage, most people cease to make any distinctions. But there is a distinction between merely perceiving words and actually perceiving the thoughts behind the words. After all, you still can perceive words when a phonograph—or writing, for that matter—has separated them from their thinker. But a sense that goes deeper than the usual word sense must come into play before I can come into a living relationship with the being that is forming the words, before I can enter through the words and transpose myself directly into the being that is doing the thinking and forming the concepts. That further step calls for the sense I would like to call the sense of thought.[28]

The twelfth sense is the *sense of the ego of the other* or the *"I"-sense*. "When we speak of the ego sense, we are referring to the ability of one person to be aware of the *I* of another."[29] We perceive that the other person is an individuality, a spiritual entity, and not an object. Rudolf Steiner explains that "When we penetrate the ego of another person with our perception, we go out of ourselves the most."[30] As we travel through each of the higher senses, we go outside of ourselves a little bit more, with the highest level of intimacy with the outer world in the sense of the ego of the other.

There have been great people throughout history who have had well-developed senses of the ego of the other. These people recognize the "I" in the other—they can see the other's "hidden truth." To me, one such person was Dr. Karl König.* In the following passage, he is described by one of his patients. The patient had arrived for her first doctor's appointment with him. After a period in the waiting room, she entered the examination room and found him seated behind his desk.

> His eyes were very big and grave. When they rested on you, they did not only see through you, they seemed to create you anew. Something dormant in yourself responded whether you wanted it to or not; you seemed to become what you really were, beneath the layers of habit, inhibition and illusion.... This peculiar gaze, I think was one of the unique characteristics in Dr. König. I would call it a "creative gaze." He not only saw what you were but what you were meant to be.... There are people who can study you, see through you, recognize the forces at work, but there are few who can "create" you. We may struggle to remind ourselves when we regard another person that a spark of the divine lives in [them] as well—indeed this is a facet of the discipline that arises from the pursuit of anthroposophy. But although this discipline no doubt clears the way to the other person, it is not necessarily an outpouring of warmth, a living flow from one person to another.... In Dr. König the gaze was a channel for the flow or warmth, it was in itself healing, for one felt one was seen in one's hidden truth, and always with respect and compassion.... I think this first grave gaze—Dr. König otherwise said little—was the initial step in healing. The medicines that followed were effective because something in the inner situation had begun to change—whereby I felt no onrush of sympathy or *Schwärmerei* for this small doctor—I only felt called up, impersonally, to my better self.[31]

---

* Dr. König was an anthroposophical physician who started the Camphill Movement during World War II. He also was a prolific author and speaker.

The Twelve Senses as Doorways into Different Worlds

We have just described each of the twelve senses. Now let us consider them as three distinct groups: the foundational senses, the middle senses, and the higher senses.

As mentioned earlier in the chapter, the twelve senses are doorways through which we may connect with three different worlds. The foundational senses allow us to make connections with the physical world. The middle senses make possible perception of the social world. The higher senses are our means of sensing the spiritual world. Rudolf Steiner explains, "Every form of life is spiritual. Even as ice is condensed water, so matter is condensed spirit. Mineral, plant, animal, or [human being]—each is a condensed form of the spirit."[32] In other words, the spiritual world is present all around us. However, it is largely veiled from us, and we are typically unable to perceive it. We can continue to develop our higher senses well into the latter periods of life. This development gives us the possibility to perceive things behind the veil.

Let us start with an exploration of the nature of the sensory phenomena perceived by the foundational senses. This is how we get information about the physical world.

Just Give Me the Cold, Hard Facts

Phenomena in the physical world are quantifiable and objective. Things can be measured and verified by another person. The four foundational senses (touch, life, self-movement, and balance) register objective, indisputable facts about the physical world.

The sense of self-movement or proprioception is also known as the "body position sense."[33] The organs of the proprioceptive sense (known as the proprioceptors) are embedded in the musculoskeletal system, which functions in a mechanical fashion. The proprioceptors provide us with information from our "joints, muscles, tendons, and ligaments."[34] Our muscles shorten and they elongate. When they contract, they generate forces that act upon our joints to bend or straighten them. The muscles attach to bones, which serve as lever arms. When the muscles contract, the bones move to change the angular position of the particular segment of the body that is being acted upon. For example, when we perform a bicep curl, our proprioceptors inform us—generally at an unconscious level—that the forearm is moving or has been moved. The result of the movement is that the hand comes closer to the upper arm. We can measure the specific angle between the forearm and the upper arm. In this way we determine, for example, whether our elbow is bent to ninety degrees or whether it is bent to ninety-five degrees. This is a very specific, quantifiable measurement!

The amount of force that a muscle generates is also measurable. If we pick up a heavy box, our muscles generate a certain amount of force, which is more than if we pick up a thimble. At first, when the baby picks up an object that is somewhat heavy for them, their arm drops down slightly. Over time, they learn to generate the correct amount of force right away, so that their arm doesn't

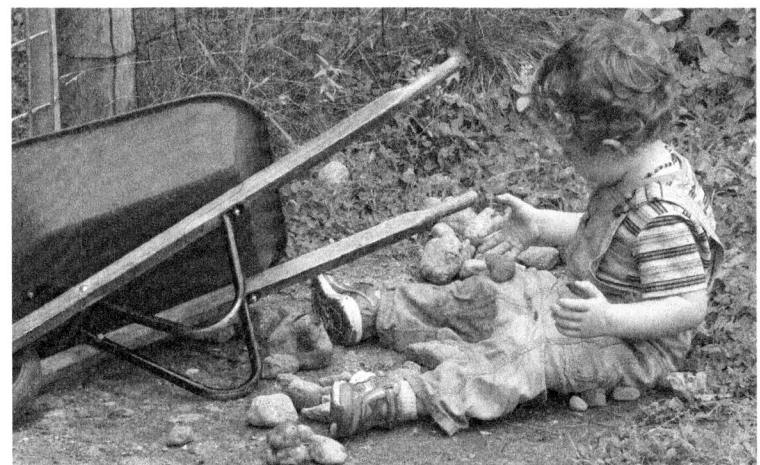

This child gathered rocks of varying sizes and weights. They sat and played with them for an extended period. They were experiencing—at an unconscious level—the forces generated by their muscles in picking up the different rocks.

FREE MOVEMENT FROM THE VERY START

dip down. It is very healthy for children to play with objects of different weights. The child perceives, for example, that a wooden block is heavier than a felted ball. Later, in school, this translates to an understanding that 100 is greater than 30. (Cognitive development is further discussed in volume 2.)

When we hang from the monkey bars, forces of traction (pulling apart) are exerted upon the joint capsules, tendons, ligaments, and muscles.

When we jump down off a rock and land on the ground, forces of compression are exerted upon the structures of our musculoskeletal system. The proprioceptors are registering these forces.

The organ of the sense of balance is the vestibular system. Through this sense we know: am I in balance or am I falling out of balance? Is my head speeding up or slowing down (perceiving forces of acceleration and deceleration)? In which position is my head—right side up, upside down, tipped sideways to the right or left, or rotated to either side? The vestibular system is responsible for giving us a basic orientation in space through which we come to understand spatial relationships in the world.

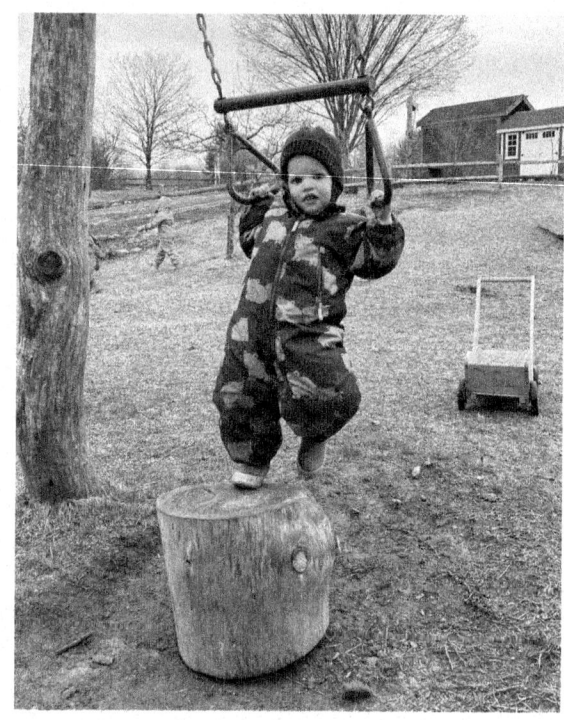

This child is experiencing a wealth of proprioceptive input as he counters the traction from the bar with the contraction of his muscles.

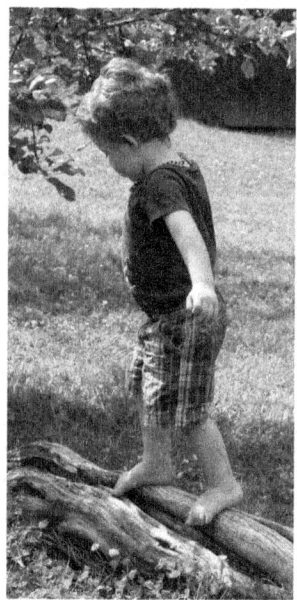

This child is experiencing—largely at an unconscious level—whether they are in balance or not.

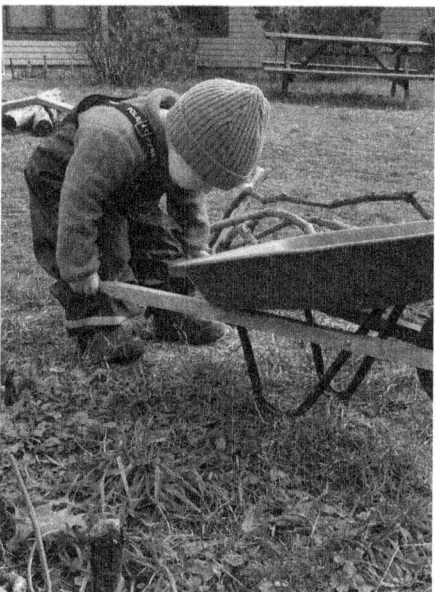

This child is keeping their balance as they bend down to lift the wheelbarrow handles.

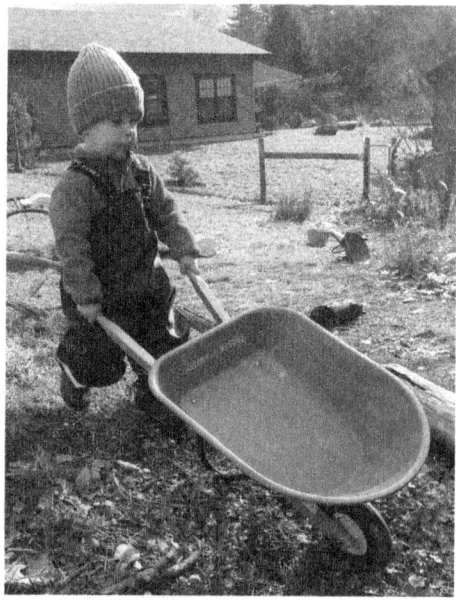

Here, the child balances their own body and also balances the wheelbarrow as they push it down the hill and maneuver around obstacles in the yard.

As mentioned above, we perceive several different earthly forces through the foundational senses: forces of gravity, acceleration and deceleration, compression, and traction. The young child is incredibly active, and their movements generate a multitude of forces.

The forces generated by the child's movements and perceived by the four foundational senses are the same earthly forces that act on other physical objects in the world. Rudolf Steiner explains that the four foundational senses are:

> pronounced inner senses; but what we perceive through them in ourselves is exactly the same as what we perceive in the world outside us. . . . Although we perceive our own movement, our own balance, in a decidedly subjective manner, this movement and this balance are nevertheless quite objective processes, for physically speaking it is a matter of indifference whether it is a block of wood that is moved, or a [person.] In the external physical world a [person] in movement is exactly the same thing to observe as a block of wood; and similarly with regard to balance. And if you take the sense of life—the same thing applies. [35]

Steiner continues that the sense of touch is also an objective process. In other words, all of the foundational senses are objective processes, which he describes as "something which has absolutely no specific connection with the content of your soul-life."[36] In other words, we typically don't respond with feelings of sympathy or antipathy to experiences of our foundational senses. We don't typically like it or not like it that our elbow is straight or bent, for example. Instead, the position of our elbow simply is a fact.

Do You Like It or Not?

In contrast, the middle senses (smell, taste, vision, and temperature) do pertain to our soul life. Our soul life includes our sympathies and our antipathies. We typically respond to sensations elicited from the middle senses by expressing whether we like them or not. When we want to know if something in the back of the refrigerator is still okay to eat, we smell it. If it smells rotten, we often express our feelings about it with a grimacing face. Similarly, with the sense of taste, we respond with characteristic statements such as, "I like that taste," or "I don't like it," or "Maybe I used to not care for that food, but I've learned to like it, and now I eat it twice a week." Regarding the sense of vision: "I like that color," or "I don't," or "Maybe I like it." With the sense of temperature, an object may feel warm to me if my hands are cold. However, if I warm my hands, the object may not feel as warm—and it could even feel cold, depending on how much I warm my hands. Yet, the temperature of the object has not changed! Our perceptions through the sense of temperature are relative to us. Additionally, I may like it that something feels cold, or not. Our feelings relate to our soul life, which Steiner describes in this passage:

> Everything in our environment cannot be counted as belonging to the soul life. . . . On the physical level, when we encounter a rose, we do not consider the rose itself to be a part of our soul life. However, if we feel joy or pleasure arising in us as we look at it, we can indeed call that a soul experience. If we meet someone and form a mental picture of that person—hair, face, expression—we do not include that in our soul life. But if we feel an interest in a person through sympathy or antipathy, or if we think of that person with love, all of these feelings must be considered soul experiences. You know that I don't like definitions; I prefer to characterize instead. I don't want to define soul life for you, since definitions accomplish little. I prefer to characterize what belongs to soul life.[37]

To reiterate, our feelings play a part in our experiences of the middle senses, and feelings are fleeting. They may even change in an instant. Today I like yellow. Tomorrow I may not like it anymore, as that color has gone out of style, or I'm simply tired of it. We can discuss these matters with each other. Unlike the foundational senses, what we perceive through the middle senses is not indisputable. We may try and convince someone that yellow looks good on them—or not.

The middle senses are social senses. We have casual conversations about our experiences of the middle senses. Whereas the physical world is a very precise, measurable, nonnegotiable, and reproducible world, the soul world has a changeable, give-and-take quality to it.

A Primal Knowing

Recall that Rudolf Steiner considers the foundational senses to be inner senses, related to the body. He explains that the middle senses show "an interplay between the outer and the inner world."[38] Steiner then considers the higher senses (hearing, word, thought, and ego of the other or "I"-sense) to be outer senses. Rudolf Steiner explains that through this group of senses, "a specific experience of what we are as part of the world-not-ourselves is conveyed to us."[39] The higher senses give us the possibility to tap into the spiritual world. Through the higher senses, we are sometimes afforded a deep knowing, perhaps even a primal knowing, which is much different than the intellectual knowledge gained by the measurement and analysis of the physical world, or the here-today-gone-tomorrow knowledge of the soul world. When we have an experience of deep wisdom, we don't mention this too often, because it can be said authentically only in profound moments. It is not parking-lot conversation. These moments often never go away—they may stay with us for the rest of our lives. We may also express this type of knowledge in its negative form—"that's not right"—meaning that something is not just or not true. These statements refer to knowledge that is universal, that transcends our worldly technical knowledge. This is a world with paradoxes, as the greatest truths can manifest in paradoxes.

The higher senses are doorways into the spiritual world, where in rare moments, we may encounter beings of a spiritual nature. We may have breakthrough moments where we experience the harmonies of the spheres through the sense of hearing—for example, when we listen to a symphony. We may perceive the living word through the sense of word—for example, when we hear an inspiring orator. In one fairy tale, the power of the creative word is illuminated. A young man must speak, but he doesn't know the words to say. Divine powers see his plight and send doves, which land on his shoulders. "The doves on his shoulders whisper rune-wise the divine words into his ear." The man understands and speaks the words. In doing so, he ushers in a new era for humanity.[40] With the sense of thought, there may be times when we may perceive living thinking. With the sense of the ego of the other we may encounter the spiritual part of another human being.

Sometimes, we confuse the mode of experiencing a sensation in one group of senses with that intended for another group of senses. Rudolf Steiner gives a specific example in his 1921 lecture series, *Man as a Being of Sense and Perception*. He describes that people can become "so firmly fixed in their middle senses, in the senses of warmth, sight, taste and smell, that they judge others, or the thoughts of others [later he includes the words of others], in accordance with these senses. Then they do not hear the thoughts of the other [person] at all, but perceive them in the same way they perceive wine or vinegar or any other food or drink."[41] He goes on to say that, in this situation, "Everything becomes subjective experience. To reduce the higher senses to the character of the lower ones is immoral."[42] In other words, through the higher senses of hearing, word, thought, and ego of the other, we have the possibility to perceive universal truths and insights from the spiritual world. When we reduce something of this stature and experience it as we would experience an odor, a taste, a color or a temperature, then we are sorely missing out on what we could be perceiving through our higher senses.

Relationship between Upper and Lower Senses

The lower senses are foundational for the development of the higher senses. Another way to think about the relationship between the lower and the higher senses is that they form four distinct pairs:

1. the sense of touch . . . . 12. the sense of the ego of the other ("I"-sense)
2. the sense of life (or well-being) . . . . 11. the sense of thought
3. the sense of self-movement . . . . 10. the sense of word
4. the sense of balance . . . . 9. the sense of hearing (or tone)

As described above, Steiner considered the lower senses to be *inner* senses, and the higher senses to be *outer* senses. In each of the four pairs, there is an inner and an outer sense. This gives the possibility of a focusing in and a focusing out—similar to what the lens of a camera does. According to Jaimen McMillan, in each pair, the peripheral and central aspect create a dynamic polarity. It is becoming aware of the movements in space between these polarities that creates the very essence and possibility of sensing.[43]

The Sense of Touch and the Sense of the Ego of the Other ("I"-Sense)

These are the two senses that Rudolf Steiner originally left out as he began by describing ten senses. Through our skin, the organ of our sense of touch, we experience the outer border of our body—the most peripheral aspect of our body. We experience our edge, and this is literally what separates us from the rest of the world and from other people. In this way our focus is inward. However, the sense of touch also offers a sophisticated means of focusing outside of ourselves. The sense of touch gives possibilities of intimacy and connection with others that are possible in no other way. For example, there has been significant study of skin-to-skin contact in the first hours after birth and its positive effect on the bonding between baby and parent. In fact, the World Health Association recommends skin-to-skin contact in the first hour after birth if medically possible.

The Sense of Life (or Well-Being) and the Sense of Thought

Through our sense of life, when we are in a healthy state, we experience a general sense of well-being. This gives us a feeling of being whole, and as such, our attention is not drawn toward or stuck in subdivisions of our bodies. Instead, we are free to venture beyond our bodily boundaries and turn our focus to the living thoughts of another person. When feeling well, we can follow the other person's thoughts well. We can meet them where they are and understand where they are coming from. On the other hand, if we have pain, or if our sense of well-being is otherwise disturbed, then we don't have the feeling of being whole. Instead, we feel disjointed, reduced to parts, and we are forced to focus on fragments of our bodies, particularly on the parts that hurt. In this case, our ability to understand may also be fragmented. When our sense of well-being is weakened, we are less connected with life around us, and we are less able to encounter the other person, focus on their thoughts, or weigh their point of view.[44]

Jaimen McMillan emphasizes that thinking is highly refined *movement*. The sense of thought in which one perceives the thoughts of another person involves following and moving with the thought shapes, patterns, and dynamics of the other's presentation of their thoughts. Comprehending another person depends on our ability to perform thought gymnastics to follow, bend, and take on new shapes in order to grasp the other's meaning. To think new thoughts, we have to be able to move in new ways. With a healthy sense of well-being, one is freer to get out of one's own body, as well as one's own entrenched thought patterns, and be more able to track the other's person's train of thought and make sense of what the other is saying.[45]

The relationship between these two senses has been especially pronounced in the children I have worked with who have had food sensitivities and environmental allergies. When the medical issues are adequately addressed, it is as if a fog lifts, and the child's perception of another's thoughts can shine through.

The Sense of Self-Movement and the Sense of Word

I have observed the relationship between the developing sense of self-movement and the developing sense of word. When I was a movement teacher in our local Waldorf school, I brought many jump rope games to the younger grades. Toward the latter part of first grade and into second and third grade, the games involved more complicated timing—running in and out of a turning rope to verses, with the children in groups of two, three, four, and so on. In order to be successful in the jump rope games, the children had to perfect their senses of self-movement. This involved reading the nonverbal cues of their partners, and adjusting the timing of their own movements accordingly. I found that these jump rope games literally wove together the social fabric of the class. For example, after mastering jump rope games, a child who formerly tended to interrupt and blurt out inappropriate words became better able to perceive the words of their peers and find their way into a conversation more nimbly.

We sometimes say that someone's words have moved us, or that we are moved to action by someone's words. Martin Luther King Jr.'s "I Have a Dream" speech is a classic example. In 2013, *Time Magazine* published a fifty-year anniversary issue featuring King's speech. People who were at the march on Washington offered memories of their experiences. One person said, "When I hear that speech—I mean this is what, 50 years later?—I still cry. It's so extraordinary, but when he finished speaking, I really had a profound sense that it was now almost inevitable. Such a force had been unleashed that history was moving. He had spoken in front of Lincoln's likeness, and I said, This is going to happen."[46] The higher senses are doorways into the spiritual world, and this person, who witnessed King's speech, sensed something of the spiritual power of the spoken word.

In my experience as a pediatric physical therapist, I have repeatedly marveled at the relationship between movement and speech. In my first job, I worked at a pediatric hospital school with children, many of whom had cerebral palsy, sometimes with severe involvement. For the children with more significant involvement, a speech therapist and I frequently did co-treatments. Our co-treatments worked out well. When I took a child out of their wheelchair and facilitated their movements, not only did the child vocalize more, but they also appeared to understand the spoken word better.

The Sense of Balance and the Sense of Hearing

Phylogenetic (having to do with evolution) studies and studies of fetal development show a close connection between the hearing and vestibular (balance) systems. Both systems share structures in the middle ear, and they also share a neurological pathway to the brain.[47]

In my study of Spacial Dynamics with Jaimen McMillan, I came to realize that both balance and hearing have strong relationships to the spaces inside and outside of the body. Balance is generally considered an inner sense. However, to successfully balance, we must simultaneously be inside our body *and* outside our body. We can't balance if we are too spatially contracted inside our bodies, and we can't balance if we are spatially too far out. We need to be in the body and simultaneously poised in the interplay of the three planes of space (up/down, right/left, and front/back) that extend beyond us. Additionally, we are balancing our body in relationship to the pull of gravity from the center of the earth and a peripheral levitational force.

In the sense of hearing, if we are spatially too far inside our bodies, we experience tinnitus, or ringing of the ears, and then we can't hear well. In contrast, if we are too far outside ourselves spatially, then our ears may be physiologically affected by sound, but we can't listen, and no real hearing takes place. Optimally, we want to listen to sounds outside our bodies—to actually have our awareness at the place from which the sounds originate. It is helpful for children to learn to listen peripherally. For example, we can take children for walks in nature. At a certain point along the walk, we can stop, have the children close their eyes, ask them if they hear any birds, and then ask them to point to where the bird's song is coming from. The sense of hearing is born of a threefold balancing act: the child's attention being drawn by the bird's song; being concurrently aware in the body; and making sense of this tug of war by dynamically connecting the two worlds and pointing.[48]

In my experience as a pediatric physical therapist, I have worked with many children who were challenged in their balance. Sometimes, in addition to balance issues, a child would have auditory discrimination issues. Again, I did not directly address the auditory issues. However, remarkably, as their balance improved, they could listen better.

I also came to understand the relationship between hearing and balance through my own personal experience. In my Spacial Dynamics training, one of our assignments was to take on something in our lives that was difficult for us and see if we could make any headway with it. My family is musical, and we often sing together at holidays. Unfortunately, I had trouble hearing the correct pitches for my part (alto). So, I chose to try and improve my singing ability for my Spacial Dynamics assignment. My husband (who is a wonderful singer) and I joined our local church choir for a year. Singing in the choir was not easy for me. I struggled. However, there was a turning point, when, for another reason, I had opportunities to improve my balance. I got a skinny balance beam, put it in our living room, and walked it every day, doing various tricks on the beam. Additionally, I learned to ride the unicycle. As my balance improved, I could perceive the space around my head clearing and opening up. As a result, I could hear the notes better, and my singing improved!

Integrating the Senses: Uniting What Is Separate

When we perform an activity or perceive something, we never just use one sense. Instead, multiple, separate sensory channels are used. The human being must unite the distinct sensory modalities. Rudolf Steiner gives the example of looking at a red ball. Steiner maintains that with the sense of self-movement we perceive the form of the ball—its roundness—and with the sense of vision, we perceive its color—red.

> You would look at a red circle in a dull and blank way if you could not perceive the red in one way and the form of the circle in quite a different way. But you do not look upon it in a blank way because you look at it from two sides, the color through the eye and the form with the help of the sense of movement, and life compels you to join the two together inwardly. There you form a judgment. . . . The things compel you to combine them inwardly and you declare yourself to be inwardly ready to combine them. Thus the function of judgment becomes an expression of your whole being.[49]

It is through our activity of uniting the disparate sensations that we can develop concepts and make judgments. Because there are twelve senses, we have a very large number of ways to unite them. Steiner describes it thus: "Now you can see the deeper meaning of our relationship to the world. If we did not have twelve senses, we would [not be able to] experience inner judgment. However, because we do have twelve senses, we have a large number of possible ways to reunite what has been separated. . . . In this way, we can see the mysterious way human beings are connected with the world."[50] Steiner goes on to say that when we unite the senses, "we participate in the inner life of things. You can, therefore, understand how immensely important it is that we educate children and develop each of the senses in balance, since we can then systematically and consciously seek the relationships between the senses and perceptions."[51] In other words, each sense has its distinct and rightful place, and ideally, all twelve should be developed in a harmonious and balanced way.

FREE MOVEMENT FROM THE VERY START

The more evenly developed and finely tuned our sensory organism is, the more avenues we have for perceiving. The more channels of sensing that we have, the more possibilities to develop capacities of understanding. Out of our comprehension, then, we are more free to act responsibly with regard to our thoughts, feelings, and deeds.

Johannes Rohen, in his book *Functional Morphology*, elaborates, "Essentially, our sensory organs and nervous system create a reproduction of the outer world through a reflective process. The more we are able to capture the object in the mirror of our consciousness, the truer the resulting image is to the object's essence. Cognition is based primarily on accurate reflections of the outer (or inner) world. We then take hold of these reflections with our thinking and pin them down with concepts."[52]

When just one of our senses experiences a challenge, we feel its effects. For example, after we go to the dentist for a procedure and a small part of our mouth is numbed, this can affect us on many levels. I remember an occasion when this happened to me, and I didn't want to go out in public afterward. Probably less than two square inches of the zone of my sense of touch had been disturbed, but I didn't feel competent to take in any other kinds of sensations—I didn't feel competent to meet the world.

9: Developmental Aspects of Sensing

A common theme runs through this book—*young children are not little adults!* In sleep, memory, and overall consciousness, young children are different than adults. Young children also don't think in the way that adults do—they don't operate from an intellectual frame of reference. They act differently than adults do. They don't reflect on what they did, nor plan out what they want to do; rather, they imitate the activities and gestures from their environments. Freya Jaffke sums this up: "Everything which the child does is done without reflection or consideration. [The child] does it out of imitation and habit."[1] These differences are discussed in detail in volume 2. This chapter discusses another related, noteworthy difference between adults and young children—that of sensing. Children have entirely different sense experiences than those of adults. To start, let us consider the act of sensing itself.

Sensing Is Not Thinking

Rudolf Steiner clarifies that "The sense-organs do not think; they perceive pictures, or rather they form pictures from external objects."[2]

Steiner explains that sensing happens before any cognitive activity occurs. "Sense is that perception through which we obtain knowledge without the help of the mental processes. Where judgment plays a role in acquiring knowledge, the term *sense* is inappropriate; *sense* is a term limited to situations where the power of judgment has not yet become active. We use a sense to perceive a color, but to make a judgment between two colors no sense is necessary."[3] In other words, we perceive different shades of orange with our sense of vision, but to decide which shade is brighter or which shade matches another color better, we must employ our judgment.

Sensing in the Young Child and the Adult: Some Big Differences

Young children do not have the same capacities for cognition that adults do. Infants and very young children engage in nearly pure perceptual processes. In contrast, the adult's tendency is to jump to a concept about what they are perceiving. In this way, adults are one often step removed from their sense perceptions. Adults sometimes try to get out of their heads—they may take a mindfulness class and work to stay focused on their perceptions. In contrast, the young child is naturally mindful. They are essentially one with what they are perceiving. There is no distance between them and the sensation, as there is in the adult. As a result, the child's sensory experiences are much more intense than those of an adult.

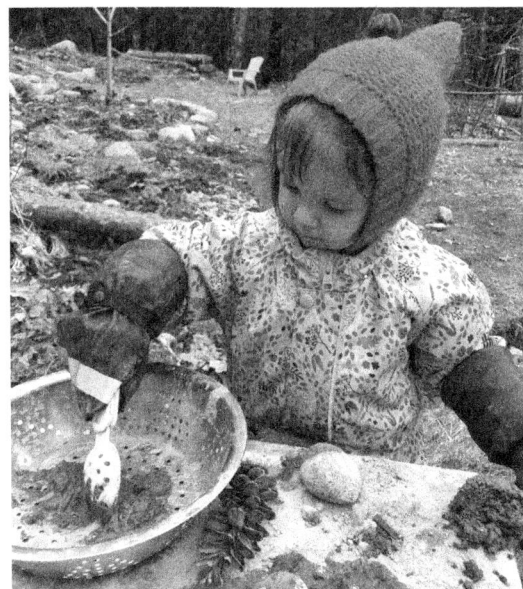

Note this child's devotion to the sensorimotor activity of stirring the mud. They are "at one" with the mud.

Georg Kühlewind addresses this difference between the young child's sensations and those of the adult. He continues that the young child's feelings are also different than those of an adult. Because the child does not rely on predetermined concepts, "everything has to be thoroughly looked at, touched, and listened to. Also this intense sense activity is still intertwined with the world of feelings, and the feelings are still partly cognitive, that is really *feeling*, feeling toward the outside, not self-feeling as in the adult. The wonder of discovery and the wonder of mental experience are still united."[4]

Dr. Michaela Glöckler further elaborates on the differences between the young child's sensations and those of the adult:

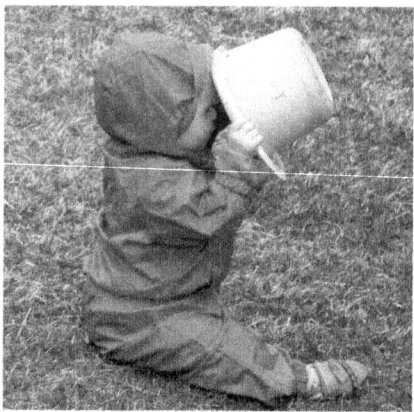

This little one shows us what Kühlewind meant when he said that for young children, "everything has to be thoroughly looked at, touched, and listened to."

> The child's perceptions of the world are very different from those of the adult, for [they see] thought-life woven around and within [their] surroundings. [The child] looks at a dark corner, for example, and sees the shadows move. [They experience] the inner meaning of darkness. Something jumps out of the darkness, and the child is frightened. [They run to the parent] who turns on the light and says there is nothing there. The child is often not understood at a deeper level, but [they are] consoled that the [parent] is strong enough to bring light into the darkness. The child has both these experiences; [they are] misunderstood and [they are] consoled at the same time.[5]

One time, I was taking a walk with my two granddaughters, who were aged three and five. It was winter, in the late afternoon. We were on a dirt road heading home. The hike had lasted a little longer than anticipated, and it was starting to get dark. One of the children sensed something coming out from the dark wooded area near the road and was frightened (I saw and sensed nothing, although I stopped to look). I had just read this passage by Dr. Glöckler the previous evening! I don't remember exactly what I said or did, but I do remember that I felt a deep connection to my grandchild. Because I understood something of the developmental nature of her sense impression, I took her sense experience seriously—and that I did this, in and of itself, was reassuring to her.

Dr. Glöckler continues, "[The child] sees the flower and experiences the inner reality of the flower; [they see] the *being* of the flower. The child experiences not only the *outlook* but also the *inlook*, the inner being or 'I am' of the object perceived."[6]

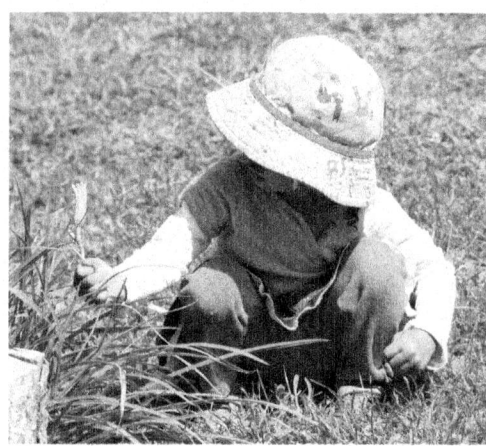

This child spent an extended period looking at the flower. Were they perceiving the flower's inner being?

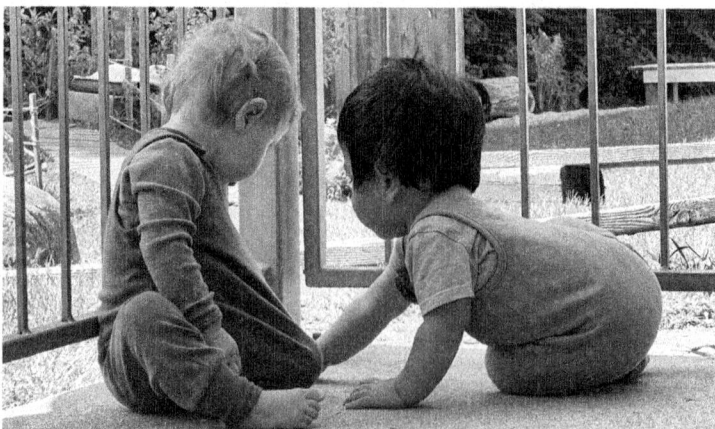

These two children have found a leaf to look at, something which would typically be overlooked by an adult. Note the reverent quality of the children's gaze.

There have been several instances when I have witnessed young babies who were mesmerized by the sunbeams streaming in through the window. The quality of their gaze was filled with awe, and I wondered what they were seeing that I could not.

Sense Fields of Activity

The sizes of the sense zones are larger in babies than they are in adults. Rudolf Steiner gives the example of the sense of taste. "An adult, who has brought taste into the sphere of consciousness; tastes with [their] tongue and decides what the taste is. A child—that is to say a baby in [their] earliest weeks—tastes with [their] whole body. The organ of taste is diffused throughout the organism. [The baby] tastes with [their] stomach, and [they continue] to taste when the nourishing juices have been taken up by the lymph vessels and transmitted to the whole organism."[7] Indeed, on more than one occasion when I have witnessed my grandchildren nursing as newborns and very young infants, I have had the impression that they were tasting the milk all the way down into their toes. In other words, the activity of the sense field in the adult has narrowed significantly. Steiner says that the baby's whole-body experience is true for all of the senses: "All that is localized in the several senses of the adult is spread out over the whole organism in the child."[8] The senses in the baby are "diffused throughout the child's organization and thus the baby has a 'generalized sensibility.'"[9]

Peter Selg states that the sensing activities of the young child operate "less through any individual sense than through generalized susceptibility to sense impressions."[10] However, in the adult, "each sense particularizes and differentiates [the human organism]. There is real differentiation."[11] In other words, as the baby's senses are diffused throughout their whole body, each sense is less specialized. The baby's senses are less differentiated from each other. However, the baby's senses are generally more sensitive than those of an adult.

The Senses Open at Birth

According to Steiner, "the human ability to perceive is radically changed already with birth."[12] Steiner explains, "An embryo has an ability to perceive that is essentially different from that of a human being who has seen the light of the world and developed a wakeful consciousness. An embryo perceives in a way that we characterize as an astral capacity to perceive. Thus the human embryo has an astral perception. Wakeful consciousness is developed only later. . . . [The embryo] perceives the emotions holding sway in its environment. You can see this in the influences exerted on the embryo by the conditions present in the womb."[13] I know a young mother who, when she was pregnant, gave her family strong boundaries regarding the topics she would discuss. She explained to them that, for the sake of the baby, she didn't want to become upset, and so certain topics were off limits. This woman had an intuitive understanding of the embryo's astral perceptual capacities and their need for a calm emotional environment in which to develop.

The embryo has an astral capacity of perception. The newborn is transitioning to a brand-new type of perception. It is helpful to remember that their consciousness at this stage is dreamlike. The dawning of perception via the senses occurs gradually, and initially, they are not awake to perceptions in the same way that an adult is.

Steiner describes that in the first few days of life, the senses are "opened": "A world opens for us that is at first not understandable."[14] The newborn does not need extra sensory stimulation. Experiencing new sensations is a full-time job for them! There are incidents of people who were born deaf or blind, and then, through a new medical procedure, were able to hear or see for the first time later in life. Their stories about what it was like to see or hear for the first time may give us of insight into what the newborn is experiencing. The stories commonly describe their amazement and total absorption in the new sense impressions.

Thus, the newborn enters a world that they do not understand. "All sense experiences are perceived by this being who as yet has no capacity for adding concept and relationship to the sensations. At this stage of life is experience without awareness of self, and without cognizing that the thing creating the sensation is somehow separate from [themself]. The newborn lives fully in the world of the experiences and is not separate from them. [Their] consciousness is completely in [their] experiences, in [their] perceptions."[15] In other words, the newborn has no context within which to place their sensations. They are united with their sensations—they have no capacity to filter any sensation.

Rudolf Steiner gives the example of a young infant's experience of a bell. When an adult or older child sees a bell, they recognize it as a bell, and they know that bells ring. They have integrated the sensations of their previous encounters with the bell—they have integrated the sound of the bell with the visual input of watching it being rung. Steiner explains that it is a different situation when a young infant first encounters a bell.

> Immediately after the birth of a human being [their] brain is not the same as it will be a few weeks or months later. The child already perceives the outer world, of course, but [their] brain is not yet an instrument capable of connecting external impressions in a definite way. By means of connecting-nerves running from one part of the brain to another, the human being learns by degrees to link together in thought what [they perceive] in the external world, but these connecting nerve-strands develop only after birth. A child will hear and see a bell, for instance, but the impression of the sound and the sight of the bell do not immediately combine to form the thought that the bell is ringing.[16]

In the above passage, Rudolf Steiner explains that basic neurological integration between different senses starts at birth. Therefore, the newborn's experience of the world is dramatically different than that of the adult. The young infant is constantly in the process of putting two and two together. They have embarked on a tremendous creative endeavor. They are creating their world through the vehicle of sensory integration. If for some reason a child (or a person of any age) is not able to sense with one of their senses, that part of the sense world doesn't exist for them. In the above example of the bell, when the child is *integrating* the visual and auditory input from the bell, neurological pathways are being made between the visual and the auditory centers of the brain. Sensory integration is described as a multistep process including: "receiving the sensory information successfully, interpreting it correctly, combining information from different senses to create a complete picture, deciding on a response based on information from all sources, [and] executing that response."[17]

The Groundbreaking Work of Dr. A. Jean Ayres

Occupational therapist A. Jean Ayres PhD ushered in a therapeutic movement for children known as sensory integrative therapy. She raised awareness of the situations faced by children and their families when a child faces challenges with sensory integration. The field has expanded significantly since its inception. When Dr. Ayres began her work in Southern California in the 1960s, she was a supportive voice for children's play at a time when America was involved in the race to the moon, and intellectual teaching in science and mathematics for children was on the uptick. Ayres contends, "Within every child there is a great inner drive to develop sensory integration."[18] She talks about the great sense of accomplishment and deep satisfaction that occurs for a child—and people of all ages—when they successfully integrate their senses. "It gives us a great deal of satisfaction to organize sensations, and even more satisfaction to respond to those sensations with adaptive responses that are more mature or more complex than anything we have done before."[19] Throughout the motor sequence, especially, we can witness babies engaged in increasingly complex motor tasks and doing things that they have never done before.

To me, one of the greatest gifts we can give our babies and young children is the opportunity for free movement, whereby they can experience the joy of movement. Here, Dr. Ayres helps us understand something of the nature of the joy of movement—or the deep satisfaction of integration. This is not a loud or boisterous experience but typically a quieter, more profound one.

In a similar vein, Rudolf Steiner speaks about loving our deeds. Author Paul Emberson explains that Steiner considers human beings to be free when they act "not out of desire, ambition, curiosity or fear, or any impulse rising from [their] bodily nature, and not out of an external social, religious or ethical constraint, but solely out of love—love of [their] own action and of [their] fellow [human beings.]"[20] In his book *The Philosophy of Spiritual Activity*,[21] Steiner sums it up: "To *live* in love of action and to *let live* in understanding of the other's volition, this is the fundamental maxim of the free [human being] [emphasis added]."[22]

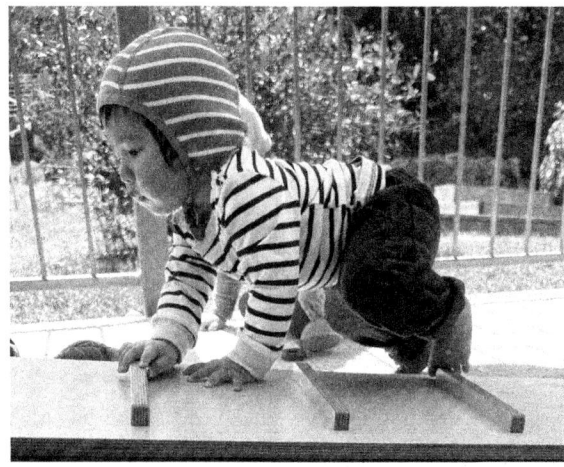

One can't claim to know another person's feelings, but to me, this child expresses something of the deep satisfaction of integration as they climb on the incline.

Adaptive Responses

The term "adaptive response" is mentioned above. Adaptive responses are the building blocks of sensory integration. As Dr. Ayres explains, "An adaptive response is a purposeful, goal-directed response to a sensory experience."[23] She gives the example of a baby seeing a toy and reaching for it. The adaptive response here is the baby's reaching. In contrast, the random, early chaotic movements of the infant's arms do not constitute adaptive responses—they are not purposeful or goal directed. As I write this chapter, I am witnessing a baby who moves around in a variety of ways: by rolling, lying on her back and pushing herself backward with her feet, lying on her tummy and pushing herself backward with her arms, and spinning around 360 degrees on her tummy. She is not yet able to belly-crawl forward. However, she uses a combination of all of these other means of locomotion to get to an object of interest. This is a more complex adaptive response than simply reaching for a toy. Over time the child's adaptive responses continue to increase in complexity.

"In an adaptive response," Dr. Ayres states, "we master a challenge and learn something new. At the same time, the formation of an adaptive response helps the brain to develop and organize itself. Most adults see this as merely play. However, play consists of the adaptive responses that make sensory integration happen. The child who learns to organize [their] play is more likely to organize [their] school work and become an organized adult."[24]

Optimally, the child chooses their tasks—tasks in which they are interested, vested, and fully engaged. When this happens, Dr. Ayres concludes, the child has tapped into their "inner drive," and she views this as a critical factor for healthy sensory integration. Another way of saying this is that the child has engaged their will.

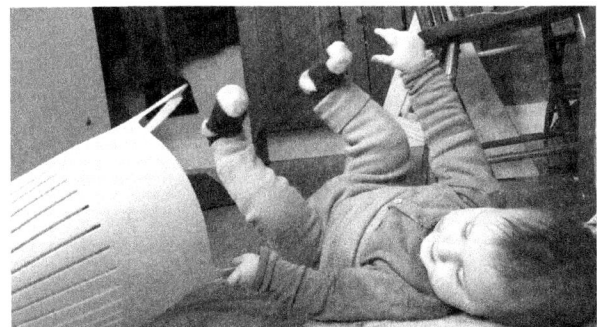 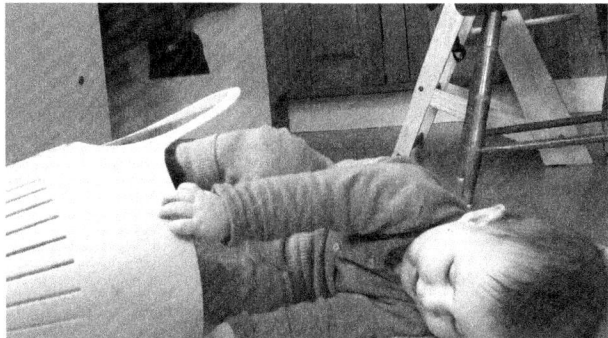

This child rolled from back to side many times, each time placing their feet inside the basket. It was as if they had purposely set themself the task of putting their feet inside the basket.

The Role of the Brain and the Ego in Sensory Integration

Dr. Ayres describes the brain as a "sensory processing machine."[25] In other words, she feels that one of the brain's essential functions is to integrate sensations. In contrast, from Rudolf Steiner's point of view, it is the higher ego of the child that integrates the sensations, and this work of the ego is *reflected* in the neurological activity and anatomical structures of the brain. The brain is not the originator of the integrative activity.

Sensory Integration

Dr. Ayres describes sensory integration as simply "the organization of sensation for use. Our senses give us information about the physical conditions of our body and the environment around us. Sensations flow into the brain like streams flowing into a lake."[26]

In processing sensory input, "the brain locates, sorts, and orders sensations—somewhat as a traffic [officer] directs moving cars. When sensations flow in a well-organized or integrated manner, the brain can use those sensations to form perception, behaviors, and learning. When the flow of sensations is disorganized, life can be like a rush-hour traffic jam."[27] The young child's movements involve a tremendous amount of sensory processing. Movements happen over time. During this time, inner and outer sensations continue to occur, and our sensory channels are constantly providing updated information, which continues to be processed and integrated.

Here is an example of an integrated sensory experience involving several sensory modalities. In the morning, when I need to take a thermos of tea with me for the day, I pour hot water from a kettle into my thermos. My arm senses the weight of the kettle as I lift it, and I see the steam coming out of its end. As I pick up the kettle, it is heavy, and I adjust my posture automatically, in order to keep my balance. I start to pour the hot water from the kettle, and my arm perceives that it is getting lighter. The tension in the muscles of my arm adjusts accordingly. Additionally, I need less stabilization from my core muscles and the rest of my body as the kettle lightens up. I hear the pitch of the pouring water changing as it fills the thermos. I see the water pouring out. I smell the aroma of the tea as the hot water touches the tea bag. In order to successfully fill the thermos, sensations from my eyes, ears, nose, inner ear, and muscles and joints must be integrated. As a result, I can accomplish a meaningful task that I have set for myself—I fill the thermos without overfilling it, and without burning myself.

When we integrate the senses, the world makes more sense to us. It becomes more ordered and predictable. We have a basic orientation to the world that makes life easier, because we don't have to keep figuring everything out. However, there can be situations where our sense experiences of the world don't add up, and this throws us off. One time, I was with my husband in our car. He was slowly backing out of a parking place, when all of a sudden he slammed on his brakes and was visibly shaken. It seemed to him for a moment that our car was moving *forward*. What had happened was that the car next to us started backing out faster than our car. My husband's reasonable interpretation was that our car going forward, and it was very disorienting.

Development of the Various Senses

Above, it was mentioned that the child's senses open at birth. How does sensory development then proceed? Does each sense develop at an equal rate? Are there any patterns of sensory development? Karl König addresses these questions in great detail. In the following passage from his book *A Living Physiology*, he describes how various sensations affect the sense of life; these sensations include "our own well-being or being unwell, such as palpitations, stomach pain or any other bodily sensation."[28] He says, "These are the first dull sensations we experience as a baby. Without them we would have no background, no fundamental sense of 'being.' They are the cradle of our daily existence."[29] Indeed, it is usually very apparent, for example, when a young baby is experiencing the sensations of digestive distress. König explains, "It is because the sense of life is not yet properly established in the infant that the organ sensations are so predominant. Hunger, thirst, wind, digestive disorders and breathing difficulties overwhelm the child's soul which becomes the plaything of these sensations. Similarly, the satisfied, warm well-being of the infant is such an all-permeating pleasure that there is hardly room for any other sensation."[30] Ways to support the sense of life in the infant and young child are covered in chapter 13.

Dr. König associates the feeling of joy with the sense of self-movement. He says, "The experience of joy grows from the realm of the sense of one's own movement. . . . Joy expresses itself in a smile. The first smile of the infant is a signal that the sense of movement has begun to develop."[31] The timing for the baby's first smile varies, but generally happens between six and eight weeks. It is noteworthy that the first smile happens at about the same time that a degree of maturation of the sense of self-movement manifests. How do we know that the sense of self-movement is maturing? We know by the quality of the baby's movements. Initially, the newborn has essentially no coordinated movement. The newborn's movements are characterized as reflexive, random, and chaotic. When the baby's movements start to have a degree of volitional control and coordination, that is a signal that the child's sense of self-movement is developing.

König notes that the development of the sense of self-movement continues for many years. Every time the child learns a new motor skill, for example when they learn to roll to their tummy, spin around on their tummy, and belly-crawl, the sense of self-movement is developing. In the older child, when they learn to jump rope, ride a bike, and play the piano, they are refining their sense of self-movement. As adults, we can continue to develop this sense indefinitely. The Spacial Dynamics exercises developed by Jaimen McMillan are specifically designed to enhance one's sense of self-movement, for example.

Summarizing the child's development of the twelve senses, Dr. König explains that "the foundations for the four lower senses [are laid down] within the first few weeks of [the child's] life."[32] The foundations of the four middle senses, as well as the sense of hearing, are laid down in the first few months. König maintains that "by about three or four months old a child can hear and see, can taste and smell, is developing [their] equilibrium, can unfold [their] sense of movement and, of course [their] sense of touch and sense of life. However, the sense of word, the sense of thought and the sense of ego [of the other] can develop only after certain other stages have been passed."[33] The specific stages to which he is referring are the stages of walking, speaking, and thinking."[34] (The three gifts of walking, speaking, and thinking will be discussed in volume 2.)

A Turning Point in Sensory Development with Standing and Walking

The child's acquisition of verticality and walking signify a milestone in sensory development. König notes that the middle senses fill our soul with sensory "impressions of the world around us,"[35] while additionally, the lower senses give us sensory information from our bodies. König maintains, "It takes the child a considerable time to distinguish between these two [inner and outer] realms of experiences, and not before the toddler has learned to stand upright and

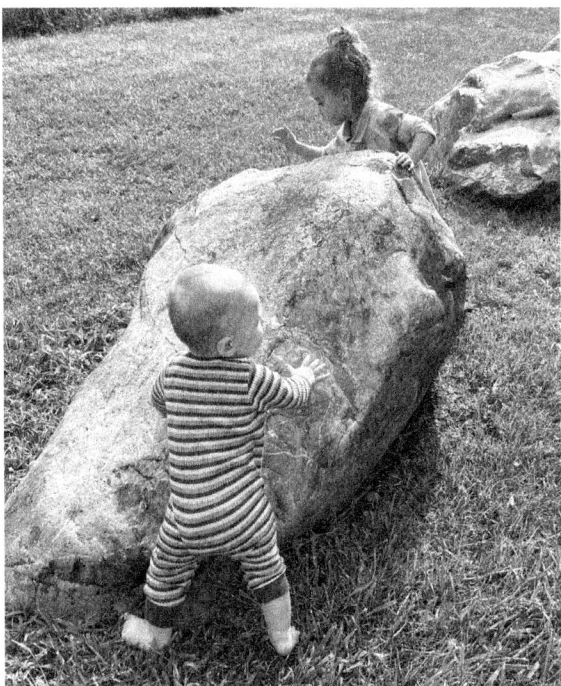

The child in the foreground is new to standing. In coming to standing, they have achieved a degree of separation from the rest of the world. Now they have the opportunity to stand on their own two feet and develop their own point of view.

to take [their] first steps [are they] able to differentiate between the one and the other. The uprightness of [the human being] draws a wall between the environment and [their] body."[36] At birth, the child is united with the world. There is no separation. The acquisition of standing and walking is a milestone in the child's separation from the world. At this pivotal stage of development, through the vehicle of the lower and middle senses, the child starts to perceive that their body is distinct from the outer world.

The Emergence of the Sense of Word

It is also at this time, when the child achieves verticality and takes their first steps, that the sense of word emerges. With the sense of word, the child perceives the meaning of the words that are spoken to them. Karl König states that walking and the emergence of this sense occur nearly simultaneously. "When the child learns to walk [they] not only [achieve] uprightness but at the same moment—I would say in the same hour—there suddenly awakens in [them] an understanding for the first few words that are spoken to [them]."[37] The child is not yet able to think at this point, "yet in spite of [their] inability to think, to contemplate any thought, [the child] understands the spoken word because [they have] unfolded [their] sense of word."[38] In *The First Three Years of the Child*, König states, "Thus, a small child does not think the meaning of the words [they acquire] but perceives it through [their] senses.[39]

The Emergence of the Sense of Thought

Rudolf Steiner relates that "Children learn to speak because they can hear and listen to what the sense of speech [or the sense of word] perceives. Their speaking then is mere imitation."[40] In other words, when the sense of word emerges with verticality and walking, then the child can perceive the words spoken to them. Because they can perceive the words of others, they then can imitate those words. They imitate the speech of those around them, and this contributes to their leaning to speak. Out of their speaking, the sense of thought emerges. According to Rudolf Steiner, "All of us are aware that children learn to speak first and only then to perceive thoughts. Indeed, speech is necessary for thought perception. . . . Observe carefully, and you will see that the sense of speech or tone [or word] develops first and provides the basis for the development of the sense of concept [or thought]."[41]

The Emergence of the Sense of the Ego of the Other (the "I"-Sense)

How does the sense of the ego of the other emerge in the growing child? Karl König explains that when the child says "I," rather than referring to themself by name, this "indicates the beginning of the development of the sense of ego [of the other]."[42] It should also be noted that, when the child says "I," this is a sign that they have developed "I"-consciousness. So, two things occur simultaneously: the beginning of "I"-consciousness and the emergence of the sense of the ego of the other. (The development of "I"-consciousness is discussed in chapter 10.) König describes that after they emerge in the young child, these three higher senses—the senses of word, thought, and the "I"-sense—have the possibility to continue to develop throughout the rest of our lives.[43]

Karl König gives the example of Helen Keller, the famous woman who was born without sight or hearing. Her story is well known to many Americans. With the help of her devoted teacher, Annie Sullivan, Helen overcame the hindrances of being born deaf and blind, and she went on to live a rich life. König calls Helen Keller's story a testament to the existence of the three highest senses. "How else would this great individual have been able to learn to express herself, to know the world, and to communicate with individuals in spite of the loss of hearing and the loss of sight if she had not been able to unfold the spiritual reality of these three highest senses?"[44]

Self-Initiated Movement in the First Hour after Birth

A significant amount of research has explored the role of newborns' senses immediately following birth. One extensive review article was published in the medical journal *ACTA Paediatrica*.[45] It found that the senses of touch, smell, taste, hearing, and smell play significant roles in the first hour after birth, when the baby is allowed to self-initiate movement. The baby is placed on the lower abdomen of the birthing parent and negotiates the journey up to the breast where they latch on, suckle, and then fall asleep. The whole process takes approximately an hour. Additionally, several primitive reflexes also play significant roles during this time, and these will be discussed in volume 2. For now, let us focus on the newborn's senses in the first hour after birth.

During skin-to-skin time immediately after birth, the newborn is sensitive to the smell of the birthing parent's colostrum, which is the first type of breastmilk. As the baby maneuvers their way up to the breast, the smell of the colostrum is considered an important guiding factor. When the baby reaches the breast, the smell further helps them root and crawl to find the nipple. The newborn has a high level of catecholamines at birth, especially for the first thirty minutes of life. Catecholamines are neurohormones associated with a decrease in pain and with an increase in memory and learning. Thus, catecholamines are thought to lessen the pain of passing through the birth canal and to help the baby remember the smell of the birth parent. Interestingly, the birth parent's sense of smell is also heightened right after birth. They are attracted to the baby's smell; thus, a chemical communication is facilitated between the child and parent.

Immediately after birth, the baby typically cries, and then has a period of relaxation, when they rest. The next stage is referred to as the awakening phase, where "the baby makes small mouth movements. They will gradually open their eyes during this stage, blinking repeatedly until the eyes are stable and focused."[46] Additionally, "During pregnancy, the nipple has become more pigmented," which makes it easier for the baby to see and find the nipple. The baby also uses their sense of vision in the first hour of life in another important way. Immediately after birth, the newborn's eyes open wide, and the pupils often enlarge. Approximately half an hour after birth the newborn searches for eye contact with the birth person. When eye contact is made, an opportunity for bonding comes into being through the phenomenon of pupillary contagion.* It is not uncommon for the birth person to "recall the first moment of eye-to-eye contact as unforgettable. The complex experiences of the newborn infant during the first hour encompass more than simply a journey to the breast; the opportunity for eye contact emphasizes the importance of parents and staff valuing instinctive behavior during this time, and the avoidance of interruptions."[47]

When the newborn reaches the chest of the birthing parent, as they maneuver their way to the breast, they often stop to rest. Here, the newborn's sense of hearing comes into play. "When lying quietly on the [birthing parent's] chest, the baby can hear the [birthing parent's] heartbeat. This familiar sound from in utero seems to comfort the newborn infant after the rapid transition to extra-uterine life."[48] The researchers also state that the baby has learned the sound of the birthing parent's voice in utero and orients to this after birth.

When the newborn reaches the breast, a phase known as familiarization begins. During this stage, which can last twenty minutes or more, the baby licks the nipple and the areola surrounding it. This serves to shape the nipple into a form more easily accessible for latching on. The baby uses their hand to massage the breast, and they move the hand from the breast to their mouth, tasting the colostrum. This massaging "increases the [birthing parent's] oxytocin† levels. During this stage, it is evident that the baby is smelling

---

* Pupillary contagion is the phenomenon in which an observer's pupil diameter changes in response to another person's pupil; Yuki Tsuji, So Kanazawa, and Masami K. Yamaguchi, "Face-Specific Pupil Contagion in Infants," *Frontiers in Psychology* 12, no., 2121 (Jan. 4, 2022).

† Oxytocin is known as the love hormone. It is important for bonding. Oxytocin also stimulates uterine contractions needed during labor, delivery, and after delivery to expel the placenta, and stimulates lactation after birth.

and tasting, and previous actions become more vigorous and more coordinated. Therefore, it is important not to interfere or introduce odors from unfamiliar hands."[49]

When the newborns are allowed to latch onto the breast in their own time and in their own way, the results are good. "During this first hour, when the unmedicated baby self-attaches, it is a perfect first breastfeeding, although the infant will continue to readjust until satisfied with the latch. The newborn infant does not need *help* to adjust the latch [emphasis in original]. Babies who self-attach during the first hour after birth have few problems with breastfeeding, latch and milk transfer. Skin-to-skin in the first hour strengthens the [birthing parent's] self-confidence, including decreasing the concerns about having enough milk. When babies are placed skin-to-skin with the [birthing parent], they have more optimal blood glucose levels. Both skin-to-skin and the suckling contribute to this effect. Thus, this reduces the risk of supplementation."[50]

In the next chapter we will look at how sensory experiences are related to the development of "I"-consciousness. We will also delve more deeply into individual senses, how to observe them in the infant and young child, and how to support their development.

10: Nourishing the Young Child's Sense Organs

The early childhood teacher is charged with supporting the development of the young child's physical body, and this includes the development of their sense organs. Rudolf Steiner emphasizes the importance of nourishing the developing child's sense organs thus: "The best way to influence the child during [their] first seven years is through the development of [their] sense organs. All the impressions they receive from the outer world are significant, and everything a child sees or hears affects [them] in terms of [their] sense organs. The sense organs, however, are not influenced by lesson-books or verbal teaching, but by means of example and imitation. *The most important thing during the first seven years is to nourish a child's sense organs* [emphasis added]."[1]

Let us begin with a general overview of ways to support the child's developing sense organs.

Supporting Sensory Development with What We Don't Do

Perhaps the simplest and most effective way to support the child as they develop their senses is to simply stop talking to them so much. The goal is for the child to have "sensory immersion" experiences—where they are totally absorbed in the experience—without our running commentaries.

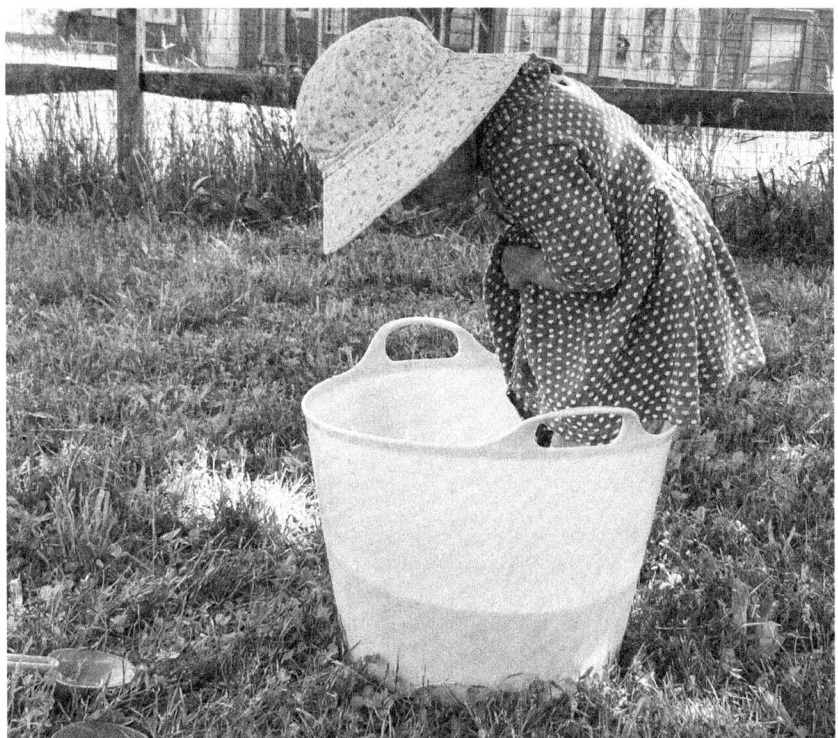

This child is completely immersed in the sensory experience of standing in the bucket of water.

FREE MOVEMENT FROM THE VERY START

Young children need time and space for their own unique sensory experiences. To accomplish this, we can refrain from evaluating or drawing conclusions about what they are experiencing. Bert Hellinger* gives a telling example: "A child goes into the yard and feels amazement at the growing things. [The parent] says, 'Look, how beautiful.' Now the child must attend to words; looking and hearing are interrupted, [their] direct engagement with what exists is replaced by value judgments. The child can no longer trust [their] own experience of being enthralled by what *is*, but must defer to an external authority, who defines what is beautiful and good [emphasis in original]."[2]

Authors Neal and Jennifer Kennerk offer additional insights:

> When the young child asks the question "why is the sky blue?", the last thing they need is a detailed explanation of atmosphere, reflection, refraction and the like. This is dead and hardening information that does nothing to nourish the soul development of the child. Since they do not have the intellectual capacity (as smart they undoubtably are) to fully understand abstract concepts, they come to mistrust their own powers of observation. The best answer, as long as it will satisfy, is "I wonder." This answer will be enough for many years. . . . These open ended answers teach young children to trust that what they see and believe is right—and this is what they need—whether it is actually correct or not. Scientific explanations should come after the child has the capacity to fully understand and engage with the information. Just because they can recite memorized facts, does not mean that they have a working relationship with the concepts. . . . *We want children to trust their own powers of observation* [emphasis added]."[3]

Johann Wolfgang von Goethe's treasured quote is worth contemplating when we are with young children.

> You must trust your senses;
> They will show you nothing false
> if your intelligence keeps you awake.
> Keep your eyes fresh and open and joyful,
> and move with sure steps, yet flexibly,
> through the fields of a world so richly endowed.[4]

The impressions from our senses are true. It is our interpretations of our sensations that can be subject to error. Rudolf Steiner addresses this: "The external world can provide correct sense perceptions, but perceptions cannot think. Thought is subject to error, however, and we human beings must have the power for accuracy of thought in us."[5]

We want to support the child to live in their pure acts of sensing, without outside influence.

The adult can witness, without interfering in a child's experience. Early childhood expert Helle Heckmann describes an instance when the children in her Danish childcare found an animal track. One child excitedly ran to Helle and told her that he and his classmates thought the tracks

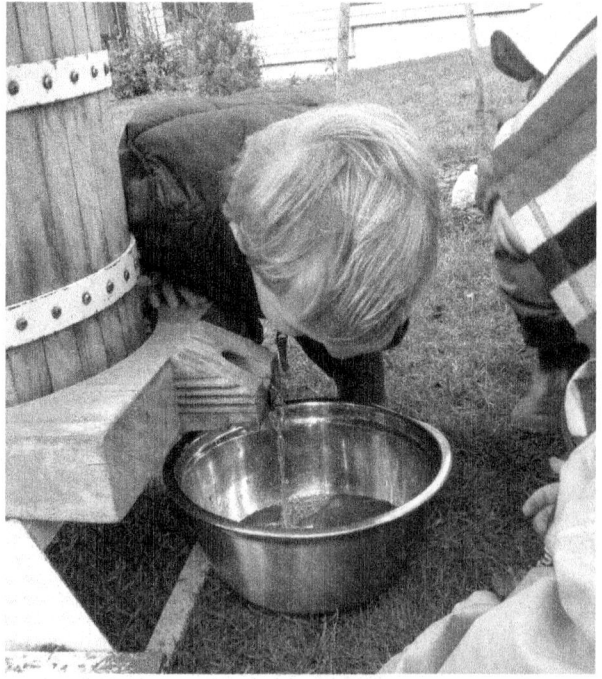

This child is free to fully experience the smell, sounds, and sights of the cider pressing without an adult's commentary. Soon, they will get to taste the cider.

---

* Bert Hellinger (1925–2019) was a German psychotherapist who developed a type of therapy known as Family Constellations.

were those of a wolf. Helle came over to the site of the tracks, where the children were talking it over. Helle explains what happened next. "In the end they are silent and turn to me. What do I have to say? I now produce a wolf-tale, which is not more than it claims to be, and which does not comment on the tracks on the ground at all. . . . When the story ends we return to the present. I leave their circle, and the children continue their exploring of nature."[6] Heckmann does not comment on the animal tracks at all. She responds to the children with a story and it satisfies them. It doesn't matter if the tracks were from a wolf or not. What matters is that the children remain open and engaged with the world around them through their sensory experiences.

Forming of the Sense Organs

How are the sense organs formed? Rudolf Steiner addresses this in a 1907 lecture: "What is the origin of the human eye? It has been formed by the light itself, and similarly the eye would degenerate if there were no light. Light is the origin of the power of sight."[7] Later, he expands this idea to include all of the senses. "All the other sense organs developed in the same way: sound formed the ear, heat the sense of heat. We would have no sense of touch if there were no hard objects. The external world moulds and forms our body."[8] In another lecture, Steiner reiterates, "The physical organs shape themselves through the influence of the physical environment. Good sight will be developed in children if their environment has the proper conditions of light and color."[9]

Let us consider the development of the physical organ of vision, the eye, in more detail. Today the incidence of myopia, or nearsightedness, in children is increasing at an alarming rate, and this is a worldwide phenomenon. In myopia, the shape of the eyeball is affected—the distance from the front to the back of the eye is longer than normal. Scientists consider myopia to be due to genetics as well as environmental factors during development. The World Health Organization addresses the environmental factors for children: "Research shows us now that spending 90 minutes outdoors is a protective factor during daylight hours for children developing myopia or short-sightedness."[10] Outdoor play is highly encouraged, where children naturally look at objects from a distance. The second key recommendation from the World Health Organization is to reduce the time spent on "near activities," such as screens. They state that device use in children is "a very strong risk factor for the development of short-sightedness."[11] Here, we see that the environment influences the way the child uses their eyes—whether for near or far vision—and this appears to be a contributing factor to developing the shape of the eyeball. Interestingly, the highest incidence of myopia has occurred in the East Asian countries, including China, where they have "implemented rigorous, highly-competitive education systems, often characterized by exposure to written homework beginning in preschool and early primary years, and extensive reliance on after-school academic activities."[12] In this region 80 to 90 percent of the population has myopia. In the United States, there is a prevalence of 42 percent. This statistic has nearly doubled in the past three decades.[13]

Similarly, we can see the impact of the languages spoken in a young child's environment upon their developing ear, the organ for the sense of hearing. People who have been exposed to a second language early in life develop "an ear" for the sounds of that language. Later in their life, they are likely able to speak it without an accent. The sounds spoken in the young child's environment were forming their ears.

Providing Authentic, Rich Sensory Environments

When we understand that young children's sense organs are formed by their sensory environment, we can take care to protect the child from overwhelming, intense sensory experiences. We can also give them opportunities for sensory experiences that are healthy and true. These can be very simple things. Regarding the sense of hearing, we can sing or play instruments rather than using recorded music. We can refrain from taking young children to public events where they would be exposed to very loud sounds. We can have them wear hats rather than hoods, as hoods often interfere with accurate auditory perception, especially localization of the sound.

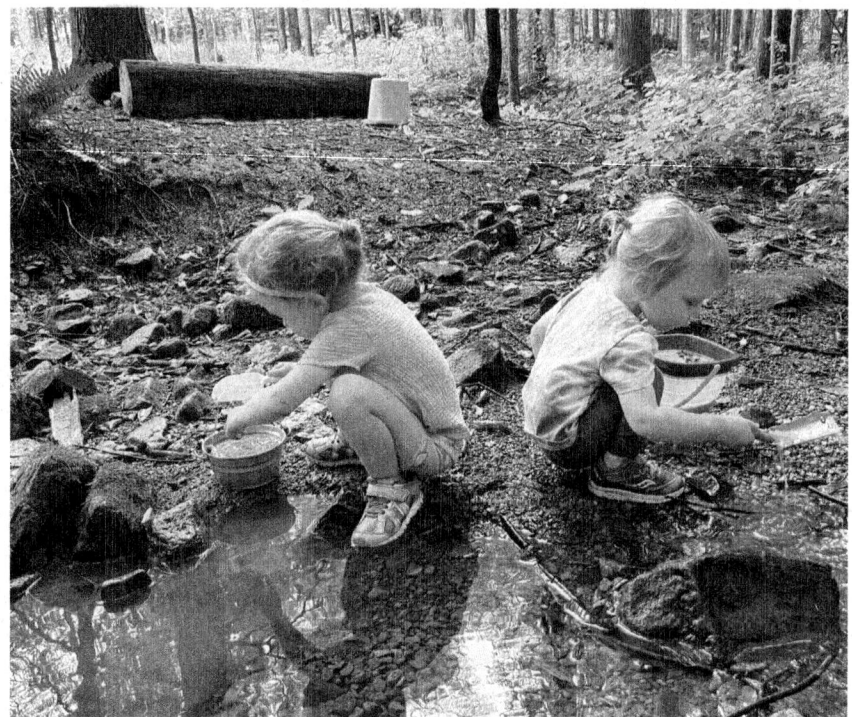

These two children are experiencing ideal natural lighting conditions, as they play in the diffuse light of the forest.

Regarding the sense of sight, as noted above, the eye develops out of the environmental conditions of light and color. Exposure to the colors found in nature—the fiery leaves of autumn and the rich colors of rocks and shells at a seashore—offer subtle variations in hues. Natural lighting is ideal. To me, there is no better lighting situation than being in the shade of a large tree, with its soft, diffuse lighting. Inside, we want to try to replicate this affect with indirect lighting coming from multiple sources, rather than the glare of direct overhead lighting.

Toys and articles made of silk, cloth, and felt that have been dyed with natural plant dyes provide colors with nuanced variation. These are generally soothing and pleasant for the developing eyes of a young child. High contrast colors can be overstimulating, especially to a young infant (high contrast colors are colors that are very different in brightness, placed right next to each other).

Here is a lovely example of how one can create a pleasant visual environment for newborns. There is a tradition of draping a soft blue and a soft pink silk above a newborn's bassinet for the first forty days, as they transition to earthly life. Dr. Michaela Glöckler explains that the combination of the soft pink and soft blue is that which comes closest to the etheric world. For many years, she recommended this in her pediatric medical practice to parents of newborns, and they found it to be a good sleep aid. Dr. Glöckler says that under such a "sky," the babies felt secure, and slept more peacefully and undisturbed than without this veil.[14] For older children, one can create a "color bath" or "color house" to play in by draping long colored silks over play stands or other furniture.

Simply cooked, unprocessed food without added chemicals offers optimal taste experiences. Some children are very sensitive to smell. They may have a hard time communicating this to us, and their aversions to certain smells may play out in seemingly unexplainable behaviors. One child's behavior was dramatically transformed when the custodians in his early childhood facility changed the cleaning products. Clothes washed in certain detergents, public bathrooms, and grade school lunchrooms can be offensive because of their smell. It is common practice for health professionals to refrain from using perfumed body products when working with patients. I advise against sprinkling rosemary or lavender oil in early childhood classrooms, as some children react to these—even if they are organic. Smells are something that one cannot avoid—we have to breathe.

Stephen Spitalny explains:

> In sensing we have an experience of the thing sensed, the thing generating the sensation, but we do not experience the sensing itself. We only experience that which is creating the sensation. Young children, through their senses, touch the creator of the thing being sensed. They connect with the creator beings and living concepts that stand behind sense impressions. Images that are filled with life and that come from life nurture and nourish the young child. The child's etheric body and [their] soul thrive through the experience of these life-enriched images, rather than a diet of electronically created images that have no origin in life.[15]

In other words, young children go deeper with their sensing than do adults. Young children perceive the spiritual archetypes which are behind the thing being sensed.

Similarly, Peter Lang touches on the importance of true images from reality for the young child:

> Children should enter a direct reciprocal relationship with the world in childhood in order to be able properly to understand it. Only by touching water do I learn what it means that water is wet. At the same time I hear it gurgling or dripping, see waves, perhaps smell the sea or the grass at the edge of a lake and thus gain an overall impression which turns—together with many other such experiences—into a complex and differentiated representation of water.[16]

Young Children Are Generally More Sensitive to Sensory Input than Adults

Infants and young children generally have heightened sensitivity, compared to the relative hyposensitivity of the adult. In order to more fully grasp the baby's general sensory sensitivity, it can be helpful to read about individuals who have overcome particular challenges with regard to their sensory organizations. These individuals can often afford us insight into the sensitive nature of particular sensory conditions. We can transfer these insights to our babies and young children, who are naturally sensitive. Of course, there are individual differences, but in general, the younger the child, the more sensitive they are to sensory input.

Jacques Lusseyran, in his book *And There Was Light*, gives us insight in how to support the sense of hearing. Lusseyran lost his sight at age eight. He credits his parents, especially his mother, for supporting him as he learned to live—and thrive—without sight. He went on to become a leader in the French Resistance in World War II. After Lusseyran lost his sight, he says that it wasn't so much that his hearing improved, but rather that he "made better use" of it.[17] After he lost his sight, he explains, "I needed to hear and hear again. I multiplied sounds to my heart's content. I rang bells. I touched walls with my fingers, explored the resonance of doors, furniture and the trunks of trees. I sang in empty rooms, I threw pebbles far off on the beach just to hear them whistle through the air and then fall. I even made my small companions repeat words to give me plenty of time to walk around them."[18] In this passage, Lusseyran recounts his full engagement in his creative, playful exploration of the sense of hearing. Whenever a child has this kind of total immersion and pleasure in their sensory experiences, one can assume that their senses are developing well!

However, sometimes the sounds in Lusseyran's environment were too much. "Sometimes the resonance, the hum of voices all around me, grew so intense that I got dizzy and put my hands over my ears, as I might have done by closing my eyes to protect myself against too much light. That is why I couldn't stand racket, useless noises or music that went on and on. A sound we don't listen to is a blow to body and spirit, because sound is not something happening outside us, but a real presence passing through us and lingering unless we have heard it fully."[19] His observations of sound "passing through us and lingering" are similar to what Rudolf Steiner describes as a young child's unity with the world. They are not yet separate from their sensations, and can not protect themselves from them. They have not yet established a buffer between themselves and the incoming sensation.

Fortunately, Jacques Lusseyran had parents who were musicians, and so he was generally spared intense, unpleasant sounds. He comments that, thankfully, his parents did not turn on the radio at supper, but engaged in conversation. He recounts his experiences of different sounds—those which were painful to him and also those he experienced as pleasing. "For a blind person, a violent and futile noise has the same effect as the beam of a search light too close to the eyes of someone who can see. It hurts. But when the world sounds clear and on pitch, it is more harmonious than poets have ever known it, or than they will ever be able to say."[20]

Supporting the Child after an Adverse Reaction to a Sensory Event

When a child has an adverse reaction to a particular sensation, we want to be aware of it, and work with the child in a respectful way. Ellyn Satter, feeding and nutrition specialist, offers insight regarding the sense of taste in babies and young children. She explains, "Children generally like what is familiar."[21] In one study, parents reported that when their children turned twelve months, their eating behavior noticeably changed. Before twelve months, the babies pretty much ate everything, but quite suddenly, when they turned twelve months, they increased their preferences for certain foods and also their dislikes of certain foods. The study states that when they turned twelve months, "they were likely to lose interest in a food after one bite."[22] However, the researchers

> found that children would taste new food, and the more often they tasted it, the more they liked it. Children might take 10, 15, or 20 tastes in as many meals before they learned to like a new food. This skepticism about new food appears in infants as young 4 to 6 months old, when they are first introduced to solid foods. The solution for the infants is the same as for older children: repeated exposure. Babies learned to like new foods when they had the opportunity to taste them over and over again. Breastfed infants, presumably because they were accustomed to tastes from their [nursing parent's] milk, were more receptive to new foods than formula-fed infants.[23]

The infants and children in this study were in no way forced to eat any food. They were offered the food, and it was up to them whether they ate it or not. The adults were responsible for which foods were offered to the child. (See chapter 4 for more on Ellyn Satter's work.)

For excessively loud and jarring noises, if the child is obviously not tolerating the sensory input, it is best to alter the environment or take the child to a less stimulating place. Additionally, we can help the child recover when they react with upset to a particular sensory event. As noted above, the sensations from the external world are literally forming the sense organs. Additionally, the child's reactions to sensations are forming their soul habits, and this directly impacts the child's physiology. Therefore, as much as possible, we want the young child to have *positive* sensory experiences. (Recall the joyful sensory experiences of Jacques Lusseyran with the sense of hearing, described above.) We want the child to be able to meet the sensations that come toward them from the world. In contrast, if the child has a particularly intense sensory experience, and they are not able to meet it, their autonomic nervous system likely goes into a fight or flight mode. This results in physiological changes in basic functions of the body such as shallow, faster breathing, increased heart rate and blood pressure, decreased digestive activity, and so on. This is not something that we want to become an established pattern for the child. With habitual, exaggerated distress, the nervous system gets used to being in fight or flight, and then it is more difficult to shift gears and calm down.

One girl, even as a baby, had difficulty with the sensory experience of having her hair washed. This lasted for several years. The parents adopted a patient, compassionate stance, and modified their procedure for washing her hair. Once they felt they had a good way of washing her hair, they committed to carrying it out consistently, and they stuck with it. One parent would sit on the edge of the bathtub, holding the child securely. The child remained dressed and a towel was wrapped around her shoulders. A washcloth was also held at the child's forehead to keep the drips out of her eyes. The other parent stood in the tub, barefoot, and slowly and gently washed the hair, telling the girl what she was going to do *before* she did it. Empty quart-sized yogurt containers had been filled with warm water and were used to rinse out the shampoo. Care was taken that the water was not too cold and not too hot. A special "bunny" towel was purchased, which was used to dry the hair. Still, the girl would verbally protest and cry. However, the parents' combined warm resolve carried the girl through the experiences. A fire in the wood stove would be made beforehand and fleeces placed in front of the stove. After the hair had been washed, the parents and the child would gather in front of the fire where one parent read a story, while the child's hair dried. The parents would comment on how shiny and pretty their daughter's hair was. Over time, the child was able to live into the sensations of having her hair washed without distress, and presently hair washing is no big deal. The girl just turned seven, and recently she was so proud that she had washed her hair by herself.

Sensation and the Development of "I"-Consciousness

Just as sensations from the environment literally form the sense organs, and the child's reactions to sensations are forming their soul habits, their sensory experiences also play a significant role in the acquisition of "I"-consciousness. At approximately the third birthday, the child refers to themself as "I," rather than as "me," or by their name. This signals that they have gained enough awareness to know that they are distinct from the rest of the world and exist as a separate individual. How do they come to know this? Rudolf Steiner explains that they realize this through sensory encounters with the world. He says the child needs to experience "resistance from the world outside" in order to recognize that they are separate from it.

In a 1912 lecture, Rudolf Steiner gives an example of one such sensory encounter—when a child accidentally knocked their head on a corner of a table. He relates:

> If you observe closely you will find that the feeling of "I" is intensified after such a thing happens. In other words, the child becomes aware of [themself] and is brought nearer to a knowledge of self. Of course, it need not always amount to an actual injury or scratch. Even when the child puts [their] hand on something there is an impact on a small scale that makes [them] aware of [themself.] You will have to conclude that a child would never develop ego-consciousness if resistance from the world outside did not make [them] aware of [themself.] The fact that there is a world external to [themself] makes possible the unfolding of ego-consciousness, the consciousness of the "I."[24]

Indeed, in free movement, the baby is continually experiencing the resistance of the earth's gravitational field and working to overcome it. Hundreds and thousands of times, the baby pushes down into the surface and their body is displaced up off the surface, as they slowly and gradually overcome the resistance of gravity and move into verticality. Here, we see a deeper purpose in the self-initiated motor sequence—the plethora of sensorimotor experiences serve to help *establish* the child's ego consciousness. It is through sensory events that we experience the resistance of the earth. We also need—and, in fact, naturally seek out—the resistance of the earth throughout our entire lives to *maintain* our ego-consciousness. For example, some people don't feel present and ready to meet the world until they have had their morning run or their morning Pilates workout. Similarly, after a period of working at a desk, our consciousness may start to dim, and we respond by getting up and walking around the building. This is usually enough to restore us so that we can return to our work.

FREE MOVEMENT FROM THE VERY START

In another lecture, Rudolf Steiner again describes the body's role in establishing "I"-consciousness.

> That is because [humans] here on the physical plane only really [feel their] Ego through contact with [their] body. You can represent it very crudely thus: If you move your finger through the air—there is nothing there! Move it further—there is still nothing. When you touch something, however, in coming against something, you know of yourself, you become aware of yourself. We are thereby made aware of our Ego. Not the Ego itself is aroused ... but the consciousness of the Ego. The opposition makes us aware of our Self.[25]

When the young child develops "I"-consciousness, they have more of a sense that they "are their own person." They "come into their own" a little more. Edmond Schoorel describes this process as becoming a "citizen of the earth." He echoes Rudolf Steiner's idea, mentioned above, that sensory experiences are crucial for this process to unfold. "To come down to earth may be the most important task children have to fulfill in the first seven years, and the senses are indispensable helpers for this purpose. Without the senses, the child will not come down to earth. The senses make it possible for the child to become a 'citizen of the earth.'"[26]

The Experiences of the Lower Senses Extend into the Soul

Each of the four foundational senses exerts a specific influence on the feeling life. Rudolf Steiner explains that "we do not directly perceive all that stirs in our body, but only what is pushed up into the soul region. One perceives the soul effects of these inner senses to a certain extent."[27] Henning Köhler, in his book *Working with Anxious, Nervous, and Depressed Children*, clarifies this statement. He says that these feelings stay under our radar of consciousness, and if they are not there, then we notice the lack thereof. The feelings "do not usually come to full consciousness. They do so only when we become aware that we don't have them."[28] Let us look at each individual foundational sense and how it manifests in the soul.

Regarding the sense of *touch*, Rudolf Steiner explains that what streams "into the soul is nothing else but being permeated with the feeling of God. Without the sense of touch, [human beings] would have no feeling for God."[29] Henning Köhler describes that "touching is the basis of the certainty we feel that something really exists. . . . Rudolf Steiner calls this certainty 'God sensing,' the sense of being permeated by 'the God substance.'"[30]

In other words, touch gives us a certainty of existence, and ultimately, existence comes from God. Köhler states very clearly: "We would have no relationship to reality if we lacked the assurance that touch gives us that we exist!"[31]

We have a common saying: "I had to pinch myself in order to know if this was *really* happening." David Brooks, in his book *The Social Animal*, relates a telling anecdote about a three-year-old boy. The boy awoke during the night and

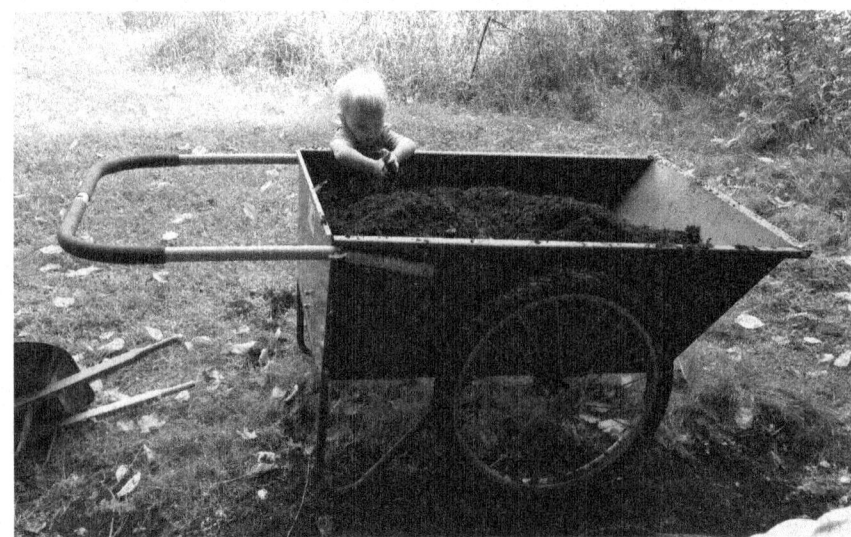

Whereas an adult typically wouldn't stop to touch the mulch in this garden cart, this child was deeply engaged in touching the mulch, and spent an extended period doing so.

called out to his mother. "'Touch me, only touch me with your finger,' the young boy pleaded. The child's mother was astonished. 'Why?' she asked. 'I'm not here,' the boy cried. 'Touch me, Mother, so that I may be here.'"[32] This child had lost his very existence, and knew that he needed more touch input in order to find himself again. Similarly, if we can't tell by sight whether if a flower is real or is silk, we touch it. Young children go around touching everything! They are trying to ascertain what is real—and that they are real!

Rudolf Steiner describes what radiates into the soul from the *life sense*. "It is the life sense normally radiating upward as a feeling of comfort that is disturbed through pain in the same way as an external sense is disturbed when a person has a hearing loss. Generally, however, the life sense is experienced in a healthy person as a feeling of being comfortable. This feeling of overall well-being, which is heightened after a good meal, and somewhat lowered by hunger, this undefined inner sense of self is the effect of the life sense that has rayed into the soul."[33]

Henning Köhler relates that the sense of life is not the same thing as vitality; rather, he refers to it as a basic sense of security.

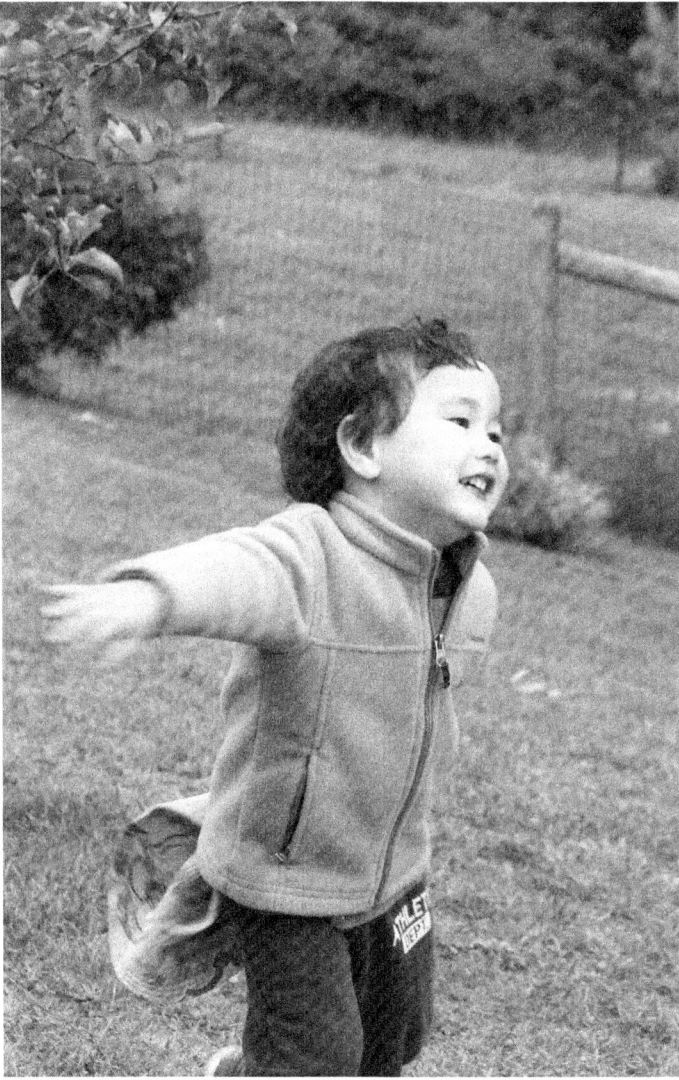

This child is running across the play yard. Their gesture gives the impression of moving with a sense of ease and freedom. Could they be experiencing themself as a free soul?

> We must not let ourselves confuse the term "life sense" with the popular concept of "vitality" as a state of wide-awakeness, liveliness, freshness. It is true that the life sense is responsible in large part for feelings of energy and freshness, but that is due to a subconscious sensing that there is peace and warmth and well-being deep down inside our bodies. ... As a rule, energy and freshness well up in the morning, after restorative sleep out of the sphere of the life sense, though that is not their only source. In the evening, when we tend to feel more settled, that sense of burgeoning vitality disappears, but without any ill effect on the basic sensation of security mediated by the life sense.[34]

Rudolf Steiner goes on to describe what radiates into the soul from the *sense of self-movement*.

> We perceive whether or how we are in motion through this sense of movement. When it is radiated into the soul, this sense results in that feeling of freedom which allows [people] to sense [themselves] as soul, namely, the experience of one's own free soul element. The fact that you

experience yourself as a free soul is due to the effects of the sense of movement. It is due to what streams into your soul from the muscular contractions and elongations.[35]

Henning Köhler makes a remarkable statement related to this feeling of being a free soul. He says that the sense of self-movement "is what gives us, even in seemingly hopeless situations, the confidence to summon up a new impulse to move on in life, to change direction, to develop initiative."[36]

In the previous chapter, we mentioned that Karl König associates the feeling of joy with the sense of self-movement. Henning Köhler agrees. He says that if a child has a challenge in the sense of self-movement, the "'sensation of being a free soul' has not developed properly. What is lacking here is that free relationship to the world, that in children, is an accompaniment of joy in motion."[37] He explains that what he means by joy in movement is "the quiet enjoyment of purposeful movement that is really pleasure in imitating. . . . All pleasure in movement has its origin in early childhood's imitative responses, and all joy in life comes from pleasure in moving—internalized pleasure in moving."[38] This is quite a statement, and it is worth pondering.

In my work as a pediatric physical therapist, I know that I have had a good session with a child when I sense that they are experiencing this quiet joy of movement. In fact, this is my goal! Emmi Pikler similarly notes the importance of joy for the infant. "The most important thing has not yet been mentioned: namely that an infant's own movements, the development of these movements and every detail of this development are a constant source of joy to [them]."[39]

When the *sense of balance* radiates into the soul, Rudolf Steiner relates,

> We feel it as inner tranquility, that inner tranquility which brings it about that when I go from one place to another I do not leave behind the being contained within my body but take it along; it remains, quietly, the same. Thus, I could fly through the air and yet quietly remain the same person. This is what makes us appear to be independent of time. I do not leave myself behind today, I am the same tomorrow. This sense of being independent of the corporeality is the inpouring of the sense of balance into the soul. It is the sensation of experiencing oneself as spirit.[40]

In this passage, Rudolf Steiner explains that through the sense of balance, we experience ourselves as spirit. As the most spiritual part of the human being is the ego, we can deduce that balance is related to one's ego. Indeed, Dr. Michaela Glöckler says that "the ego power is the power of balance."[41] It has been my experience that balance pulls in the ego forces of the child (or person of any age.) When a child is successfully engaged in a balance activity, they are more fully present and more themself. It is not possible for silly, frenetic behaviors to coexist when a child is fully engaged in a balancing activity.

11: The Forming of the Body Image

In middle school, when my girlfriends and I would buy new jeans, they would be stiff, ill-fitting, uncomfortable, and unpleasant to wear. In those days, the fabric of jeans didn't have spandex, and we didn't wear leggings. We used different strategies to break in our jeans. Many of us would repeatedly wash and dry them until they softened up. One classmate would wash her jeans, put them on when they were still wet, and let them dry on her. She thought this helped the jeans more quickly find the form of her body and speed up the breaking-in process. Similarly, when the newborn dons the garment of their earthly body, it's not broken in. To the newborn, their body is something entirely foreign, and it is not uncommon for their experiences in the body to be uncomfortable. Like a pair of broken-in jeans, we want the child's body to become a nice, cozy place where the child wants to be. We want them to take up residence in their physicality. This is a process that takes time. In fact, it takes approximately seven years. In this chapter, we will explore how the four foundational senses contribute to the child's coming into their body and making it their own.

Embodiment of a Unique Space

Newborns do not have the ability to orient their bodies in space. They do not yet have the consciousness that they have a body which takes up a unique space that is theirs alone to occupy, let alone how to orient their body in relationship to the surrounding spaces of the environment. Here is an example of how this can manifest in a young child. On one occasion, an eighteen-month-old wanted to sit on a little bench at a child-sized picnic table and join the family to eat watermelon. She stood behind the bench, saying, "Uh, uh, uh." It was a tight spot, and her parent perceived that the child was informing her that she couldn't figure out how to get her body to the bench. The parent gestured to her in a way that said, "Come around here in front of the bench, and you can sit down." This was just enough of a cue for the child to successfully maneuver her body between the picnic table and the bench and sit down. This is an example of a time when a young child didn't quite have enough body awareness to know where her body was in relation to the objects in the environment, and so she had trouble navigating in a small space.

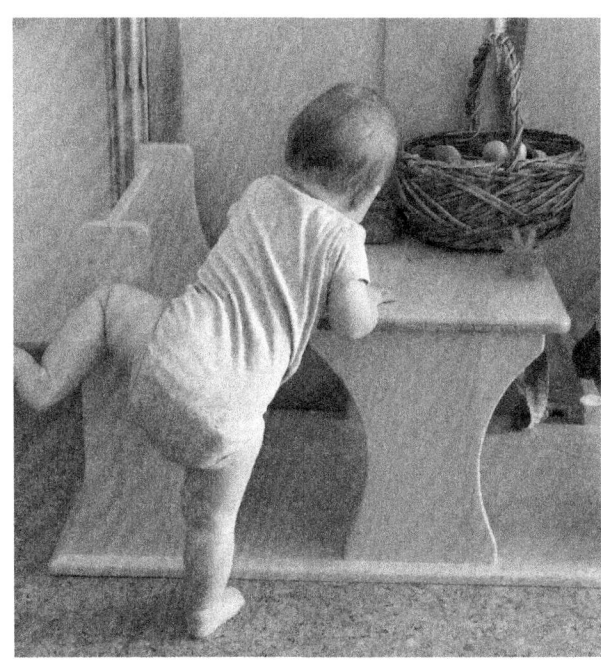

This child is attempting to climb into the feeding bench, and they can't quite position their body correctly in order to do so. They tried for several days and then succeeded.

An essential task, then, in the first months and years of life is to come to understand (at an unconscious level) that the body takes up space and has spatial attributes. A signpost that this process is well underway is the classic game of peek-a-boo. A. Jean Ayres comments that the child "can hide and reappear because [they know]

FREE MOVEMENT FROM THE VERY START

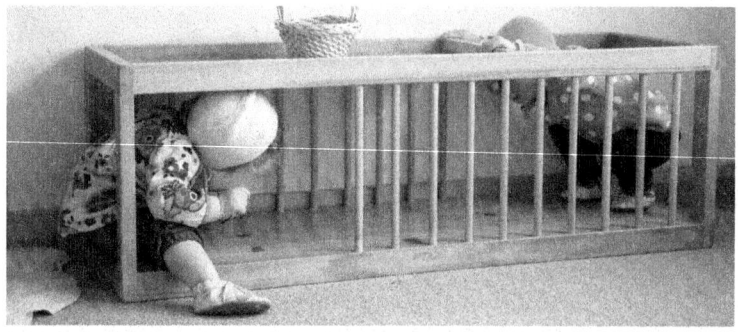

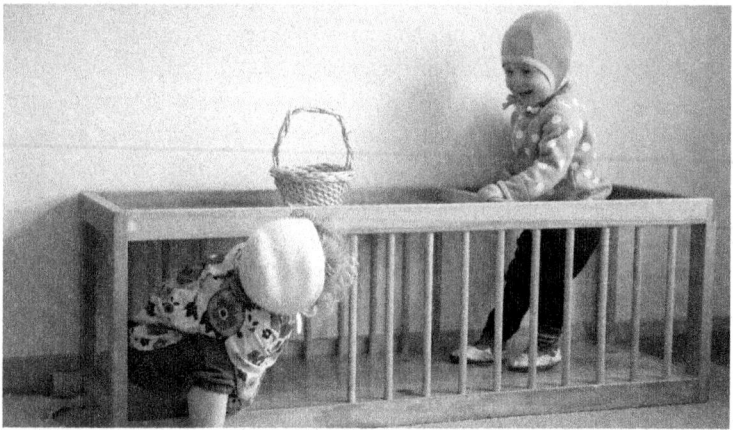

These two children have self-initiated peek-a-boo while playing in the labyrinth.

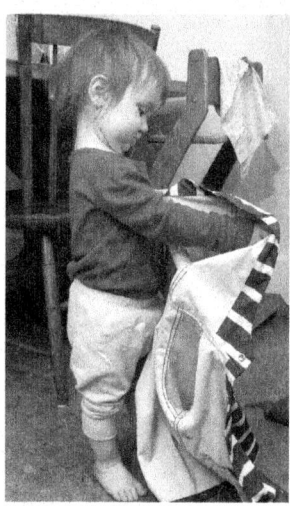

Dressing oneself requires a considerable degree of body scheme, as well as a good amount of motor planning and coordination. This child is attempting to put on a raincoat. They tried for an extended period in all manner of ways before dropping the coat and running off.

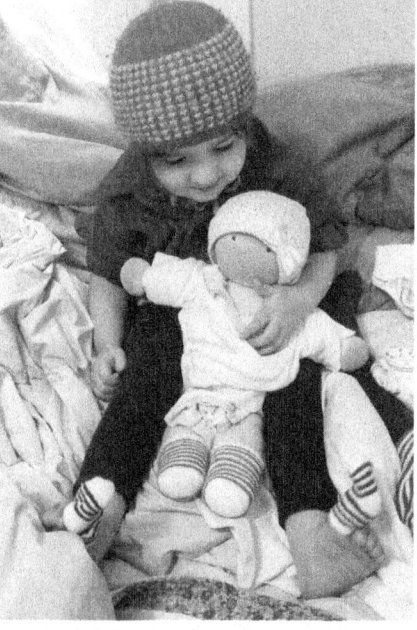

Dressing dolls is a universal activity of young children. It requires knowledge of the various body parts transposed to the doll. This child has dressed a doll, and also dressed their own toes in matching socks.

the dimensions of [their] body, and peek-a-boo is an important activity" at this stage of development.[1] My youngest grandchild, at fourteen months, self-initiated peek-a-boo games very frequently. When I wiped her mouth at the end of a meal, she would take the napkin and initiate a game, covering her own face for several repetitions and then covering my face. Once, during a period of free play, she found a napkin and played a game of peek-a-boo with herself, and it obviously gave her great pleasure. She continued peek-a-boo for months, and the games became more elaborate.

The four foundational senses (touch, life, self-movement, and balance) are a significant means by which the child comes to understand the spatial features of their physical bodies. This can be described as developing one's body image. As Karl König puts it, "body image is nothing more than these four senses put together."[2]

Gay Lloyd Pinder,* a renowned pediatric speech and language pathologist, explains that body discovery—or the development of body scheme—requires a stable head. The baby begins to know their body relationships because they have a point of stability from which to orient.[3] (The importance of a stable head will be further discussed in volume 2.)

I recently witnessed my 20-month-old granddaughter "dressing" her dolly. I watched with quiet awe, knowing that she was entering into a new stage of development with her body image. It is very helpful for the

---

* Gay Lloyd Pinder PhD, CCC-SLP is also a certified instructor in Neurodevelopmental Treatment (NDT). She teaches in the United States as well as internationally.

child at this age to have doll clothing that is loose fitting—even sleeveless. My granddaughter attempted to put the doll's leg into the arm hole. She stuck with this activity for an extended period before moving on to something else. I sensed no frustration in her as she played, even though she never got the doll's leg into the arm hole.

If we have gained or lost a significant amount of weight in a relatively short period of time, we may not have a good sense of the spatial parameters of our bodies. For example, if we have recently given birth, we may mistakenly think that we can't squeeze through a tight spot when indeed we can fit through the space. Young children are growing, and their body sizes are changing rapidly. They constantly need to be updating their emerging body images. When teenagers are in the middle of a growth spurt, they sometimes experience a temporary period of incoordination. This is because they haven't yet accommodated to their new body parameters.

The Spatial Parameters of the Body

Through experiences with the sense of touch, we perceive the border of our body. The sense of well-being gives us the sense that our body has contents—that it occupies the inner space, enclosed by our skin. Through the sense of self-movement—or proprioception—we perceive that our body has parts that move in relationship to each other. Through the sense of balance we perceive the position of our head in space and whether we are in balance or falling out of balance. Typically, we do not have a conscious awareness of these features of the body given to us via sensations arising from the four foundational senses. Yet, they are critical for coordinated movement and to feel at home in the body. One doesn't feel at ease in the world unless one has this anchoring in the body.

Initially, young infants experience discrete sensations. For example, through the sense of touch, the infant may feel the different parts of their head touching the floor as they lie on their back and turn their head from side to side. Through the sense of life, they may feel satiated after a nursing or bottle-feeding. Through the sense of self-movement, they may experience the position of their arms when they push down into the surface and rise up onto straight arms when in prone. Through the sense of balance, they may experience that they are starting to fall when they shift their weight to reach for a toy that is just out of their reach. Initially, the sensations are fragmented. Gradually, they are integrated and become ordered. They serve to orient the child to their bodies. Over time, the four foundational senses combine to develop a body image, as mentioned above. The ultimate goal is to establish the body as a unified whole, rather than as disparate parts.

Here is an example of what can happen when one loses a spatial parameter of part of the body. As I write this chapter, I am recovering from a surgery to one of my fingers. Following the surgery, my finger was numb for several hours, during which time I returned home. I couldn't perceive the border of my finger. I couldn't tell where it ended and the world began. I could move it, but I couldn't perceive how it was moving. As a result, I was clumsy and I compensated with vision, i.e., I had to look at my finger to see what it was doing. I tried to type, but made too many mistakes to continue. During the period of numbness, it was as if my finger didn't belong to me any longer. I lost the feeing of the wholeness of my body, which was quite disconcerting.

Becoming Acquainted with the Body

As noted by Karl König, above, experiences in the four foundational senses weave together the child's body image or body scheme. In the infant, experiences of touch, well-being, self-movement, and balance occur during two major activities: caregiving activities and free movement activities. Let us consider the caregiving first. Dr. Judit Falk explains that the child comes into relationship with their body "by everything that is done to [their] body when [they are] touched, held, fed, nursed, [and so on]."[4] When the child is actively engaged in caregiving activities, this especially supports the baby to come to understand the spatial attributes of their bodies. For example, the baby has opportunities to come to know the various parts of their body when they participate in bathing, drying off, and dressing.

A second way that the child comes to know their body is through their own free movements. Indeed, the child who negotiates the gross motor sequence of their own accord has a plethora of opportunities for finely graded sensory experiences. They are free to choose the different types, frequencies, and intensities of sensation according to their own sensory preferences and needs. We want the child to have positive experiences in their bodies, and giving them the control to grade their own sensory experiences makes this more likely.

The gross motor sequence offers an abundance of deep tactile input through which the baby comes to experience the border of their body. This is especially true when the baby is in the horizontal positions of supine, side-lying, and prone. For example, when they lie on their backs on a firm surface, the weight of the body presses into the floor, and the floor exerts an equal amount of counterpressure back up into the body. Playing in these horizontal positions, as well as rolling and belly-crawling, give wonderful deep pressure touch input. The higher developmental positions offer less deep pressure input, because a smaller area of the body is in contact with the floor. A child who seeks deep pressure touch can stay in the horizontal positions and activities for a longer time before moving into the higher developmental positions. Additionally, once they are in the higher positions, they can come back down to the lower positions to satisfy their need for deep touch. (The sense of touch is discussed in further detail in chapter 12.)

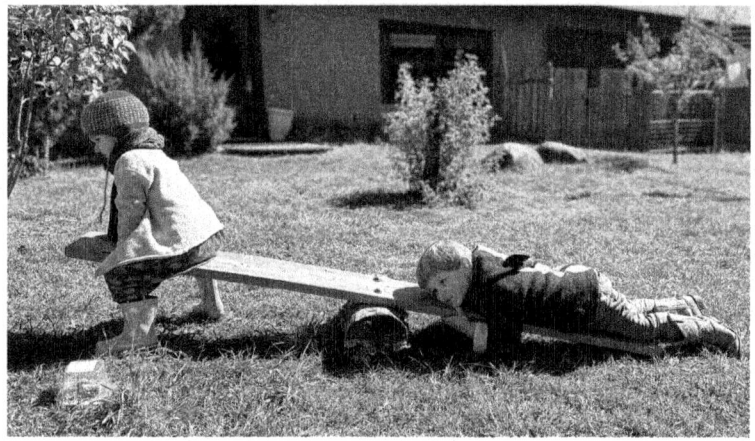

This child has chosen to stop and rest on the teeter-totter. They are listening to their inner cues.

With free movement, the child can move as much as they want. When they get tired, they can stop. This is an optimal situation for the sense of life to develop, and it is a key factor for learning to self-regulate. When someone else is encouraging the child to move, they aren't as able to listen to the internal messages that inform them of fatigue, and so they may miss the body cues telling them to stop and rest.

If the child is in baby equipment, their movements are restricted, and they can't get physically tired in the same way as when they are able to move freely. For the healthy development of the sense of life, we want the child to "give it their all" and get good and tired out. Then, they can rest better. Similarly, we want them to get good and hungry, enjoy their food, and then feel satiated. (The sense of life is further discussed in chapter 13.)

The sense of self-movement (proprioception) provides the child with perceptions of their own movements. The child refines the sense of self-movement by moving freely and practicing variations of movements as often as they wish. Periods of free, uninterrupted movement allow the child to properly register the proprioceptive feedback necessary for the development of coordinated movement. When an adult encourages a child to move, the child is not as able to attend to this inner proprioceptive sensing. (The sense of self-movement is further discussed in chapter 14.)

When the child moves of their own accord without outside commentary, they are also more able to properly "listen to" the vestibular feedback that is necessary for the development of healthy balance. Please note that these sensory experiences are largely at an unconscious level. Nonetheless, sensory perceptions are taking place at this level, and it is necessary that they occur in this way for healthy sensory development to ensue.

The child is also free to satisfy their vestibular needs with just the right amount of movement. For example, rolling across the floor provides a hefty amount of vestibular input, and in free movement, the baby can roll as much or as little as they determine. Many adults get dizzy when they roll across the floor. The baby who seeks out vestibular input may use rolling as a means of locomotion to travel long distances in the house for months. Other babies, with a lower threshold for vestibular input, may never roll all the way across the floor, but instead just roll from supine to side-lying and back again, and from supine to prone and back again. Each child can satisfy their individual sensory preferences with self-initiated movement. As soon as they begin to walk, some children self-initiate spinning around in circles and appear to enjoy making themselves dizzy. Other children refrain from seeking out this type of intense vestibular input, but may teach themselves to swing on a swing quite early and seek out much swinging thereafter.

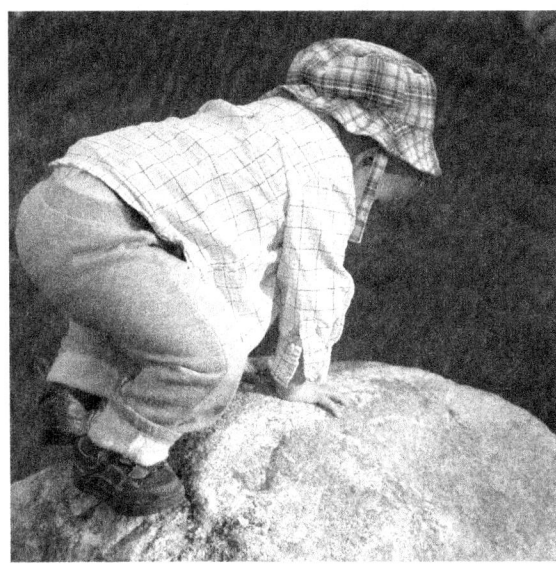

The senses of self-movement and balance are employed when climbing onto a rock.

When we witness different children seeking out such a wide range of sensory experiences, we may marvel at how the individuality of each child expresses itself so uniquely in their sensory preferences. We can come to understand that we cannot teach children to develop their foundational senses of touch, life, self-movement, and balance. These tasks are theirs alone to do. Rudolf Steiner sums it up beautifully: "Basically, there is no education other than self-education, whatever the level may be. . . . Every education is self-education, and as teachers we can only provide the environment for the child's own self-education. We have to provide the most favorable conditions in which, through our agency, the child can educate [themself] in accordance with [their] own destiny."[5] What are the most favorable conditions for the self-education of the child's basic sensory systems? The complementary combination of respectful caregiving and free motor exploration supports the development of the child's four bodily senses. In this way, we can offer them the conditions whereby their self-education of these four senses can unfold in a healthy way.

When the Body Scheme Is Established

The body scheme develops gradually over the first seven years. When it is fully established, subtle changes may be noted in the child's abilities. For example, let us look at the child's ability as it manifests in a circle game.

With the very early circle games, for the three- and four-year-olds especially, the children will hover "like a bunch of grapes" (as Freya Jaffka put it) around the teacher as the teacher moves in the circle game. The children aren't able to hold the form of a circle because they don't have the spatial foundation to do so. As the child approaches the seventh birthday, they know, largely at an unconscious level, that they have an inside and an outside space. The ring of a circle game also has an inside and an outside space. When the children intuitively know the inside and the outside of their own bodily forms, they can transfer this knowledge to the form of the ring. Only at the end of the first seven years is it realistic for the teacher to expect that the children are able to arrange themselves in and maintain the form of a circle. It usually takes well into first grade for this to be accomplished with ease. Until such time, the teacher invisibly "holds" the form of the circle with their own space, as a potential form, into which the children can live. There is no need to impose one's will upon the children and verbally cue them to correct the spacing. One can employ gesture to some extent. However, the form of the circle will emerge in its own good time.

Sense Experiences Are Multifactorial Events

In the next chapter, we will continue with an exploration of the sense of touch. In the chapters that follow, we will also look at the senses of life, self-movement, and balance. However, before we begin, it is helpful to understand that every sensory experience involves input from more than one sense alone. One time, I observed a young girl repeatedly rotating her head to the right, stopping, and then rotating it to the left and stopping. Her hair had just been washed, and was still wet. It swung out and tapped against her face with each turn of the head. She performed this movement quite quickly for a dozen or so repetitions, and then she stopped. Several sensory modalities were involved in this activity. Her vestibular system was sensing the acceleration and deceleration of her head movement. Her tactile system was perceiving the touch—it was almost a slap—of her hair as it contacted her face. Her hair was colder than her face was, and her sense of temperature perceived this. Her sense of proprioception was noticing the movement that her neck was making, and she was keeping her balance throughout the maneuver. She was sensing how dizzy she was getting, and she stopped before she became too dizzy—before she would have lost her balance.

12: The Sense of Touch

The sense of touch is the first of the foundational senses. As has been mentioned, it is through the sense of touch that we experience the edge of our bodies. We typically think that we discern different textures through the sense of touch, however Rudolf Steiner disputes this. He says that, through the sense of touch alone, we don't perceive anything of the object that touches us, only its effect upon our skin. In a 1920 lecture he says, "You perceive nothing of the object, however; you sense only the effect upon yourself, the change in yourself. A hard object pushes your organs far back into you. You perceive this resistance as a change in your own organism when you perceive by means of the sense of touch."[1] Later, in a 1921 lecture he sums it up: "When you touch something, the experience you have is an inner experience. You do not feel this chalk; roughly speaking, what you feel is the impact of the chalk on your skin."[2]

Dear reader, please find an object in your environment, something like a hairbrush. In order to isolate your experience of the sense of touch, place the palm of your hand over the bristles and hold it there without moving. You will feel small, discrete points on the palm of your hand. You are feeling the impact of the bristle tips pressing into your palm. If you then move your palm over the bristles, you will perceive their prickly texture. Similarly, if you place your palm over the back side of the brush and hold it there, you will feel a larger area of the palm of your hand. You are feeling the impact of the back side of the brush pressing into your palm. If you move your palm over the back of the brush, you will ascertain its smoothness. Movement of the hand is required to feel the prickly or smooth texture. Through the singular sensation coming from the sense of touch, you only feel the various parts of your palm, depending on how much of it is in contact with the hairbrush—you feel the border of a part of your body. Through the entirety of the sense of touch we may feel bounded, enclosed.

If we don't have a good feeling of where the boundary of our body is, it can affect our functioning in the world. When I worked as a physical therapist in home health care for a few years, one of my jobs was to remove patients' staples after knee replacement surgeries. Of course, I had to wear gloves for sanitary reasons, but they often didn't fit me well. I remember wanting to take off the gloves so that I could feel the edges of my fingers better, which would have made the task a lot easier. A similar situation occurs when we try to find something in our bag or backpack with gloves on. We often remove our gloves as it is easier to locate the object with our bare skin.

The organ of the sense of touch is the skin. There are two types of touch input—deep pressure touch and light touch. Light touch tends to be "alerting," in physical therapy terms. When I was in college, during the summers, I worked at a camp for children with special needs. The head girls' counselor would come into our counselors' cabin every morning to wake us up. It was often difficult for us to wake up in the mornings. However, one morning a daddy longlegs spider happened to crawl across my face. This was light touch input. I was instantly awake! In contrast, deep pressure—or more firm pressure—tends to be calming. We can observe children seeking out deep pressure when they press their bodies into other people or into objects. I know a woman whose bed was up against the wall when she was a child. She would slide her body down between the bed and the wall and then tuck herself in between the mattress and the box springs. This position gave her a good dose of deep pressure. She did this every night before wiggling back up on top of the mattress, where she fell asleep. The deep pressure was the calming influence that she needed in order to go to sleep. I know another boy who has this same practice of tucking himself in between the box springs, the mattress, and the wall every day when he comes home from grade school. The deep pressure assists him in the transition from school to home. In each of these cases, the child self-initiated this activity—intuitively knowing how to meet their own tactile needs.

Henning Köhler speaks about how the sense of touch may be transformed in a mature individual: "The sense of touch has the task of bringing about a healthy, mobile balance between too great and too little impressionability, between openness and boundedness, between sympathy and antipathy. When it is well-developed, its metamorphosed functioning as the regulator of a soul/spiritual relationship to the world makes it possible for an unthreatened selfhood to take profoundly participating interest in what surrounds it."[3]

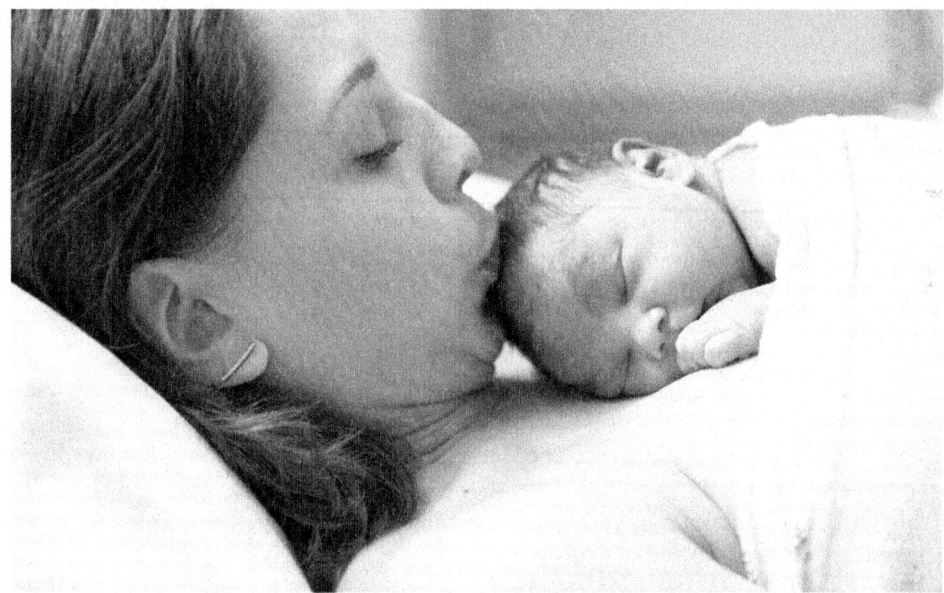

This newborn and parent are engaged in skin-to-skin contact in the first hour after birth.

The Effects of Skin-to-Skin Contact Immediately after Birth

The sense of touch plays an important role at the very beginning of life. Skin-to-skin contact immediately after birth has been studied at length, and its many physiological benefits have been well established: "Whether premature or full-term, [newborns] who have SSC [skin-to-skin contact] with their [birthing parent] have better and more stable physiological functioning than newborns who do not have SSC. SSC is associated with the regulation of newborns' temperature, heart rate, respiration, and gastrointestinal adaptation."[4] Skin-to-skin contact for the birthing parent also has favorable outcomes, including "earlier expulsion of the placenta, reduced bleeding, increased breastfeeding self-efficacy* and lowered maternal stress levels."[5]

Skin-to-skin contact is possible when no medical intervention is needed for either party immediately after birth—whether vaginal or Cesarean deliveries. In some of the families that I have worked with, when the birthing parent experienced a medical emergency during or after the birth, the other parent engaged in

---

* Breastfeeding self-efficacy refers to the birthing parent's belief in their ability to breastfeed—including, for example, the belief that they have enough milk to nourish their baby.

skin-to-skin contact with the baby. Later, when it was appropriate, the birthing parent had skin-to-skin time with the baby.

Skin-to-skin contact immediately after birth affects both parties on an emotional level. Our skin, the organ of the sense of touch, literally separates us from each other, and it is also a means of intimacy, a way of uniting us with loved ones. The research demonstrates a link between skin-to-skin contact in the first hour after birth and bonding. Oxytocin, known as the love hormone, "plays a major role in the developing [birthing parent]/infant relationship. . . . Oxytocin is increased by touch, gentle pressure, and warmth during SSC, as well as breastfeeding. In SSC, increases in oxytocin in one member of the dyad influences increases in the other, and their responses become synchronized, facilitating social connectedness."[6] That skin-to-skin time immediately after birth is associated with earlier discharge of the placenta and less bleeding makes sense, as oxytocin is also shown to stimulate uterine contractions. Oxytocin also plays a role in lactation.

In the 2019 study mentioned above, the authors state, "A systematic review of [the birthing parent's] experiences of skin-to-skin contact includes overwhelming feelings of love, a natural experience that taught them how to be a [parent], improved self-esteem, and a way of knowing and understanding the infant. We have noticed that this simple act of the staff handing over the newborn infant to the [birthing parent] supports early parental confidence."[7]

The emotional effects of skin-to-skin contact can be far reaching. In one longitudinal study, the birthing parents who had participated in skin-to-skin time with their babies immediately after birth "were rated as 'less rough' when latching and stimulating their babies during breastfeeding at day 4 postpartum. Skin-to-skin time was also linked to improved [birthing parent]/infant mutuality one year later. Skin-to-skin contact after birth also positively influenced the infant's self-regulation at one year."[8] Skin-to-skin time appears to help get the relationship off to a good start and establish favorable habits.

Skin-to-skin contact can also continue over time. One crawling baby had skin-to-skin time with his father every day when his dad came home from work. His dad would lie down on the floor in the living room, and the baby would crawl over, pull up his dad's shirt and lie on his bare chest. It was a calming and bonding activity for both parent and child. Older children also can seek out emotional connection through the sense of touch. One summer my grandchildren—then four and six years old—went on vacation and were away from me for ten days. When they came home, the children were eager to reconnect with me. It was remarkable how much contact they sought out with me through the sense of touch.

Traditional touching games such as "The Moon is Round" and "This Little Piggie" are other ways for us to connect through the sense of touch with very young children. When my second granddaughter was three years old, she performed "The Moon is Round" with care and sensitivity with her new little sister, then a month old. It was a nice way for the two siblings to connect. There are also many lovely touching games created by Wilma Ellersiek, which I also recommend.[9]

How Does the Child Respond to Our Touch?

When we care for a baby or young child—when we wipe their mouth after feeding them, when we bathe and dress them, when we put cream on their faces—we touch the child. Anna Tardos reveals the importance of this tactile experience for the child. She says, "The general wellbeing of the toddler depends in high measure upon the way [they are] being touched by the adult."[10] This is perhaps even more true for the infant. In general, the young child is exquisitely aware of the manner in which we touch them. Are we being careful? Are we rushing? Are we paying attention? Do we want to be doing this? Are we confident? Do we let the child know ahead of time that we are going to touch them, so the touch experience is not unexpected? Do we approach them from the front? Perhaps the most important of all of these questions to ask ourselves is: Are we noticing the child's response to our touch? We want the child's touch experiences to be pleasant. We want them to be able to *meet our touch*. If the child winces back and withdraws from our touch, they are not meeting our touch, and we need to alter it. The child's *response* to our touch is key. Even when we think that we are touching the child in a pleasant manner, we don't really know unless we observe the child's responses from moment to moment.

I once mentored a caregiver of toddlers who believed that she was touching the children in a respectful manner, and who wanted to do so. She was concerned that the children were not engaging with her in the way she wanted. She spent one week simply observing how she touched the children without any attempt to change her practices. She soon realized that she was frequently approaching them from behind, and she was also tickling them. Prior to her observations, she had no awareness of this. The following week she began approaching the children from the front and she stopped tickling them. Her interactions with the children improved dramatically.

Different children like to be touched differently—there is a wide range in children's touch preferences. Some children snuggle up close to us and press against us. Others, not so much. Some children love to be hugged, and they initiate hugging. Other children grin and bear it, or they may even run away. Additionally, a child's touch preference can change over time—sometimes in an instant. A child may not appear to like to be touched. However, when they are in charge of the touch—for example, when they can freely initiate snuggling and also end it—they may seek out and appear to enjoy considerable touch input.

If the parent discovers a mismatch with their child in terms of touch preferences, it is very helpful if the parent takes this into consideration during tactile interactions with their child. For example, a parent may enjoy and seek out a lot of touch, whereas the child may want much less, or vice versa. In my work with children and their parents, this issue is not uncommon. Often, it is a delicate one for the parent and it brings up a lot of feelings. However, once the sensory component is understood and addressed, it usually mitigates the parent's distress.

We also touch a child with our gaze. It is helpful to notice how the child is responding to the way we look at them and to the frequency of our looking. For example, is the child meeting our gaze? Are they relaxed or are they tensing up? Like physical touching, we want the child's visual touching experience to be pleasant for them, and so we adapt our gaze accordingly. There are many ways of looking at another person. We can look at a person in an evaluative manner—as a person in charge of quality control in manufacturing would look, i.e., we size them up. We can look at someone and indicate in a no-nonsense fashion that they should do something or stop doing something—we can direct them with our eyes. We can cast a glance—as if our gaze rides a wave—across the play yard to see if all is well. We can also look because we are drawn to look. When we first see someone that we later fall in love with, we often say that we couldn't keep our eyes off them. Sometimes there is a meeting between our gaze and that of the other person, and something profound passes between us. When a parent first holds their infant, immediately after the child's birth, it is not uncommon for the newborn to gaze deeply into the parent's eyes, and the parent remembers this as an extraordinary experience. There is a time and place for each type of looking. For example, if a child is injured, it is appropriate to look in an evaluative manner to see if medical attention should be sought. What is important is that we observe the child's response to our gaze and change our gaze accordingly. How we interact visually with a child affects our budding relationship with them.

We say that someone's words "touched us" or were "very touching." The way we speak to an infant is also a touch experience for them. When I observed the caregivers with the children at Lóczy, I was impressed by the beautiful, soothing quality of the caregivers' speech, and it seemed to me that their speech had a positive impact on the children—their words seemed to be a healing balm surrounding the children with a protective sheathing. According to Rudolf Steiner, "The kind words spoken to us have a direct effect on us, just as color affects our eyes directly. The love living in the other's soul is borne into your soul on the wings of the words."[11]

Speaking in a considerate, interested, and respectful manner, the caregivers were using language to orient the children—they were letting the children know what they were going to do before it happened. The caregivers did not use language to teach the children intellectual concepts.

Touch Input during the Child's Free Movements

I recommend that infants be laid on firm, horizontal surfaces, as opposed to soft, semi-reclined surfaces. It is helpful to remember that the development of the sense of touch is not a passive process! The child's ego is actively involved in each healthy sensory experience, including touch experiences. As mentioned above, for the healthy development of the sense of touch, we want the child to be able to meet our touch, and so we alter our touch so that the child can meet it. In this way, the ego can be active. How does this manifest for a child who is playing on the floor? The floor is actually pushing up into the child's body, and the child meets that incoming sensation by subtly pushing out from the inside of their body to the edge of their skin. A firm, horizontal surface provides the best opportunity for the child to achieve this. On a horizontal surface, the pressure from the floor is equally distributed, so that the baby can feel each part of the body evenly. This is not the case in a reclined sitting posture, such as in an infant seat, where the pressure is focused on the buttocks and sacrum. A firm surface gives the child something to push against and makes it easier to move on the surface. In this

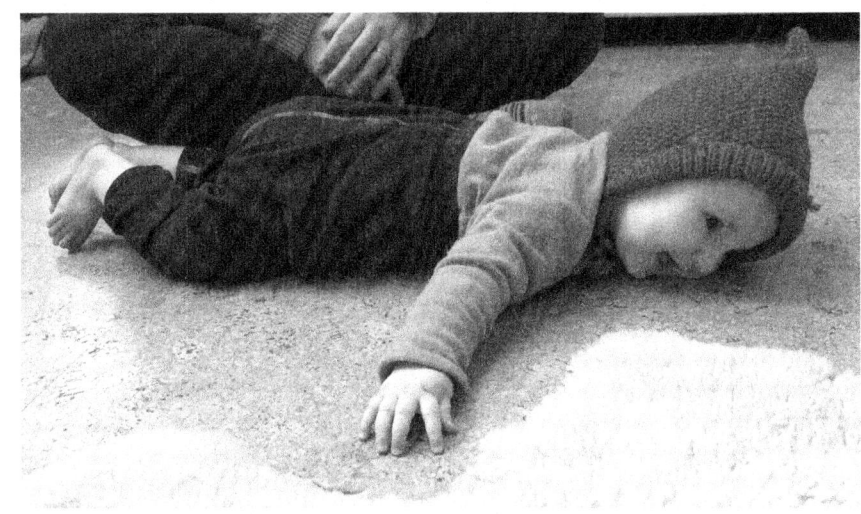

This is one of the first times this baby rolled onto their belly.
They lay on their tummy for an extended period, smiling and kicking their feet.
It was as if they wanted to savor the sensations that the new position provided.
They were actively meeting the incoming touch sensations from the floor.

way the child can alter their touch sensations, and the tactile input can occur over more areas of the body, depending on the child's stage of motor development. For example, when the child begins to roll to each side, they receive touch input to the sides of the body. With a soft surface, the baby's body sinks into the surface. They tend to stay in one position because it is difficult to move in this situation, hence the touch experiences are more limited and more static.

According to Pikler's research, babies, if given opportunities for free movement, will commence crawling on hands and knees anywhere from 8.5 to 12 months (with an average of 10 months). This means that they will spend anywhere from 8.5 to 12 months in the horizontal positions and activities (supine, side-lying, prone, rolling, and belly-crawling.) Offering rich opportunities for tactile input from the surface, horizontal activities provide the baby with optimal circumstances to develop the sense of touch and establish the boundary of their body. When they begin to crawl on hands and knees, the amount of full body tactile input is reduced. What is especially nice about self-initiated movement is that the child can spend as long as they want in the horizontal activities, satisfying their need for tactile input. Additionally, they can return to the horizontal positions as often as they want, after having progressed to hands-and-knees crawling and beyond.

FREE MOVEMENT FROM THE VERY START

The horizontal positions and activities allow various options for different parts of the skin to touch the floor. For example, while lying on the back with the legs on the floor, the infant experiences deep touch sensation primarily at the back of the head and upper back, the buttocks, and the heels. This input to the heels is very helpful for future walking, as it sets the stage for a good heel strike.

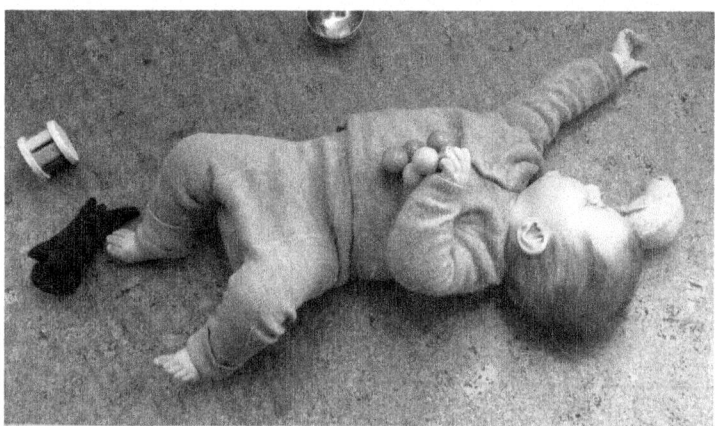

This baby is pushing into the floor with their heels and sliding their body backward across the floor. This activity gives substantial deep pressure to the heels and backside.

In contrast, let us consider what happens when the child is placed into a piece of baby equipment such as a saucer. Here, their tactile experiences are markedly different. The touch input is not received via a firm, horizontal surface, and so it is not distributed evenly throughout the body. Additionally, the child is not able to move freely in the device to change where they are receiving the touch input—the scope of the touch input is narrowed, and it is static. Specifically, in the saucer, they receive deep pressure primarily through the balls of the feet and the crotch. They also receive deep pressure through small portions of the trunk and forearms when they lean against the surrounding tray. Bearing weight through the balls of the feet with the heels up off the surface can contribute to a future toe-walking pattern.

In free movement, the baby will also lie on their back with their legs in the air, so that they no longer receive input to the heels from the floor. However, now the low back comes into contact with the floor, building up the sense of the boundary of that part of the body.

When the baby belly-crawls, they receive deep pressure input to the front side of their bodies, and when they roll, they receive deep pressure input to every side of their body.

When we go for a massage, we may say to the masseuse, "Oh that's the spot. Please stay there." Or, "No, the spot is a little to the right." Similarly, when they baby plays on the floor, they are free to satisfy their tactile needs very specifically because nuanced types of tactile sensations are possible there. The child is in charge of the amount and the location of their touch experiences by the positions and activities they choose. In essence, on the floor, the child can give themselves a satisfying massage.

Once, when I was observing in a kindergarten classroom, a child climbed up onto the large lunch table, lay her back, pushed her body into the surface of the table, and then rolled repeatedly from side to side. She appeared to enjoy this. She was seeking deep pressure from essentially the only available hard surface in the classroom, as the majority of the floor was covered with

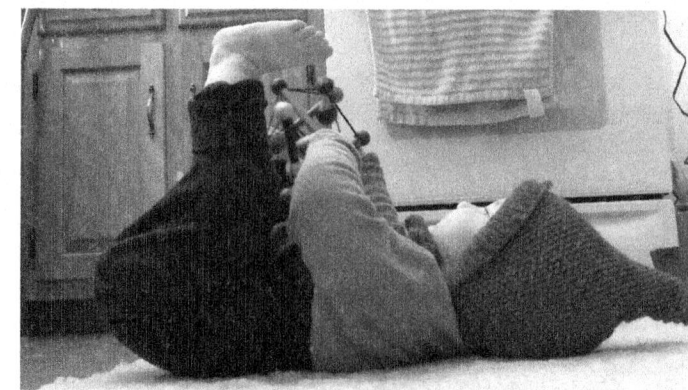

This baby's feet and bottom are up off the floor, and they are receiving deep pressure input to the low back.

a thick, braided rug. This is a more obvious example of what the baby does all the time when they are playing and moving on the floor. The teacher was concerned that lying on the table was not an appropriate behavior, a reasonable concern. My response was to ask if there could be another way for this child to nourish her tactile system. The teacher thereafter offered a touching game (to all of the children) every day at one of the transitions and cleared out an area of the room so the child could have access to the wooden floor. Additionally, the child's parent hung up a cloth hammock at home. With these interventions, she stopped lying on the lunch table.

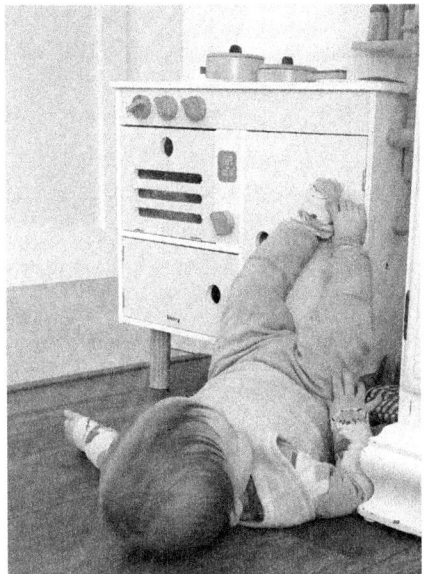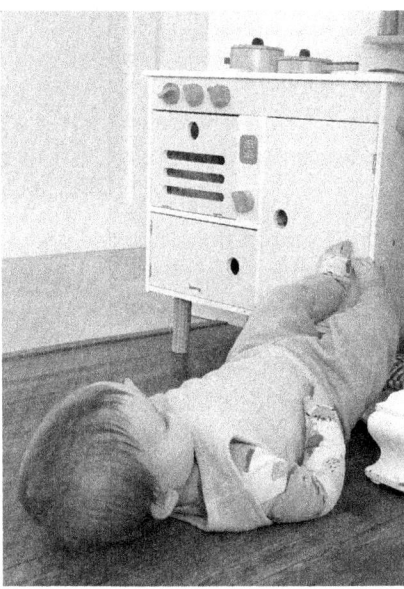

This baby frequently pushed off the toy stove with their feet at this stage of development. In doing so, they were receiving a good amount of deep pressure on the backside.

By the end of their time spent in the horizontal positions and activities, the child has had a plethora of deep pressure experiences from the floor to almost every possible part of their skin. This includes input into the fisted hand, the open palm, the heel of the hand, the sides of the hand, the different fingers, and, to a lesser degree, the back of the hand. Such tactile input

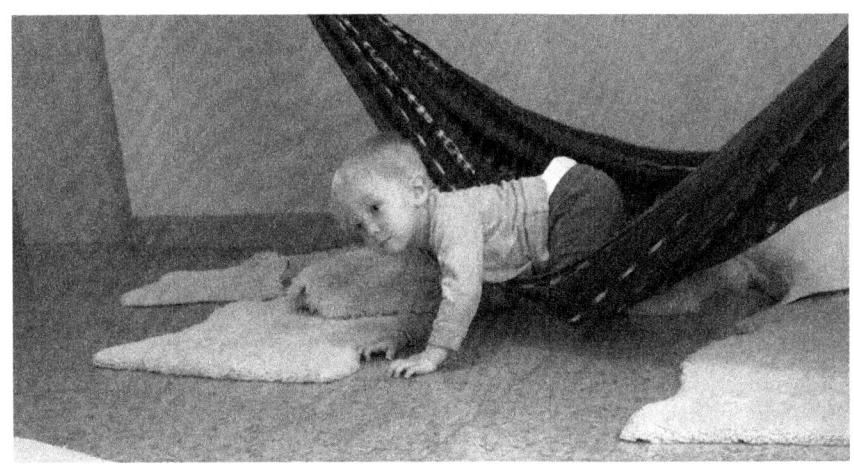

A hammock provides a plethora of deep pressure input. It also provides a significant amount of proprioceptive and vestibular input when children climb in and out of the movable structure.

favorably influences the development of the hand. For example, when the thumb starts to receive more tactile sensation from the floor, the child's awareness of their thumb increases, and they start to use it more. (Fine and gross motor development are further discussed in chapter 7.)

Other Opportunities from the Environment for Tactile Sensation

At Sophia's Hearth, we have a cloth hammock (not a net hammock) that can be put up and taken down in a corner of the room. There are two sturdy hooks in the studs of the walls, and there are fleeces underneath. The hammock is adjustable and is placed low to the ground for the toddlers. One morning, during the indoor free play period, a 24-month-old boy played in the hammock the whole time. He negotiated the hammock in a variety of ways. He climbed in and repeatedly opened and closed the hammock over himself—it was as if he was playing peek-a-boo with himself. He also climbed in and out, climbed in and purposely fell out onto the fleeces, wiggled his body inside the hammock to make it move, lay on his belly over the hammock and gently pushed himself forward and backward with his feet, and on and on.

Young children seemingly want to touch everything in their environment. This starts very young. Babies, playing on the floor, stroke their toys, bat at them, and slide them along the floor. They pick up their toys, transfer them from hand to hand, drop them, and shake them. All these actions involve touching the toys. Therefore, we can provide healthy touch opportunities for the child through the particular toys and objects we select for them. Natural materials provide rich touch opportunities for discernment. For example, when a child rubs their hand over a wooden toy, they may perceive the subtle grain of the wood, whereas plastic toys are typically of uniform consistency. Children also receive touch sensation from the clothes they wear and also from the clothes their caregivers wear. Natural fibers generally provide pleasing touch experiences.

Tactile opportunities are plentiful outdoors. Young children have been playing in sand and mud for a long time! Playing in water at the beach or swimming pool offers a significant degree of deep pressure, especially when the child is old enough to swim underwater. Planting mullein or lamb's ear in the yard provides an opportunity for the children to touch soft, velvety plants. At Sophia's Hearth, we have also planted blue globe thistles so that the children have opportunities for a stronger touch experience.

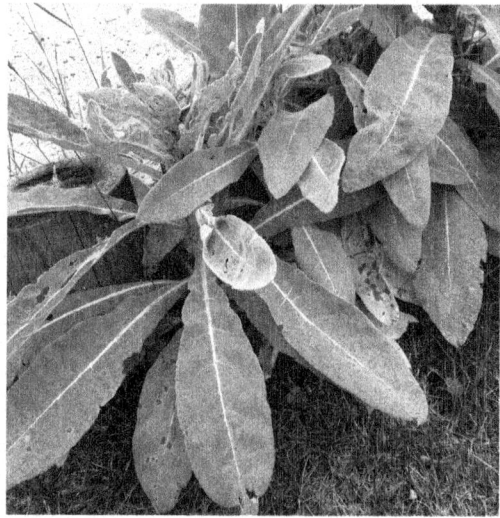

Mullein plant.

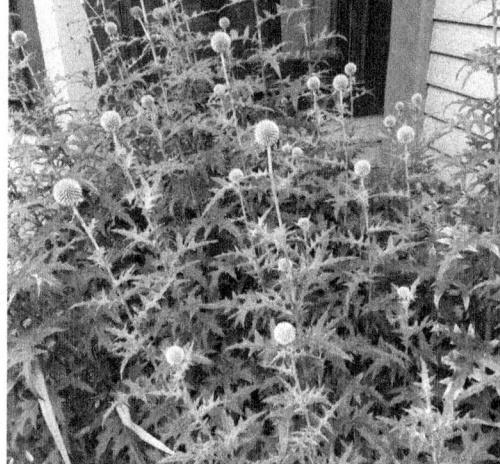

Blue globe thistles.

It is helpful to dress the children appropriately so they may better take part in tactile experiences outdoors.

The children can also receive tactile input from each other.

In another example, a grandmother was cooking supper for her grandchildren. The four- and six-year-olds were starting to get a little out of themselves. The grandmother noticed this and moved the baby out of the way of the commotion. She continued to watch the older children but did not intervene. The two older children soon remedied the situation themselves when they invented the "tangle wangle game." In this game, they were lying on the kitchen floor and they squeezed up next to each other, enjoying making up as many configurations of their body contact as they could think of. They would lie on top of each other, side by side,

Chapter 12: The Sense of Touch

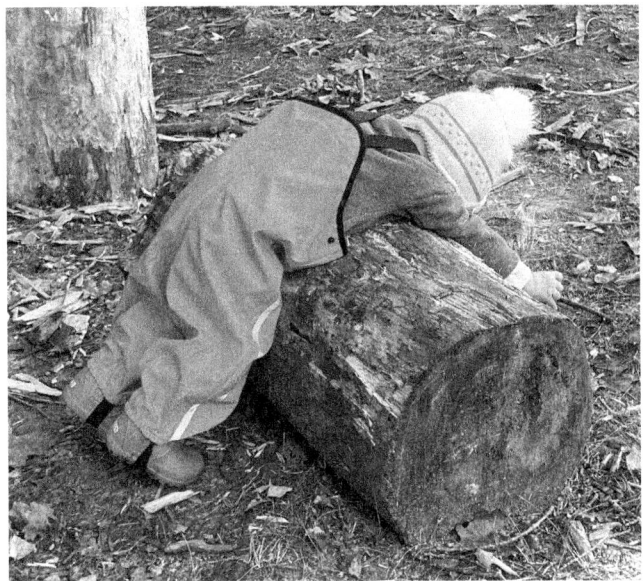 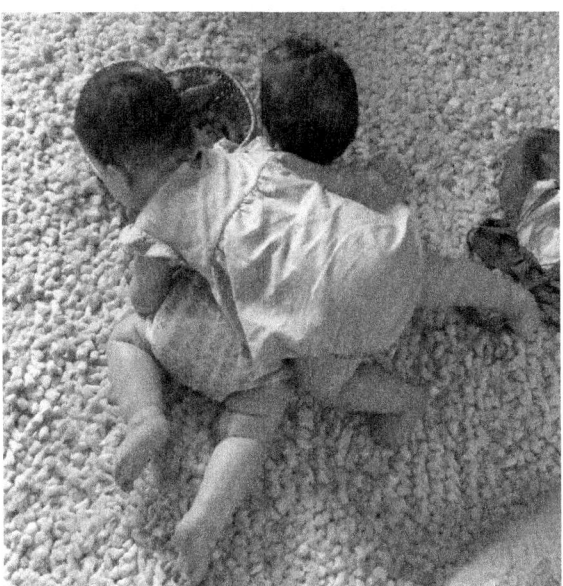

This child, well-equipped in a rain suit to lie on the stump on a chilly day, is experiencing deep pressure on their front side.

These twins frequently give each other a good amount of deep pressure input.

or back to back. These activities provided them with deep pressure and also proprioceptive input. This type of behavior is indicative of children with healthy developing sensory systems, in that they know how to nourish their own systems with what they need.

It is also not uncommon for children start to get "out of themselves" and need assistance to come back into themselves—inside the border of their body. In this case, they often respond well to being held firmly, yet gently, and perhaps being sung to. This tends to work better if the adult nips it in the bud—if the adult can respond before the child gets too far out of themselves. The adult must have no hint of irritation when holding the child.

In addition to touching games, mentioned earlier in the chapter, adults can also offer tactile experiences through imaginative activities. Paula Sousa, our childcare director at Sophia's Hearth, has created a lovely image for the children that allows her to offer deep pressure touch. She tells the story of some ponies who are galloping outside in the rain. The farmer calls them in to the barn to be dried off and brushed. The children gallop around the room and then come to the "barn," where she has an assortment of massage tools and brushes. (We have found that the children prefer horse massage tools from equestrian shops.) Paula brushes the children who come to her. They are free to enter into the activity as they choose. The ones who could potentially be more reticent often "come to the farmer" out of imitation of the other children and because they are able to live into the image that Paula has created for them.

Sensory Preferences and the Sense of Touch

Each child has unique sensory preferences—their own individual sensory signature, if you will. An eighteen-month-old from the East Coast went on vacation to Southern California. He started to walk across a lawn of thick, spongy grass that is characteristic of the area, lost his balance, and fell forward to land in the prone position. He smiled, laughed, stood up, and repeated the scenario five or six times. The activity provided a plethora of pleasing tactile, vestibular, and proprioceptive sensations to him. Through the skin he experienced the edge of his body against the grass, through the vestibular system he experienced falling through space, and through the proprioceptive system he experienced the contractions of his muscles as he braced for the fall and then stood back up again. Another child may have become upset with these particular sensory events, yet this child reveled in them.

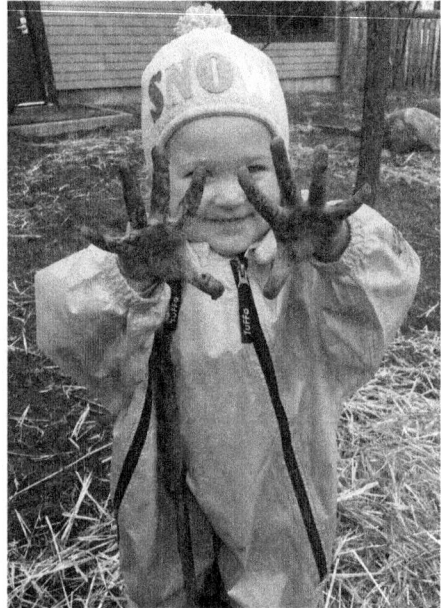

This child's hands were muddy at the end of the outdoor play period.

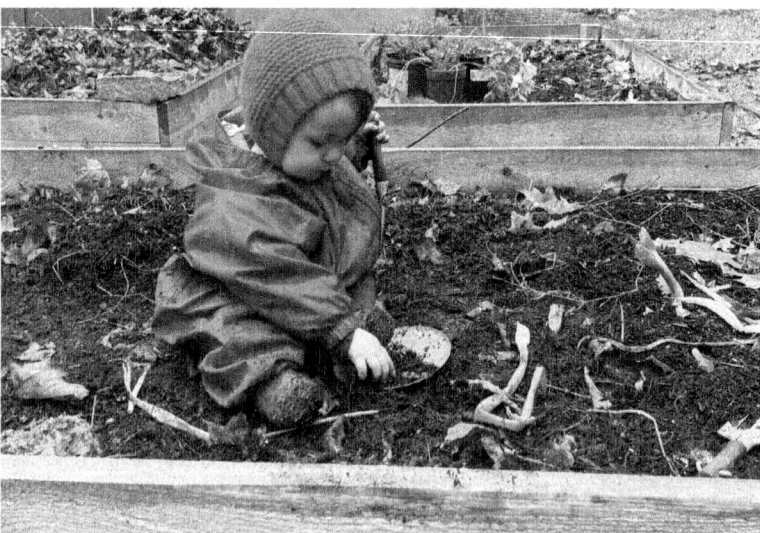

This child would routinely climb in and sit down to play in the raised garden bed. In warmer weather, they would often rub the soil all over their bare limbs. This happened so frequently that the parents refrained from planting one of their raised beds so that their child could satisfy their tactile needs. This child sought out significantly more tactile input than the child in the photo on the left.

For some babies, the experience of grass can be an intense tactile event. I recall watching one baby, who was just starting to crawl, move off the blanket into the grass and then stop suddenly. She obviously did not like the feeling of the grass against her skin, as she winced back and grimaced. However, she wanted a toy that was further out on the grass, and so she ventured forth. This is a good example of how children can initially be averse to a new sensation, but then expand their tolerance level for the sensation through a self-initiated action.

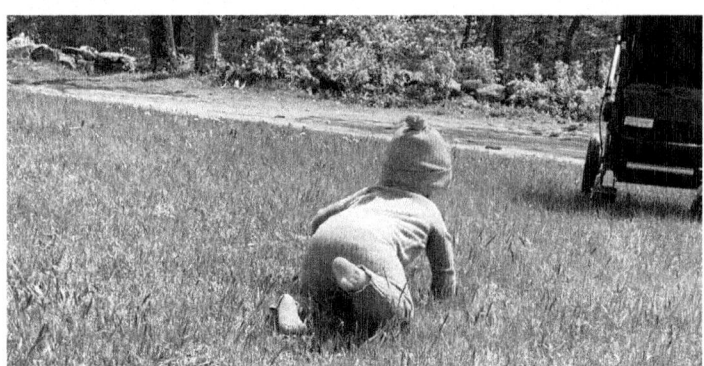
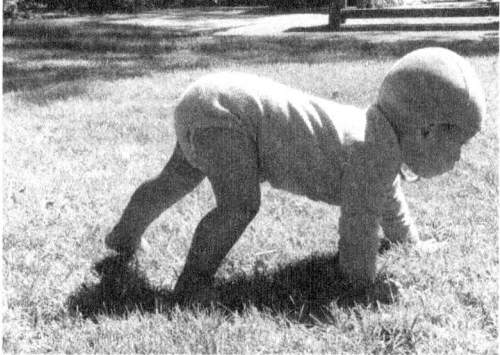

Above, left: This photo was taken in the spring. The child's grandmother regularly cared for them and would put a blanket outside each day. Mostly, the baby would stay on the blanket; they appeared to not like the feel of the grass. However, on the day this photo was taken, they saw their stroller and headed toward it, where they could pull to stand. While crawling on the grass, they paused a few times, pulling their hands back when they touched the grass, but the stroller was so inviting that they continued until they reached it. Above, right: Some children who are sensitive to the feel of the grass avoid contact with it by bear-walking.

Observing children over time can help us come to know their sensory preferences. This is valuable information, as we can consciously set up their environments with this in mind. The child is free to partake of the sensory opportunities for as long as they choose to, or to avoid them altogether. A group setting is nice, because some children who may not initially choose to take part in a particular sensory activity may be drawn into it by imitating the other children. One summer at Sophia's Hearth, the staff created a "mud bog" by adding water to a large dirt area. One little girl was happy just to watch, and her teachers did not urge her to join the other children. One day, after several days of watching, she too—gingerly at first—entered the mud bog.

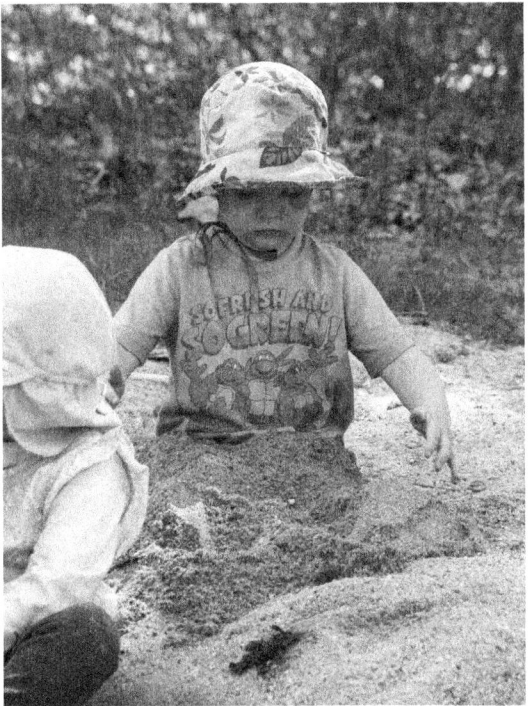

This child has buried their legs in the sand, receiving a good amount of deep pressure.

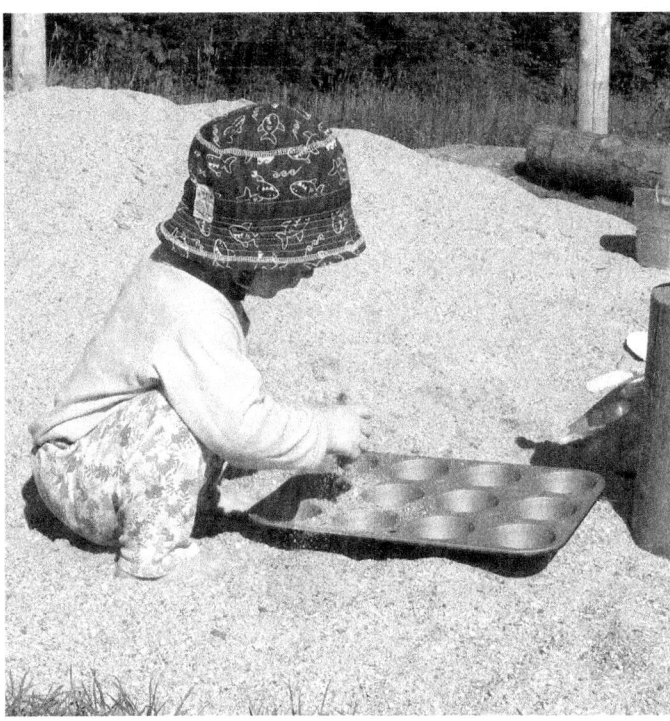

This child has relatively less contact with the sand—only with their bare feet and hands—as they make "sand cupcakes."

Caring for the Skin

We can support the sense of touch by caring for its organ, the skin. We can protect the child's skin from too much sun, wind, and cold with appropriate hats, clothing, awnings, and sunscreen. We can refrain from using harsh soaps, and on some occasions, it is fine to wash infants and young children with just water. On one occasion, I worked with a very fair preschool child who was having challenges with her sense of touch. The family was going to the ocean for the summer, and I recommended that they buy her a wetsuit to protect her from the elements. The mother told me, later, that the wetsuit made all the difference in the child's ability to partake of the beach experience.

13: The Sense of Life

Karl König explains, "The sense of life gives us the experience of the well-being or being unwell of our body—the flow of our blood [and] the flow of the fluids within our body, the movements of the inner organs, the sensations which the organs give us or which we sometimes do not even experience at all."[1] In another place he adds, "All of this is experienced as a kind of well-being so long as we are well. The sense of life for us is a 'happy sense,' a happy experience."[2] According to Henning Köhler, "Rudolf Steiner once described this as a state of 'feeling comforted and comfortable through and through,' of a being at home in oneself that is a fundamental orientation in life; all other later orientations build on this."[3]

It follows that when there is a disturbance in our physiology—such as heart palpitations, digestive cramping, pain, or illness—this has "a disorienting effect on the sense of life."[4] Steiner likens these physiological distresses to what the loss of hearing is to the sense of hearing.

The impressions given by the sense of life, known in the medical literature as the interoceptive system, are important. If a child has a decreased sensitivity to pain, this can be a serious situation. The child may have a medical condition, but not be able to perceive this and communicate it to their parent so care can be provided. It is not uncommon for children to have environmental allergies, food sensitivities, or both. These conditions grate on the sense of life, often making it difficult to feel a deep-down sense of well-being. In this case, focusing on any disturbing sensations such as malaise and fatigue can be overwhelming, and the child does everything they can not to feel them.

Here is a not-uncommon example of such a child. A four-year-old boy had environmental allergies. At preschool, he played well during free play time, and his behavior did not stand out. However, rest time was very difficult, as was sitting still and listening to a story. The boy was unable to still his body, and all manner of restless, silly, fidgety behaviors manifested. The child was paying attention to the world when he was playing, and this was fine. But when he was asked to come to quiet, his attention was drawn inward, and he experienced the feeling of "being unwell" in the body, as mentioned by Dr. König, above. It was as if it was simply not possible for this child to feel "comforted and comfortable through and through." His behavior was a compensation for this.

Compare this to our experience after an injury, such as a sprained ankle. During the day, we can often manage pretty well, because we are attending to things outside our body, but when we try and go to sleep, the discomfort of the injury becomes front and center in our awareness and we can't get to sleep. In these situations where there are physiological challenges, working with a skilled, appropriate medical provider is invaluable.

The Inner Volume Space of the Body
THE SENSE OF LIFE AND OCCUPYING THE SPACE OF OUR BODY

And now, let us focus on the spatial parameter that the sense of life gives us—a feeling that we take up the space inside the border of our skin, a feeling that we have an inner volume. This space is also known as the body space. From a spatial point of view, the way the child develops their sense of life is by filling up their body space. This is a process which takes seven years to fully complete if all goes well. Karl König explains, "By means

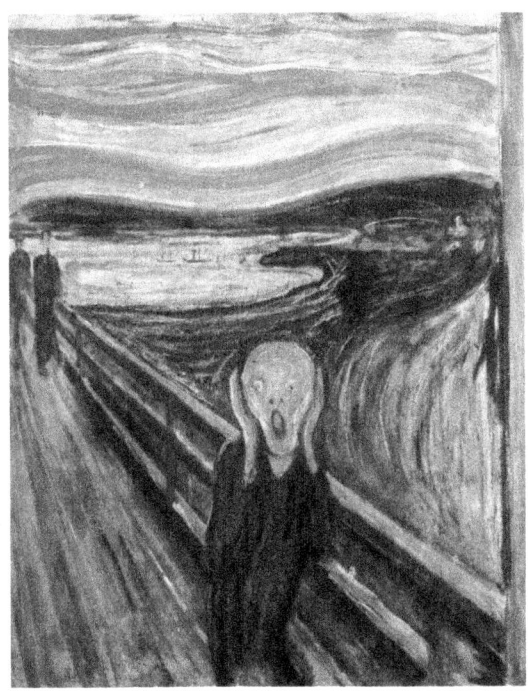

The Scream by Edvard Munch.

of the sense of life, the human being learns to experience [themself] as a 'complete within-ness' and senses [themself] as a 'bodily self, filling space.'"[5] He goes on to say that "In normal circumstances our bodily organization is experienced as a unity. We experience this wholeness as our own existence filling space. That I can call the body 'my' body, that I identify 'myself' with this body is the result of the sense of life. The body becomes mine through the sense of life. That I and my body are 'one' is an experience we must attribute to the sense of life."[6]

In contrast, if the sense of life doesn't develop properly, "The child's soul experiences [their] body as not belonging to [them], but as part of the world. ... What should have become the child's experience of [their] *own* body does not happen; instead the body becomes a part which, like a suitcase, the soul has to carry around, but not an instrument on which [they] can play and express [themself.]"[7] Unfortunately, this is not an unusual situation in our world today. It is not uncommon for an adult to become exhausted and depleted, and to feel like they are "just dragging their body around," trying to get through the day. To me, the classic painting *The Scream*, by Norwegian artist Edvard Munch, illustrates a person in such a state. I saw the original painting when I was a few years out of college, and it left a haunting impression on me. Years later, when I studied the sense of life, I related the figure in the painting to a person with a severely challenged sense of life. The figure's inner space appears hollowed out and nearly void.

CAREGIVING AND THE SENSE OF LIFE

Here is an anecdote of a child who did not experience his body as his own. A three-and-a-half-year-old boy—I will call him Johnny—was crying and crying with obvious deep distress. Even though he said "I" at the time, he did not refer to his foot as "his." Instead, he repeated, "Johnny's foot is cold. Johnny doesn't have his sock on." We might say he was *beside himself*. Rather than being *in his skin*, he wasn't inhabiting his body space, his inner volume space.

The boy was referring to his foot as an object, something that did not belong to him. The remedy for such a child, who is estranged from their body, is to tend to the child's bodily needs, in a respectful, caring manner. It would have not been helpful to expect that this child, because of his age, *should* have been able to find his own sock and put it on by himself. His behavior was telling us that his sense of life was challenged, and that he needed to be lovingly attended to. He needed this type of assistance in order to come into relationship with his body space.

Not only is this type of caregiving helpful for older children who are challenged in their sense of life, but it is also beneficial for *every* infant, baby, and young child, as they develop their sense of life. Respectful caregiving was championed by Dr. Emmi Pikler, and it made such a difference in the children's lives who were in her care at the children's home, as described in the early chapters of this book. Many of these little ones had experienced trauma, such as the loss of a parent. A common trauma response, spatially, is to start to withdraw from the body space, as Johnny did in the above example. The exquisite, respectful caregiving that these children received at the children's home served to help them come back into their bodies and continue the process of filling their body spaces.

FREE MOVEMENT FROM THE VERY START

Henning Köhler also recognizes the importance of quality caregiving. Regarding the sense of life, he says, "We should avoid making the mistake here of thinking that a dutiful carrying out of hygienic and medical rules and regulations could suffice in nurturing the development of the life sense. Duty is not the issue here. The real need is for a relaxed reverential devotion to nourishing and warming acts of bodily care; they must be done with true inner participation. Caring for the life sense is not at all the same thing as bodycare. . . . We educate the life sense by letting children experience goodness as a bodily condition."[8] Dr. Pikler recognized the nuances of caregiving mentioned here. When she opened the children's home, she first hired registered nurses to care for the children. However, after three months, she fired them all, as they were carrying out the *duties* of caregiving. Pikler replaced the registered nurses with young women who had no prior training and who genuinely liked babies. Dr. Pikler then instructed these women in the *art* of caregiving.

OTHER WAYS TO SUPPORT THE SPACE DEFINED BY THE SENSE OF LIFE

When I was in kindergarten, my teacher got a roll of white paper, cut a piece for each child in our class, and taped it to the floor. She had us lie down on our papers. She then drew the outline of each of our bodies around us, and we used crayons to fill in our outlines. I remember this experience as profoundly satisfying. I took my paper home and enjoyed looking at it repeatedly over time. In my practice with children who have challenges in their senses of life, I have found this activity beneficial for them also. I find that it gives the child an experience of the entirety of their body space, a space that is theirs alone to occupy.

Similarly, I have found a therapeutic Spacial Dynamics technique, called the Silhouette, to be helpful for supporting the sense of life. In the Silhouette, the person has "a simultaneous experience of the form of the entire body."[9] The individual parts often disappear "while the entire form, the gestalt, appears as an entity in itself."[10] To perform the Silhouette, the adult rests their hands gently on the child's head, at the top center. The adult then slowly traces the silhouette of the child's body—going down the sides of the head, behind the ears, to the neck, shoulders, outside of the upper arms, turning at the elbow to continue down the inside of the forearm and onto the palmar surface of the hands, giving a slight pull on the fingers. The adult continues to trace the remainder of the body, traveling down the sides of the chest, waist, and hips, continuing along the outside surfaces of the thighs, knees, and lower legs, below and behind the ankle bone, and along and off the outside edge of the feet, giving slight pressure to the end of the toes.

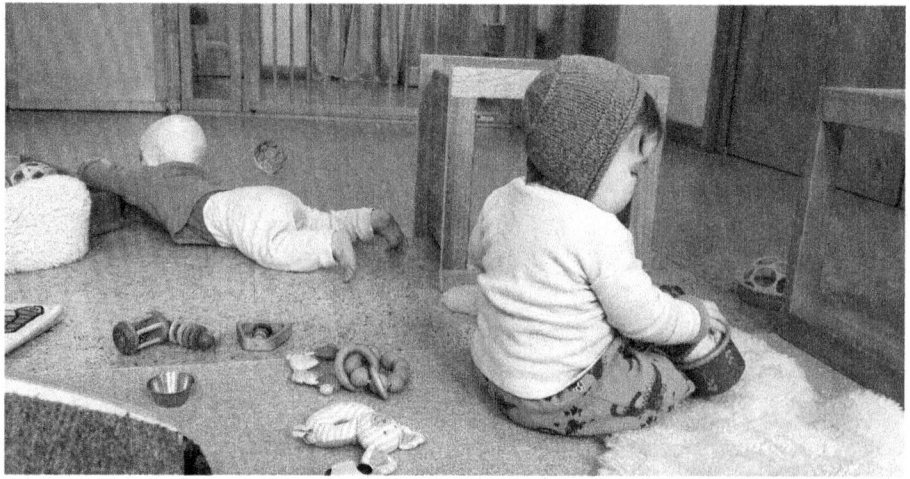

When young children wear hats during their waking hours, it provides a sheathing around their heads, contributing to the feeling of the body as a whole, rather than as separate parts. To prevent potential risk of suffocation and overheating, it is recommended that infants sleep without hats.

The Autonomic Nervous System

THE ORGAN FOR THE SENSE OF LIFE

Karl König states that the organ for the sense of life is the autonomic nervous system.[11] The autonomic nervous system is a division of the nervous system that operates without conscious control. It "influences the activity of most tissues and organ systems in the body. ... The regulation of blood pressure, gastrointestinal responses to food, contraction of the urinary bladder, focusing of the eyes, and thermoregulation are just a few" of its many functions."[12]

The autonomic nervous system has two main divisions: the sympathetic and the parasympathetic systems. The sympathetic activity is well known as the fight-or-flight response. We move into this state when we perceive that we are in danger, and physiological changes ensue to prepare our bodies to fight or flee. Our heart races, our blood pressure goes up, our pupils dilate, we perspire, the hair on our arms and the back of our necks stands up, and we feel a surge of adrenaline.[13] Additionally, our breathing becomes shallow and faster. It is not the time to digest our lunch! When we are about to get into a fight, our digestion stops. In a person who is in the sympathetic state, "there is too much energy in the system, and the [person] is flooded."[14] The person is on red alert—scanning the environment for the source of the danger. This level of consciousness is exactly the opposite of the natural dreamy state of young children.

In the parasympathetic state, these physiological conditions reverse. The heart rate slows, the blood pressure lowers, and digestion readily occurs. In fact, the parasympathetic state is classically known as the "rest and digest" state. Also, in the parasympathetic state, the breath slows and deepens, and the diaphragm is engaged.

A common technique for helping adults come into a parasympathetic state is to work with the breath, specifically enhancing the exhalation phase over the inhalation phase so that one blows out longer than one breathes in. Please note that it is best to avoid making breath work conscious in young children. However, there are many other ways to address breathing in the young child. First and foremost, one can pay attention and notice how the children are breathing and when their breathing changes. When does the child's breathing get faster, slower, deeper, or shallower? I have often observed changes in children's breathing during puppet shows, for example. I have also observed that asking children to take a deep breath is counterproductive. When they do this, they almost always shrug their shoulders, using the upper lobes of the lungs, and *not* the diaphragm. This is the opposite of what we want if we want to help them come into a parasympathetic state. Better to incorporate images of blowing out candles in verses and games, as well as the actual activities of blowing out candles and blowing white fluffy dandelion spheres, pinwheels, bubbles, and so on. In these activities, children naturally extend their exhalation. Following a good blowing out, one will naturally breathe in deeply (engaging the diaphragm) and effortlessly, without shrugging the shoulders. With activities, one is not making the breath conscious in the children. Instead, the children are focused on the dandelion or the pinwheel or the bubbles.

Anthroposophical physician Dr. Gerald Karnow also speaks about breathing. He says, "To learn how to activate the breathing needs to be part of our [early childhood] training. Educators become soul artists in learning how to appropriately speed up or slow down the child's breathing."[15]

THE POLYVAGAL THEORY

Much research has been performed on the autonomic nervous system. Stephen W. Porges began researching the vagus nerve in 1969. Decades later, in 1994, he proposed the polyvagal theory. This describes a threefold path of autonomic nervous system response. It gives a neurophysiological framework by which to understand a person's behavior. The polyvagal theory has become widely used in the clinical setting, especially for individuals who have experienced trauma. According to this theory, "every response is an action in service of survival."[16]

FREE MOVEMENT FROM THE VERY START

Specifically, in the parasympathetic branch of the autonomic nervous system, there are two pathways. These are known as the ventral vagal and the dorsal vagal pathways. Both travel within a single nerve, the vagus nerve. The vagus nerve has become well known to the public in recent years. It is the longest of the twelve cranial nerves. It is well named, as "vagus," in Latin, means wandering. When a person is in the ventral vagal state, "the system is regulated, open to connection, and the [person] is ready to engage."[17] In contrast, when a person is in the dorsal vagal state, "there is not enough energy to run the system: The system is drained, and the [person] is numbed."[18] When we perceive that we are in danger, we go into the sympathetic state, employing the strategies of fight and flight. However, when we perceive that we are in *extreme* danger, we use the dorsal vagal path. This is the "path of last resort."[19] It is an extreme response, in that we shut down physiologically. We use stillness "as a survival response, conserving energy to take us out of connection, out of awareness, and into a protective state of collapse. When we feel frozen, numb, or 'not here,' the dorsal vagus has taken control. The term 'scared to death' fits the dorsal vagal experience."[20]

SIGNS OF A HEALTHY AUTONOMIC NERVOUS SYSTEM

A healthy autonomic nervous system is flexible and resilient. It is not characterized by always being in a regulated state. It is appropriate to go into a dorsal vagal state when one is in extreme danger. It is similarly good to respond to moderate danger with a sympathetic response of fight or flight. And it is healthy to be in a ventral vagal state during safe social interactions, for example, when a child is engaging in respectful caregiving with a loving adult, as in the Pikler caregiving. The sign of a healthy autonomic nervous system is being able to shift gears according to the situation at hand. Expert Deb Dana explains: "A nervous system that brings qualities of well-being still dysregulates, but rather than remaining stuck in a survival response, it finds its way back to regulation through flexibility and resilience."[21] The questions to ask when considering the health of the sense of life in a developing child include: Can the child become alert and engaged in a task that they are interested in? Can they settle down and go to sleep? How easily do they recover from an experience that is a jolt to them? Depending on their age, can they sometimes regulate on their own? Can they also engage in co-regulation and be soothed when they do go into fight or flight? In other words, does the child get stuck in a dysregulated state, or can they shift their state of regulation, with help from an adult as needed? We want to give infants and young children a plethora of experiences in the ventral vagal state so that this becomes well known to them. In this way, they are more able return to this state when they inevitably become dysregulated.

Supporting the Child to Develop a Healthy Sense of Life
HELPING THE CHILD TO MEET THE WORLD

It is noteworthy that in order to co-regulate, both parties have to feel safe with each other, and they "have to find a way into connection and regulate with each other."[22] Here is one such incident. A family with a two-year-old girl had some people over for supper. It was a little louder than the girl was used to, and she did not know everyone well. The girl wanted to be seated right up next to her mother—closer than was usually the case. During the meal, she periodically touched her mother's arm, and said, "Mama." Every time she did this, her mother calmly and lovingly responded by saying the child's name back to her. The mother was very attuned to the feelings and needs of her daughter, and as a result, the girl was able to use her mother's calm state to co-regulate. Here the mother needed to have facility with her own autonomic nervous system, and be able to keep herself regulated, for her daughter's sake (and her own!).

In this example, the mother was helping her daughter successfully participate in the meal with the guests. The mother was helping her daughter meet the world. We meet the world well when our state of regulation matches what the situation calls for. With very young children, we sometimes need to assist them to wake up, but usually they need our help to calm down.

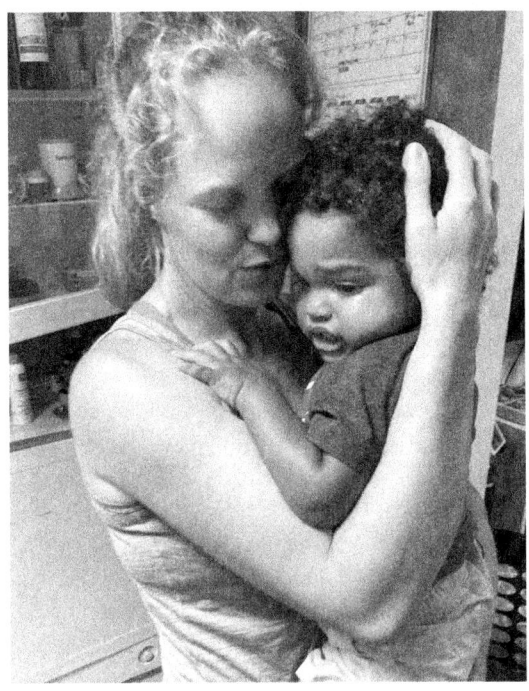

This child just had a minor injury, and their mother is helping them to soothe. This is a lovely example of co-regulation.

It's not that we want to overprotect our children and spare them from every potential stressor. However, the children are establishing soul habits in response to their environment that are foundational for their futures. "Early life experiences are fundamental in shaping both the development of the stress response system and how an individual responds to stress across the lifespan."[23] It is not helpful if a child's habitual pattern becomes one of sustained fight or flight. During fight or flight, the adrenal glands produce and release the powerful hormone cortisol, also known as the stress hormone. Cortisol is very beneficial in activating the appropriate physiological responses in order to face a stressful event, however, prolonged high levels of cortisol are detrimental to health and well-being.

How can we support the developing child to meet the world well? Our ability to support the child starts with careful observation. One of our previous master teachers at Sophia's Hearth was very attuned to the children's gestures. As such, she greeted each child differently every morning. She welcomed one older baby with wide open arms, a big smile, and a warm hello. The boy would come toward her and they would engage in a hug, and then he would go off to play. In contrast, when another girl arrived, the teacher would say hello to the parent who dropped her off, and then say something like, "It's nice to have Susie here today." She said this so the girl could hear her, but without directly addressing the child and without giving her eye contact. The mother of the girl noticed the different greetings, was concerned on behalf of her child, and spoke to the teacher about it. The teacher responded that, out of her initial observations of the girl, she felt that direct eye contact and a direct greeting would be too much. The teacher stressed that she was equally happy to have both children join the class every morning, but intentionally modified her greeting so the girl could be successful in the transition. Indeed, the girl did come into the room and soon began playing—there was no upset. She was not overwhelmed during the transition with behaviors of clinging to the parent and backing away from the teacher. Upon consideration, the parent of the girl agreed that the teacher's approach was what her daughter needed.

Here is an example of how an adult thought ahead and created specific environmental conditions to help two children successfully meet a potentially stressful situation while staying regulated. The adult changed the world so that the children could meet it well and thus experience well-being. During the pandemic, a grandmother was caring for her two grandchildren, ages two and four. The children had been home for an extended period and had not been out in public much. A friend of the grandmother was expected to come to the house and drop something off. The grandmother anticipated that the children might experience some degree of anxiety upon the arrival of the "stranger." She didn't want the children to run back to their bedroom when the friend arrived—she wanted them to stay near her so they could have exposure to a healthy social encounter. So, the grandmother created a "cozy house" in the kitchen with long colored silks for the roof and fleeces on the floor. (The kitchen was right near the front door.) She had the children settled on the floor of the cozy house, with a blanket over them, and was reading to them when the friend rang the doorbell. The grandmother went to the door, and the children were free to stay inside the cozy house or to come out to meet the friend and interact. There was no pressure for them to engage with the visitor. In this way, the children could meet the situation with self-initiated activity. One of the children stayed inside the cozy house until the very end of the visit and then peeked out, and the other child came out and spoke to the visitor for a short period. Both children were successful in staying regulated. The next time a visitor came over to the house, the children knew ahead of time, and they built their own cozy house. This routine happened several more times, and the children gradually grew more at ease. After a while, the cozy house was no longer needed.

THE ADULT'S ATTITUDE SUPPORTS THE DEVELOPING SENSE OF LIFE

The underlying attitude of the adults in these examples is a belief in the child's ability to meet a potentially stressful situation with support. The adults recognize the many small steps involved in a larger process of the child's coming into relationship with the wide world, and that this process unfolds over time and hopefully builds with each step. The adult supports the child by breaking down the world into bite-sized pieces so that, ultimately, the child can digest the world and receive nourishment from it. The adults themselves have faced the many challenges and heartbreaks of life—they have come to operate out of an attitude of, "I can handle what comes towards me in life. I can keep myself together, without falling to pieces. I can roll with it." My father, who had faced hardship during the depression, was a farmer, and the weather was often on his mind. I remember times as a child when we were in dire need of rain in order to make a crop. My father's response always was, "We'll take it as it comes." He lived a long, rich life of ninety-eight years. This attitude of the adult, which lives in the invisible part of the child's environment, is nonetheless tangible and reassuring for young children. Additionally, we help the child develop the sense of life by knowing our children well through our nuanced observations of their states. We recognize when the child is facing something that feels dangerous to them—when their autonomic nervous system is at risk of reacting with fight or flight. We support them with our realistic expectations of them and through the kind, compassionate, and confident way we help them co-regulate during these types of situations.

A RHYTHMIC ROUTINE SUPPORTS THE DEVELOPING SENSE OF LIFE

A rhythmical routine provides conditions for the child to get good and hungry and then feel satiated with a good meal, and also for the child to get good and tired out and then experience restful sleep. Experiencing these polarities is very healthy for the sense of life. Predictability arises through a rhythmic regularity in the day's sequences. This helps the child know what to expect and therefore to more readily meet the events of the day. We want the child to "go for it" and to "give it their all"—at whatever stage of development they are in. In this way, they are meeting the world well. At Sophia's Hearth, we get the snowplows out for the children when it snows. (The snowplows are pictured in appendix 4.) An older three-year-old in our childcare characteristically had difficulty settling down at rest time. One snowy day, this child plowed the snow for the entire time he was outside. Later, during rest time, he told his caregiver, "I plowed the snow! Now I'm going to sleep, and when I wake up, I'm going to plow the snow again!" That day he went to sleep easily and slept deeply.

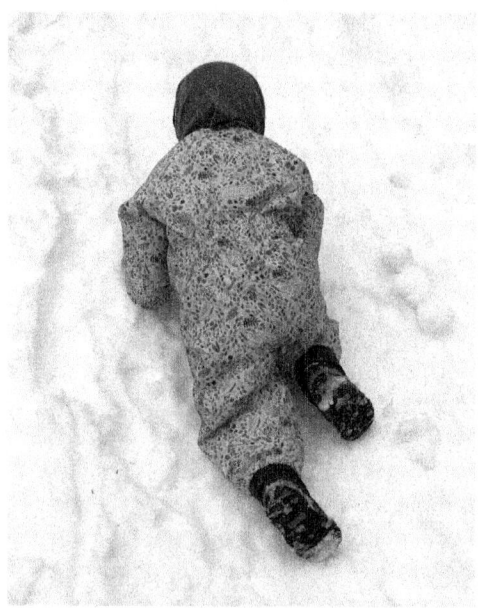

This child is climbing up a steep hill in the snow and then sliding down on their bottom. After playing outside in this way, they worked up a good appetite, had a hearty lunch, and easily went down for a nap.

OPPORTUNITIES FOR INNER SENSING TO SUPPORT THE DEVELOPING SENSE OF LIFE

The sense of life is in its element when children (or people of any age) are sensing their inner bodily state. Children involved in self-initiated activity will characteristically pause in the middle of their play and take a rest when needed. This is very healthy behavior! How many times do we as adults push ourselves too far, without listening to the inner state of our bodies, and then get sick?

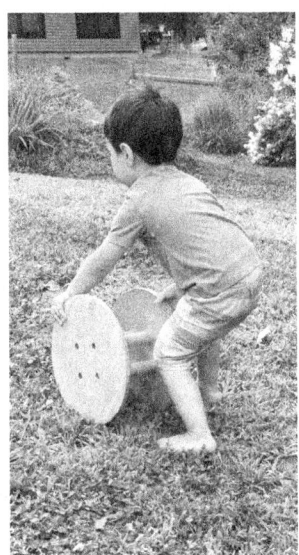 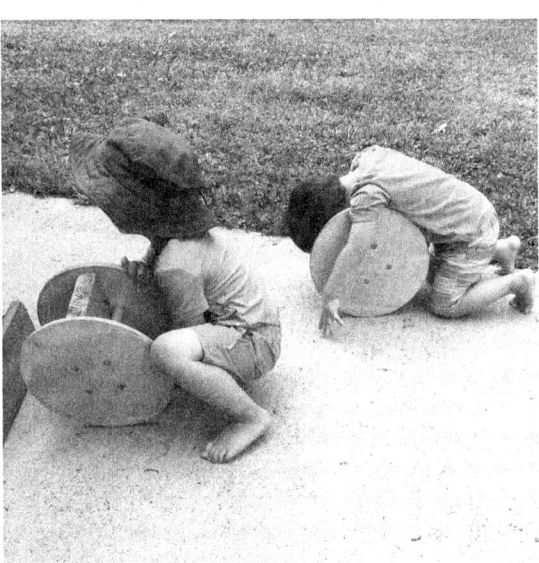

One afternoon, the children were pushing the round stools across the play yard. After a period of time, they rested. They were listening to the inner states of their bodies.

Inner sensing is enhanced when the child's motivation is internal—when they are not acting because an adult is encouraging them—when they are not performing a task to please an adult. When they do something out of their own initiative, they are more able to notice and act on their inner cues.

I once observed a crawling baby, who had just recently achieved pulling to stand. The baby was trying to climb onto her older sibling's seated scooter. She pulled to stand and was attempting to lift her leg over the seat. However, the scooter had wheels, and it moved just as she lifted her leg. She let out a vocalization, which had meaning to the effect of "Oh wow! This is unstable and I am in danger!" She automatically perceived that she had started to lose her balance, but then caught herself and didn't fall to the floor. Then she lowered herself down to the floor and crawled away. This is a good example of a situation where a child self-regulated—she experienced a degree of dysregulation, yet she managed the situation on her own, and she recovered. Additionally, she also was developing judgment regarding her abilities—I did not see her try to get on the scooter again for several months. (Later on, she did master climbing onto the scooter.)

States of Regulation

SENSORY DEFENSIVENESS, A STATE OF DYSREGULATION

Sometimes children (and people of any age) perceive sensory input as dangerous, and they respond with a fight-or-flight response—when, in actuality, there is no danger and their response is out of proportion to the actual event. This condition is known as sensory defensiveness, sensory hypersensitivity, or over-reactivity. In a young child, fighting may manifest as hitting and kicking, for example. Fleeing may manifest as pulling back, looking away, or running away and hiding. An older child may have a more sophisticated response and say something like, "My mom doesn't want me to do that." The sense involved in most sensory defensiveness is tactile. Defensiveness occurs in other senses as well. For example, I have had several of the clients in my private practice react defensively to the color green. Additionally, some people are defensive to certain smells. I know an adult who had to go to a motel one night because skunk smell had invaded his house. There are children who are unable to use a public restroom or eat in the school lunchroom because the smells are too offensive to them. There are also children who are defensive to the sound of a hair dryer or a blender, for example. Sensory defensiveness is a problem with regulation. It is a problem in the sense of life.

Most pediatric occupational therapists and some pediatric physical therapists are trained in ways to mitigate sensory defensiveness in children.

SENSORY DISCRIMINATION, A STATE OF REGULATION

The developing child is learning to discriminate. During discrimination, the salient qualities of sensory input are detected, and differences between sensations are noticed. For example, a child discriminates when they can tell whether they are speaking in a loud voice or not, whether this toy is heavier than that toy, and whether "five" rhymes with "hive." "Sensory discrimination develops with neurological maturation. As a child matures, [they respond] less protectively to every sensation and [become] more discriminatory about what is happening in [their] body and in [their] environment."[24]

When children (or people of any age) are engaged in sensory discrimination, different neurological circuits, which are distinct from those involved in a fight-or-flight response, are active. Facilitating use of the discriminatory circuitry can support a person to recover more easily when they do go into a fight or flight response. Many techniques have been developed to support people who are recovering from post-traumatic stress syndrome. If a person becomes triggered and responds with a fight or flight response, one of the techniques to assist them in recovering from the triggered state is to use a 5-4-3-2-1 grounding technique. In this technique, you notice five things in your environment with the sense of sight, four things with the sense of touch, three with the sense of hearing, two with the sense of smell, and one with the sense of taste. These tasks all involve sensory discrimination, which switches the neurological circuitry. I was a movement education teacher in the younger grades for five years in a Waldorf school, and I used sensory discrimination to help my older students regulate. For example, I would ask the third grade class to listen for two different sounds as they walked through the halls, and they would tell me the sounds that they heard after the transition. This engagement in sensory discrimination helped the children stay regulated. These types of activities are generally appropriate for children over seven, because they are explicit methods and do not entail working out of imitation. (Working out of imitation will be covered in detail in volume 2.)

PLAY INVOLVES BOTH UP-REGULATION AND DOWN-REGULATION

When young children become deeply engaged in play, they naturally discriminate. For example, when children build structures and designs with blocks, they distinguish between the different colors, shapes, and sizes of the blocks. In this way, play builds capacities for self-regulation.

Stephen Porges PhD, who is mentioned above as the originator of the polyvagal theory, has written about the inherent benefits of play for regulation. In his article "Play as a Neural Exercise: Insights from the Polyvagal Theory," he questions a common assumption about learning. He says, "From an educator's perspective, play is the antithesis of learning; play steals the precious time that could be dedicated to learning. This perspective is based on assumptions derived from learning theories that were outlined by behaviorists about 100 years ago. What if this perspective, prevalent in our society, is outdated? What if play, rather than displacing learning experiences, actually provides a neural exercise that would facilitate learning?"[25]

Indeed, for many years now, as schools have been forced to teach so the children perform well on standardized tests, recess has been limited and even eliminated in grade schools across the United States. In the above-mentioned article, Porges describes how play is a means for the child to learn to quickly and efficiently regulate, and he states that this ability to regulate is "as important as IQ and motivation in predicting classroom performance."[26]

When young children play with each other, things happen unexpectedly. The play can feel comfortably exciting, and then it can quickly cross over to feeling dangerous. I recently watched two children, ages four and six, playing together. They were playing an animal game, and the older child made a scary face and snarled. After a couple of times, the younger child was obviously distressed and told the older child to stop it. The older child stopped and resumed her normal affect. Their play then evolved into something

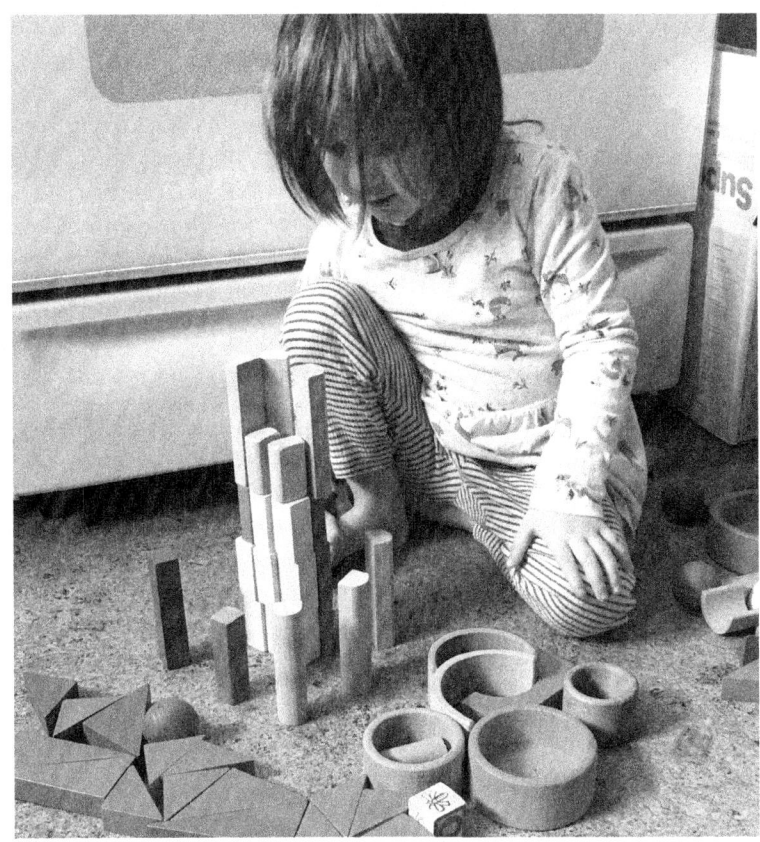

This child spent an extended period carefully creating patterns and structures with the blocks. They were discriminating between the various shapes and colors.

else. In this situation, the younger child was becoming scared and was on the verge of entering into a fight or flight condition. However, she managed to act, instead of react, and told the older one to stop. After the older child stopped, the younger child realized that the danger was gone and quickly downregulated to a calm, settled state. In this particular interaction, the children successfully resolved the issue on their own, although, of course, sometimes an adult is needed. Additionally, over time, I have seen children learn to recognize another child's stress and to offer help for them to recover from such "mini jolts." Essentially, what is happening is that the regulatory system of the child is being exercised. Just as fevers exercise the immune system, so do such interactions in play exercise the autonomic nervous system. Ultimately, these successful stress and recovery experiences serve to strengthen the sense of life. In this way, the child learns to *bounce back*. They learn to meet what comes toward them from the world with *resilience*.

The jack-in-the-box is a classic toy in which young children typically experience excitement as they anticipate Jack popping up. The growing excitement surges when Jack pops up, and then it resolves. Hide-and-seek is another game with a similar pattern of excitement.

Stephen Porges interprets play from the polyvagal theory's perspective: "The process of play is about active inhibition of the neural circuit that promotes fight/flight behaviors. Play functions as a neural exercise that improves the efficiency of the neural circuit that can instantaneously downregulate fight/flight behaviors."[27] He goes on to say that this type of neural nimbleness can translate to other situations. For example, in the classroom setting, it can support learning.

In the baby, perhaps the first game that exercises this neural circuitry is the classic game of peek-a-boo. The child typically experiences a degree of excitement when the adult's face is covered. Then, when the adult's face returns, along with a warm yet matter-of-fact tone of voice, the child recovers to a well-regulated state. It is very helpful if the adult doesn't overdo the exciting aspect of the game, so that the game doesn't become too stimulating for the child. In fact, the adult doesn't need to teach the baby to play peek-a-boo! The child will come to this game by themselves, in their own time. One can imagine that the child self-initiates peek-a-boo at the most opportune time for them—when their autonomic nervous system has matured enough to successfully manage the excitement of the game.

Our Spatial Configuration and the Sense of Life
THE SPATIAL COMPONENT OF MEETING THE WORLD

Let us consider sensory defensiveness through the lens of how a person lives in the spaces in and around their bodies. I am indebted to Jaimen McMillan, founder and director of the Spacial Dynamics Institute, for introducing me to the spatial phenomenon of sensory defensiveness. I have personally found it to be invaluable in my work with young children and their families. Earlier in the chapter, we spoke at length about the body space, or the inner volume space. Living into this space—fully embodying it—is the cornerstone of health and well-being. The young child is coming to inhabit the body space through the healthy development of the four foundational senses, as well as through the experience of the primitive reflexes. (The spatial development of the child in relation to the integration of the primitive reflexes will be discussed in volume 2.)

In addition to the body space, the personal space is another developing space in the young child. The personal space extends about an arm's length in front of and around the body. When people shake hands, they naturally shake at the border of their personal space. Some people shake hands close to their bodies, and some farther out in front of their bodies. These distances reflect the degree to which an individual's personal space is filled out. The personal space varies between each person, and it also changes over time—even from moment to moment—for the same individual.

The personal space serves as a protective buffer. When this space is thoroughly filled out, the person appears robust and "plumped up" in a healthy way. When this space is collapsed and shrunken, the person can be characterized as "pinched" or "drawn." Recall the figure in Edvard Munch's painting *The Scream*. The person with compromised personal space may feel as if they have "been through the wringer," "run over by a truck," or "flattened." If the personal space is not filled out, its buffering activity does not function well. As a result, the sensations from the environment literally come in toward the body too closely—and this causes distress. It can also happen that when something from the environment comes in too close and invades the personal space, the personal space does not withstand the assault and collapses, and the person experiences upset. Here is a simple example. A grown friend of mine was at a picnic. Unfortunately, a bee flew up under his shirt. Even though he didn't get stung, he ripped off his shirt and ran. He would have very likely been able to stay regulated if the bee was simply in the vicinity, but when it got that close, his personal space collapsed, and he reacted with flight.

Another friend recounted to me what happens to him when he walks through the terminal of a major airport. He experiences the noises and the lights as jarring and piercing. He describes these auditory and visual sensations as literally entering his body. This is not an uncommon occurrence for people. From a spatial point of view, what is happening is a collapse of the buffer space surrounding the body—in which case it can't do its job of shielding the person against the invading sensations. Failed buffer spaces are the spatial explanation for sensory defensiveness.

HOW DOES THE PERSONAL SPACE DEVELOP IN THE GROWING CHILD?

The personal space is an enlivened space. We imbue our personal space with our own substance. It is literally a part of us. We intuitively perceive this space as ours, and we don't like it if people come into our personal space uninvited. There is a reason for the expression "Get out of my face." The socially acceptable distances that we keep from other people stem from the typical parameters of people's personal spaces, and these differ from culture to culture.

The development of the personal space happens over time, and its maturity does not come to full fruition until after puberty. A crawling baby will come right up close to your face. This reflects that they do not yet have a well-established personal space. The infant begins to enliven the space in front of their body as they find their hands and look at them, and later when they play with toys in this position. They continue to build up their personal space when playing in prone on elbows and prone on extended arms, and when crawling. In these activities, especially, they come to an intimate relationship with the space in front of their bodies.

These babies are continuing to develop their personal space in the prone positions.

Very young children often become attached to a particular doll or a stuffed animal. The child imbues the doll with their spatial substance. When they hold and carry a doll around, they typically hold it in front of themselves, and this serves to enhance the personal space of the child. In this way, they may better meet a new or questionable situation because they have a little extra spatial padding around them.

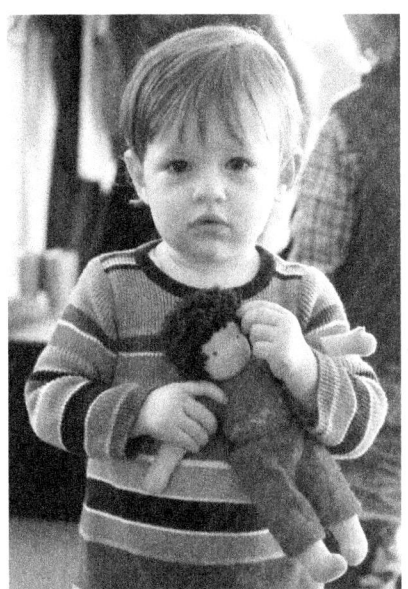

This child is attached to their dolly and carries it around frequently.

It is helpful to note that too many stuffed animals or dolls can be overwhelming to a child. If a child is not attaching to one, or more, of their dolls or stuffed animals, then it is often better to put most of them away, so the child's space is not cluttered. When a child's environment is too full of objects to which they do not bond, they may be practicing being scattered instead of the stillness that comes with being able to take in what is around them. Instead of inadvertent indifference, a child will practice attachment and caring, along with spatial sharing and expansion.[28] One mother described her child as detached when she was eighteen months old. The child had a plethora of stuffed animals and did not play with any of them. A friend of the family cleaned out her room, leaving only a few carefully selected toys and one special doll. That evening, when the parents put their daughter to bed, it was striking to them how she reached out and brought this doll close to her. With her arms still around the doll, she fell asleep. She continued to sleep with the doll until she was fourteen! The mother noticed that her daughter formed more connections with other people and objects after the clutter was removed.

Young children naturally want to play dress-up. This is a healthy activity for the sense of life, as the puffy clothing and extra sheaths of capes, vests, and hats can help them fill out the buffer space, so that the inner volume space is protected and kept sovereign. As an adult, I once had a small part in a play—just a few lines. I had never been in a play before, and I was experiencing some anxiety. Fortunately, they dressed me up as an older, slightly overweight male—literally stuffing a pillow under my shirt. This extra padding did the trick. It served as my protective buffer. I was able to live into this space, and I had no stage fright during the performance. We can tell children stories about birds who puff themselves up with their feathers or porcupines who puff themselves up with their quills in order to successfully scare off a predator.

In general, dressing infants and young children in layers supports them to fill out their personal space. (However, one would not want a child to become overheated or dressed such that the layers would inhibit their movements.) Indeed, young children who need extra protection often wisely know what they need, and pull down the brims of their hats when they feel a little threatened. Older students sometimes insist on wearing bulky hoodies, even in warmer weather. Wrapping up preschool and kindergarten-aged children in "burrito wraps" or "cocoons" are also good opportunities for enhancing their personal spaces. It can be helpful to have the child arrive early to school and cocoon them, letting them stay in the cocoon for a period of time before the other children arrive. This helps build up a protective sheathing around the child, and thus they are better prepared to meet their classmates. Similarly, sleep sacks provide extra sheathing for infants.

It is also helpful to provide young children with "plumping stations" or "sheathing stations." These are protected places where the child can go to regroup and reconfigure their personal space. The early childhood teacher can prepare a couple of special spaces in the classroom where it is understood that this is a place for a child to be alone when they want to be—perhaps in a bottom cupboard with the door removed and with a colored silk covering the opening, or perhaps in a dog bed covered with a small comforter. At home, a similar space can be created. Children are naturally drawn to these small, cozy spaces. One parent, who grew up in the tropics, got a mosquito net and placed it over her child's bed. In this way, the child felt more settled and could go to sleep more easily. Old-fashioned canopy beds also serve this purpose.

THE PERSONAL SPACE IS TENUOUS IN THE YOUNG CHILD

Two-year-olds have established a degree of personal space. However, it is fragile and fleeting. For example, if a two-year-old initiates a game of catch with an adult, the child may hold their arms out straight in front of their body to catch the ball. However, chances are that when the ball is thrown, they will physically wince away from the incoming ball. In addition to the physical movement of pulling back, the personal space will also shrink back. The child typically blinks, unaware, for a moment, of what has happened. When they "come to," they find the ball on the floor. This is also described as a startle reaction. (The startle reaction will be discussed in more detail in volume 2.) In order to help the child keep continuous expansion of their personal space and stay present throughout the activity, we need to "change the world" so that the child can successfully meet it. For example, we could come closer to the child and very gently toss the ball to them, or we could sit down on the floor and gently roll it to them. We want to engage with the child in a manner that allows the child to succeed in keeping their personal space intact. In this way, the child doesn't "practice" a pattern of collapsing their personal space, which is an unhelpful gesture.

In my pediatric physical therapy practice, I have worked with many older children to help them learn to catch a ball with "alligator hands." (The child holds their hands such that the bottom hand is palm up and the top hand is palm down.) When the ball comes to them, the alligator's hands bite the ball, instead of the ball biting the child, i.e., instead of their personal space collapsing in on them. The child stands with their hands showing the place where they want to catch the ball, which is at the border of their personal space. The therapist stands relatively close to the child and gently tosses the ball right into the child's hands, so they can catch it and remain fully present, without any receding gesture of their personal space. Over time the therapist steps back and makes the catch more and more difficult, carefully watching that the child continues to keep their personal space intact. The child eventually learns to *step toward* the incoming ball and catch it. Once a child learns the spatial gesture of maintaining their personal space during a game of catch, that gesture can transfer to other situations—including social situations, where they can "hold their ground."

One can learn to perceive the dynamic changes in the personal space of a child in day-to-day circumstances. The adult supports the child by noticing what environmental situations cause their personal space to recede. Common causes include too much eye contact, pointing a camera at them, criticizing—and also praising—them, and simply directing too much attention at them. I recall an incident of young child who was an early walker. She and her mother were at the post office, waiting in line. A well-meaning stranger addressed the child with a compliment, and the child quickly disappeared into the folds of the mother's skirt. It was too much input coming toward the child—she couldn't meet the situation, her personal space collapsed, and her whole body withdrew. Luckily, she could take cover right away.

When the infant and young child are subject to quickly changing, abrupt, erratic movements, this can negatively affect the child's budding personal space. When I was a child, my sisters and I would take a balloon, rub it on our clothes to make static electricity, stick it to our clothes, and then walk around the house, trying to keep the balloon from falling off. If we moved slowly and carefully, the balloon would stay attached. If we moved too quickly or abruptly, it would fall off. This is a good image to have in mind when we pick up and carry young infants—we want to move them in a manner that will keep their personal space intact, as it is tenuous and incomplete. When young children go into "bounce houses,"* they can become "out of themselves." With all of the sudden and unexpected movement—especially when there are other children present—their personal space becomes "unglued," and they "can't hold themselves together."

Here is an example of a situation where a child initially was not able to meet what was coming toward her from the world. A parent brought her child to see a pediatric therapist because the child was experiencing selective mutism. The girl did not speak at school or in public. If she had to communicate, she would whisper to one special friend or to her mother in order that the confidant would speak for her. The parent and the teacher were dealing with this condition by asking the child direct questions and encouraging her to respond, and they felt she was not making progress.

When the child came to see the therapist, the therapist did not ask direct questions of the child, nor did she give the child too much eye contact. The therapist did not stand opposite the child, but instead stood at the child's side, and created activities that the child could do out in front of the two of them. In other words, the therapist did not direct any gesture in toward the child's body. She consciously did not put the child's personal space in jeopardy of receding by putting the child "on the spot." The remarkable thing was that the child spontaneously spoke three times to the therapist during the first session. The child did not need many visits to the therapist. The therapist explained the phenomenon of personal space to the parent and the teacher, and how to change the world so that the child could meet it at the border of her personal space, without any wincing back. It did not take long before the child was speaking freely at school.

Inconsistent Sensory Sensitivity

I recently spoke to the mother of a child who experiences auditory sensitivities. She said that her child could sometimes tolerate certain noises with no problem, and yet at other times, she could not tolerate the same noise or a similar level of noise. This is not uncommon, and it can be confusing to parents. It is helpful to

---

* Bounce houses are inflatable structures, resembling castles or other such buildings, made for the purpose of letting children jump inside them.

understand that when children—and people of any age—are interested and actively engaged, their ego forces are active, and they are meeting the world well. As a result, the child perks up, they plump up, and they are protected from sensory overwhelm. Similarly, people who routinely get car sick when they are the passenger don't get sick when they are the driver. As the driver, their ego forces are engaged, as opposed to being in the passive stance of the passenger.

The Movement Gestalt and Sensory Sensitivity

Jaimen McMillan characterizes the *spatial gestalt* as the shifting forms and dynamics of movement which surround a person's physical body. Included in the spatial gestalt are the many individual dynamic paths of movement on and around the body. McMillan refers to these as streams. (The streams are discussed further in volume 2.) They are also known as etheric or life force currents. The streams undergo development and can be influenced for better or worse throughout the course of one's life. As adults, we can learn to consciously influence and change them. This typically takes a movement training, done over a period of time. One example is the Spacial Dynamics training. Why would one want to cultivate awareness of one's streams and achieve facility in changing them? The streams have archetypal directions and forms that are life-enhancing when care is taken that they are properly developed. When the streams have poor form or even a reversed direction, there can be negative effects on a person in body, soul, and spirit. Proper use of the streams will result in positive functional movement patterns. When one can learn to establish the archetypal patterns of the streams, one's life can unfold in new ways. The streams have a relationship with the personal space, and the personal space is also included in the spatial gestalt. The spatial gestalt is an entirety. It is the totality of the way the person lives in their space. If any single part of the gestalt develops or changes, the whole of the gestalt is affected, either positively or negatively.[29]

A mother whose child had a high degree of tactile defensiveness brought her in to see a pediatric therapist. Getting dressed every morning was an ordeal, and the girl could only tolerate wearing a couple of outfits. The therapist tried deep pressure, as this is the classic treatment for tactile defensiveness. Deep pressure often mitigates sensory defensiveness (including tactile, auditory, and olfactory defensiveness, etc.) This is because deep pressure is generally calming and can help the child move out of the fight-or-flight state.

However, this child was unable to tolerate deep pressure, so the therapist addressed the child's spatial gestalt with a number of specially designed activities. What finally unlocked the tactile defensiveness was handstands! The girl was very interested in learning to do handstands, and she practiced for extended periods every day until she mastered them. When one successfully achieves a handstand, the archetypal forms and directions of the arm and leg streams are established. Prior to this, the directions of the child's arm and leg streams were reversed. In this case, mastery of handstands reconfigured the child's entire spatial gestalt, including the buffer space peripheral to the physical body. The buffer space could then carry out its protective function, and the tactile defensiveness resolved.

Another parent brought in his very young child, who had severe auditory defensiveness. She couldn't tolerate certain noises, such as a blender or a vacuum cleaner, and would scream for over an hour if triggered. The child was also a severe toe-walker. The therapist addressed the toe-walking first. As soon as her heels came down and she walked with a good heel strike, her balance improved and the noise sensitivity abated and ultimately ceased. In order to walk with the heels down, the archetypal patterns and directions of the streams of the legs must be established. Prior to this, the leg streams were moving in the opposite direction. In this case, the establishment of a proper gait pattern reconfigured the child's entire spatial gestalt. As a result, the personal space as well as the space around the child's head were enhanced. These buffer spaces could then perform their protective function, and the noise sensitivity ceased.

14: The Sense of Self-Movement

At birth, the baby is able to move every muscle in their body, but their movements are far from coordinated. Development of the sense of *self-movement* plays a key role for the development of healthy, fluid movement. What has helped me the most to understand the nuances of the sense of self-movement, and especially how to support its development and work with a child who is experiencing a challenge in this sense, is my study of Spacial Dynamics under the tutelage of Jaimen McMillan. In fact, the exercises and activities of Spacial Dynamics are specifically designed to support the development of the sense of self-movement. Therefore, I am grateful to Jaimen McMillan for much of the content of this chapter, especially the relationship of the sense of self-movement to the countermovement and the life force streams that are discussed later in the chapter.

The sense of self-movement is also commonly referred to as the sense of proprioception, and sometimes as the sense of position. It is the third of the four foundational senses, and like the others, it is largely outside of our awareness. With the sense of self-movement, we perceive the movements of our own body parts in relationship to each other, without having to look at them. The famous British neurologist and author Oliver Sacks describes proprioception as "a vital sense which tells us the position of our limbs, informing us exactly of all their movements. It is indispensable for our motor control, for any movement we make and even for the maintenance of our posture at every second. If it is cut off even momentarily we collapse."[1] Thanks to this sense, we can tell if our elbow is bent or straight, or if it is bending or straightening, for example. However, we usually aren't aware of the movement or the position of our elbow. We simply use our arm. In order to have coordinated movement, the awareness of what our arm is doing is necessary—it is just that this is usually under the radar of consciousness.

When there is an immaturity or a challenge in the sense of self-movement, we use vision as a compensation. This is what babies do when they initially start to grasp—they don't yet have a well-developed sense of self-movement, and so they look at their hand in order to know what it's doing and therefore to accomplish what they want to do. For the same reason, babies also look at their feet when they lie on their backs and play with toys with their feet. Early in life, the child gets the feedback of what their hands and feet are doing largely from their eyes instead of from the proprioceptive sense organs, which are embedded into the muscles, tendons, and joints. The proprioceptive organs in the muscles are known as muscle spindles, those in the tendons as Golgi tendon organs, and those in the joints as joint receptors.

We can better understand a particular sense by learning what a person goes through when they have difficulty with that sense. I once worked with a woman who had had a stroke. She had lost proprioception in one leg—she couldn't feel its position or how it was moving. However, she could still move the leg—there was no paralysis. Yet, in normal daily function, her movements were awkward and very challenging for her. To stand, she had to look at her leg and pay full and continuous attention to it. This is similar to what the baby does when they first use their hand, as mentioned above. The woman needed a walker in order to walk. She also did everything she could to avoid moving. It was exhausting for her to pay such close attention to her leg. Her family did not understand why she was so anxious and hesitant to move. After all, her leg was not paralyzed—why was she withdrawing? I explained that her behavior was understandable. Sensorially, she didn't have "a leg to stand on." She wasn't grounded in her body, and this had a huge impact on her emotional life.

We can perhaps have an inkling of what it was like for this woman if we imagine a situation when we are confined for an extended period of time—perhaps when we must remain sitting on a long airplane ride or at a meditation retreat—and our leg falls asleep. When we stand up and aren't able to feel our leg, it is very disconcerting.

The Remarkable Story of Ian Waterman

It is very rare for a person to suffer a complete loss of proprioception. However, this is what happened to a young man named Ian Waterman, who lived in Great Britain, in 1971. He was nineteen years old. He cut his hand, got the stomach flu, and suffered an inflammation of the sensory nerves for the senses of touch and proprioception supplying his entire body below his neck. He lost these sensations permanently. In his book written with Ian, *Pride and a Daily Marathon*, author and neurologist Jonathan Cole describes the remarkable way that Ian learned to compensate for his condition and how it affected his life.[2] I highly recommended this book for its unique insights into the sense of proprioception. The loss of proprioception presented as Ian's biggest challenge. Although the loss of the sense of touch was also complete, Ian was able to compensate to some degree for this with his sense of temperature and sense of life (which registers pain and muscle fatigue), which were still intact, thankfully.

Here is an incident relating how Ian compensated for the lack of touch sensations with the sense of temperature:

> The nights were the worst. He would lie awake for hours. Once a young nurse came and sat by his bed, holding his hand as they chatted away. Occasionally she would disappear to see to someone else, or do a round, but she always came back. Ian remembers her as tall with dark hair and a kind face, but most of all he remembers her warm hands holding his. Contact was desperately important even though he could feel only the warmth. Her simple human kindness counted for more than all the talk and bustle he received from others.[3]

Initially, after the sensory loss, Ian reacted the same way as the woman who had had the stroke. There was no paralysis, but he didn't want to move. Cole describes the situation:

> [Ian] could not feel anything [via the sense of touch] with his arms, his legs or his body. That was frightening enough, but he had no awareness of their position either. It wasn't that the muscular power was affected, since he could make an arm move. But he had no ability to control the speed or direction of the movement. Any movement happened in a totally unexpected way. It was pointless to try.[4]

Cole also relates that Ian felt that it was dangerous to move. For example, when he initially tried to sit up, he ended up falling out of bed. Several times, he inadvertently hit family and friends who were visiting him, because he couldn't control his limbs. Similarly, one time he inadvertently knocked over a physiotherapist who was working with him. Ian required total care for many months. Here we see how crucial an intact sense of proprioception is for any degree of coordinated movement. All movement is a sensorimotor process, and the sensory component is by far the most important aspect of the process. Here, also, we can notice the important relationship between the sense of self-movement and the will.

The Sense of Proprioception, Impossible to Comprehend

Cole goes on to relate how utterly indescribable Ian's condition was to him and to others, including many of the doctors and physiotherapists. Ian's condition was so rare, and, as was mentioned previously, input from the sense of proprioception is usually not in our consciousness. We take it for granted. We don't think about it or talk about it.

[Ian] was further handicapped by problems of communication and comprehension. These perceptions of movement and posture, and of sensation, are so intimate, so essential to us, that they seem scarcely to reach our thinking selves: and words to express them are lacking.... Though the problems are more profound than we think, we can at least imagine what it is like to be blind and perhaps deaf. Ian's loss is beyond words and almost beyond imagination.[5]

The fact that words don't exist for this condition speaks volumes to our lack of awareness of it.

Here is a telling anecdote from when Ian was first in the hospital:

The family would visit, and his brother was puzzled at how Ian would "waste sweets." They would put one in his hand, and when he tried to put it in his mouth the arm would come up away from his head and throw the sweet behind him. Meringues were crushed in his hand. They all saw it without knowing why.[6]

Characteristic Feelings Arising from the Sense of Proprioception and Its Loss

Ian experienced powerful feelings during his arduous rehabilitation. He wrote poems at this time, and typically destroyed them afterwards. Only one poem remains. "What is striking," notes Jonathan Cole, "apart from the fact that it obviously originated in his work experience [Ian was a butcher before his loss of sensation], is its equation of lack of movement with lack of life."[7] Here is an excerpt from Ian Waterman's poem, "Living Death":

> Turned every two hours
> Like a joint of meat.
> Basted with lotions.
> Unmoving like a statue [...]
> What use an active brain
> Without mobility?[8]

Henning Köhler talks about a person's soul state when there are disruptions in the sense of proprioception. He describes these disturbances in the sense of proprioception as manifesting "a depressed state of mind."[9] As mentioned in chapter 10, Rudolf Steiner credits the development of the sense of self-movement with our experience of ourselves as free souls: "It is due to what streams into your soul from the muscular contractions and elongations."[10] It follows that if one is not properly sensing one's muscular contractions and elongations, then one would lack an experience of oneself as a free soul, as "Living Death" so poignantly relates. Ian did not experience himself as a free soul, and it is logical that he would feel depressed. Understandably, this period of Ian's rehabilitation was a difficult time of adjustment for him.

Ian's Rehabilitation

When Ian was first learning to stand and walk, he often fell. In fact, falling was inevitable if he was going to learn to walk, and so, "he had to learn to fall correctly. To fall tensely was to risk greater injury and pain, and once he hurt his back."[11] This passage could easily describe babies as they journey from their initial horizontal position of back-lying all the way up into standing and walking. It is inevitable that the child will fall along the way. Sometimes they may fall all the way to the ground, and sometimes they may start to fall, but catch themselves. It is important that they, too, learn to fall correctly.

Despite all of the formidable trials, Ian demonstrated remarkable tenacity and resilience in his recovery. He explained that he was too proud to give up—hence the first word in the title of his biography (*Pride and a Daily Marathon*). He learned to sit, use utensils, and feed himself. He learned to perform his self-care activities, and, remarkably, he learned to walk without an assistive devise. He learned these things through exquisite planning and utter and complete mental concentration. Therefore, "any interruption was disastrous. If he sneezed, he fell over in a heap, and he quickly learnt to sit or lie down until the sneeze had passed. He could not walk and daydream at the same time."[12] Also, if the lights went out so that he couldn't see his limbs, he was incapacitated. He slept with a light on so that he could visually orient himself to the positions of his limbs as soon as he woke up.

As Ian got better at planning and visually monitoring his movements, the quality of his movements did improve somewhat, but he never achieved the graceful, coordinated movements that he had before his sensory loss. As a butcher, he had developed a high degree of coordination and skill.

Ultimately, Ian did get his life back. He accomplished functional movements, though they appeared stiff and awkward. He studied for a new profession, held down a desk job, and was well liked and accepted at work. He was known for his sense of humor. Additionally, he had two happy marriages. (His first wife died of cancer.)

Automatic Movements

For the typical person with intact proprioception, the vast majority of our movements are automatic. When we learn a new skill, for example when we learn to tie our shoes, initially it may be difficult and we must pay close attention to what we are doing. But after we have learned the skill, the task becomes automatic—and easy. We can tie our shoes while thinking of something else, and even while looking at something else.

When babies are born, they haven't yet developed a repertoire of automatic skills. Karl König explains that "We can only come to a fundamental understanding of motor activity when we begin to look at it as a musical process."[13] Dr. König explains that throughout the entire gross motor sequence, babies are "developing their instruments for the music of movement."[14] He describes the musical instrument of the body as similar to a violin or cello. The child is also tasked with developing their muscle tone, which König describes as the tension on the strings—the tendons and muscles—of the instrument. If the movement is stiff, the tension of the strings is too much. If the movement is floppy, the tension of the strings is too slack. When the muscle tone and the instrument are tuned, "then motor activity can begin to play on this instrument; melodies or movement patterns begin to develop."[15] König goes on to say that, optimally, we continue to learn and master new melodies, or new movement patterns, on our bodily instruments throughout our lives. Recall that in chapter 3, Julian de Ajuriaguerra observes that in order for harmonious movement to occur, there must be a fluid attunement of the opposing muscle groups. He refers to this phenomenon as a "kinetic melody."

In Ian Waterman's case, unfortunately, because of the complete lack of proprioception, he was not able to master new melodies on his bodily instrument. The loss of the sense of proprioception resulted in a complete lack of automatic movements, and all of Ian's movements required a high degree of consciousness as well as constant visual monitoring. This takes an incredible amount of effort! For Ian, each day was a marathon—the second part of his biography's title. At the end of his rehabilitation period,

> despite all his effort to relearn movements, his repertoire and daily routines remained very different from other people's. All movements still had to be under conscious control and continuous visual inspection. Without thought there was no movement. His actions for the day, for any day, reflected his thoughts for the day. These thoughts were the result of nearly three years' experimentation: three years of thinking all day, every day—thinking how to get by while still having some mental energy available to do more than just get by, for he wanted not just to function but to live.[16]

When Ian achieved a new task, it did not become automatic. Instead, he had to maintain the same degree of effort every subsequent time he performed it. In addition to being physically challenging, this must have been emotionally difficult for Ian, as the people around him, for the most part, did not have "the faintest idea how hard it was for him."[17]

The Countermovement

Ian's account of how he managed his life without automatic movements begins, "If someone said reach for something I knew I couldn't simply do it but had to move an arm and then a leg in the opposite way to compensate."[18] Later, he says, "This need to concentrate was total. I cannot emphasize enough the effort needed to build up in my mind every move and countermove."[19] Here is an example of what Ian had to consider in order to perform the seemingly simple task of shifting the location of an object that he was holding: "If he wants to move an object he is holding from his side to the front of him, he first has to think that he must lean back a little to prevent the extra weight in front from pulling him over."[20]

Professional violinist Hiroko Matsukawa has observed that she naturally employs the countermovement. She related to me that playing the violin sometimes involves quick shifts of the fingers when going from a low note to a high note, and this can be challenging. She said that to be successful in reaching the high notes, she has to ground herself spatially—she has to descend into the depths in equal measure.[21]

Coordinated movement is the signpost of a healthy sense of proprioception, and underlying the coordination is an innate facility with the countermovement. Partner dancers are masters of the countermovement. The old joke is that Ginger Rogers did everything that Fred Astaire did, only backward and in heels. Let us consider the differences between the movements of a dancer and those of Ian Waterman. Dancers, classically, have well-developed senses of proprioception, whereas Ian's sense of proprioception was absent. The dancer is not operating out of their head. Instead, the dancer is sensing out beyond their limbs, perceiving the movement cues of the partner, and then responding accordingly. Their movements are peripherally led. In contrast, Ian's movements were centrally led. He had to direct his movements via his thoughts. He was thinking constantly. The dancer is "thinking" with their limbs, not with their head. Dancers characteristically have graceful, efficient movements. In contrast, Ian's movements were characterized as slow, stiff, and having a lack of fluidity.

It would be a fair statement to say that the dancer's movements are enlivening to them and typically give them joy. I personally can attest to this. I studied dance from early grade school through college. In college, my coursework was primarily in the scientific fields of study. However, I made sure that I took a dance class every semester, and I also joined a performing dance club. The dancing fed me and literally gave me energy, which I needed to balance out the extensive amount of studying that I did. Unfortunately, Ian's movements did not give him energy. Instead, at the end of the day, he felt like he had run a marathon.

Rudolf Steiner and the Role of the Countermovement in the Sense of Self-Movement

Rudolf Steiner speaks about the countermovement in relation to the sense of self-movement or proprioception: "If we stretch out an arm, for example, destroying the balance through this change of position, the balance is immediately restored because the astral body is in a state of equilibrium. In proportion as we stretch out an arm the astral current streams in the opposite direction, thereby re-adjusting the balance. With every physical change of position, even merely blinking, the astral current in the organism moves in the opposite direction. In this inner experience of a process of equalization the sense of movement manifests itself."[22]

Rudolf Steiner proposes that with every movement, with every change of position in one of the segments of the body—even in the blinking of an eye—our balance is disturbed and must be equalized. What restores our balance is that an "astral" stream flows back in the opposite direction of the physical movement. This happens in the astral body. (The astral body is discussed in greater depth in volume 2.) Our ability to sense our own movements comes about through the inner experience of this astral countermovement. Rudolf Steiner explains that this inner experience is largely unconscious or subconscious. The Spacial Dynamics exercises invented by Jaimen McMillan, designed to develop one's sense of self-movement, explore the countermovement in great depth. The student of Spacial Dynamics learns to "stay awake in the dream" and perceive the countermovement—thus

FREE MOVEMENT FROM THE VERY START

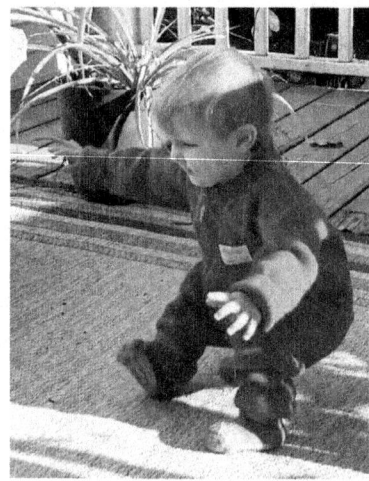

This child is new to walking. They have exaggerated the "down" gesture, and down they go!

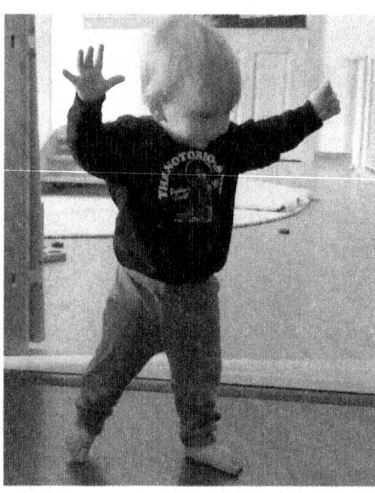

This child is also new to walking. They have an exaggeration of the upward forces, resulting in the arms flying up.

bringing what is normally unconscious or subconscious into "day" consciousness.[23]

It is noteworthy that perception of the countermovement typically occurs in a dream state of consciousness—in an unconscious or subconscious state. During the first three years of life, children are naturally in a dream state of consciousness, and this is when an incredible amount of development occurs in the sense of self-movement—they are constantly developing their coordination and learning new motor skills. It follows, then, that babies and toddlers are primed to be sensing the countermovement.

This is perhaps most apparent in a child who is just learning to walk. The child's legs are in relationship with the supporting surface. The direction of the gesture of the leg is out, away from the body, into the surface—the leg is raying out. In contrast, the gesture of the countermovement is back in, toward the body. With each step, the child is "measuring" the strength and the constancy of the two gestures. They are sensing the two opposing forces. This is a type of kinetic listening, and it is best not to interrupt them, for their ability to "listen" to these complementary forces is what make their steps successful. If the two gestures are equal, when the child steps and puts weight on the leg, it will hold them. If the child steps onto the leg and exaggerates the pushing down, the outgoing force is stronger, and they plop down on their bottom. If the child steps onto the leg and they don't push down enough, the incoming, upward force is stronger. Their arms elevate, they wobble, and may also fall. Over time and with practice, the child learns to balance the two gestures and they become more sure-footed. It is this type of invisible spatial activity that is responsible for the development of motor skills. Although we are not typically aware of this invisible activity, it is possible to develop the capacity to observe it.[24]

Several years ago, I had a remarkable experience of "staying awake in the dream," in which I perceived the countermovement. I had had an extensive knee surgery and had been on crutches for six weeks. I was not able to bear any weight through my leg during this time. When I finally was able to step onto my leg, I felt a gesture moving away from my foot down to the center of the earth. As the same time, I perceived a gesture coming back toward me from the earth. This was the countermovement. I felt profoundly welcomed by what was coming toward me from the earth, and it occurred to me in that moment that perhaps this is what it is like for the baby when they take their first steps. The gesture out and away from my leg was equally matched by the countermovement coming back toward me, and my leg held me.

Resistance and the Countermovement

The countermovement must be successfully dealt with for healthy movement to ensue. I remember watching an older two-year-old peel a carrot for the first time. It was a complex task, but he really wanted to peel that carrot! He was holding the carrot with his left hand and had the peeler in his right hand. He moved the peeler down the shaft of the carrot, away from his body. He had to have just the right amount of force (in toward his body) in order to stabilize the carrot against the outgoing peeling motion. This took some doing, but the boy made the appropriate adjustments and was successful. He was fully engaged with this task for an extended period. In this activity, he was working against resistance. Activities that involve resistance offer increased potential for an inner sensing of the countermovement, and hence for the development of the sense of self-movement.

Other examples of moving against resistance include walking uphill, walking through snow, or through water at the beach. The amount of resistance needs to be just the right amount—not too much and not too little. If it is too little, then the child has difficulty perceiving the countermovement, and these types of movements are often not satisfying and not performed well. However, resistance is counterproductive if it is too much, because then the child strains, which works against achieving fluid movement. For a toddler, walking on a slight incline, as opposed to a steep hill, gives a more appropriate amount of resistance. For a crawling baby, crawling on and off the Pikler box, over firm pillows on the floor, and up hills outside provide rich opportunities to develop the sense of proprioception, as these activities give more proprioceptive input than crawling on a level surface. Similarly, climbing on the Pikler wooden structures (shown in appendix 3) provides wonderful opportunities for the child to develop the proprioceptive system. Playing in wet sand gives more resistance than dry sand. For an older child, sawing, rasping, and hammering all involve moving against resistance. Also, for older children, playing with magnets is a wonderful activity for experiencing resistance in a fine motor activity.

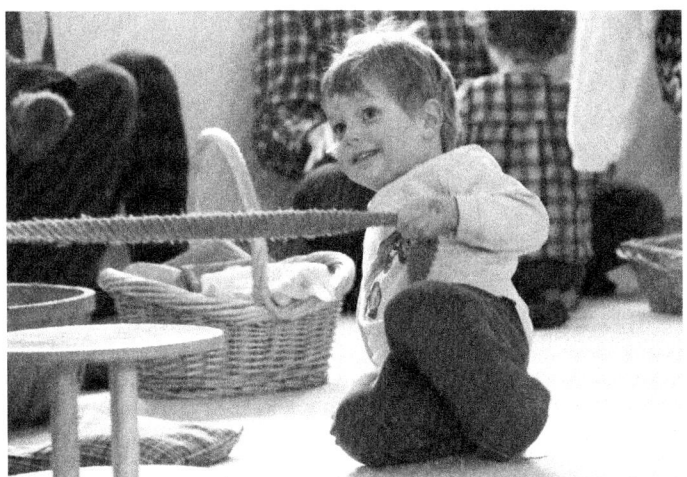

This child is getting a good amount of resistance, pulling on the knitted band.

Children who have decreased sensitivity to proprioceptive input naturally seek out activities that require increased resistance, as this affords them better opportunities to feel the countermovement. As a movement therapist trained in Spacial Dynamics, Marita Tulloch worked with a middle school boy who had significant challenges in his sense of proprioception. The boy was having a difficult time socially because he was perceived as too rough. For example, he would pat his classmates on the back, but was unable to tell how hard he was patting them, and it was perceived as too hard. The boy was awkward and broke things. When writing with a pencil, he pressed very hard into the paper and often broke the lead or tore the paper. What helped the student the most was learning to balance on top of a large wooden telephone cable spool (about four feet in diameter) and roll it forward. After he learned to maneuver the spool, the therapist added playing toss and catch with a weighted medicine ball while he was maneuvering the spool. In this way, the boy learned to master the countermovement. When he threw the ball, he had to counterbalance the throw with a slight backward shift of his core. When he caught the ball, he had to counterbalance the catch with a slight forward shift of his core. For some people, this activity would have been too much. However, this boy needed a very high degree of proprioceptive input, and the activity met him.[25]

We all have our proprioceptive likes and dislikes, and this manifests in some of the mundane details of life. For example, people often have a favorite type of pen or pencil because it gives them just the right amount of resistance to satisfy their proprioceptive preferences. The boy who is mentioned above needed a very sturdy, sizable pencil.

Here is an example of an elderly woman who was at the other end of the proprioceptive preference continuum. The woman was in the middle of a health crisis, and she wanted to change her will. The family arranged for a notary public to come to the house so that she could sign the appropriate document. The woman would not sign the paper until her family found her preferred writing utensil—a slender, fine, felt-tipped pen. This pen provided the right amount of proprioceptive input to match the refined capacity of her proprioceptive system. Any other writing utensil for her was simply out of the question.

Supporting the Child's Developing Sense of Self-Movement

As mentioned previously, sensing (largely at an unconscious level) the countermovement is the means by which we develop the ability to sense our own movements. We support the development of the baby's proprioceptive capacities by giving them extended periods of self-initiated movement in which we refrain from unnecessarily interrupting them. In this way, they can better stay in the dream consciousness, in which the sensations of the countermovement naturally arise. Also, during self-initiated movement time, the child is free to choose activities that best suit them—that best provide them with the optimal resistance in order for them to sense the countermovement—as this is a highly individual matter.

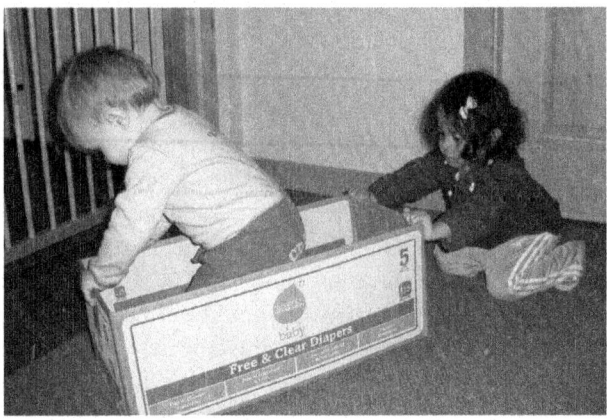

This child self-initiated giving their classmate a ride in a cardboard box. This activity involved a significant amount of resistance, something many of the other children choose not to do.

The child needs lots of time to practice sensing the countermovement. Hence, they need lots of time for free movement. We support the child's developing sense of proprioception by letting them move entirely out of their own initiative from the very start. We also support this by giving them a firm, horizontal surface upon which to move. One important thing that the baby is learning—at an unconscious level—is that pushing against something propels their body in the opposite direction. This is key for the development of the sense of proprioception. It's more difficult to move on a soft surface than on a firm surface. If the child pushes against a soft surface, the start of the push depresses the soft surface rather than propelling them in the opposite direction, and so the child doesn't get the optimal feedback of the countermovement. Similarly, the baby does not receive optimal feedback of the countermovement when one props them up or holds them up before they can manage a position on their own because, in this way, we are unnaturally influencing the forces and counterforces of the child's movements.

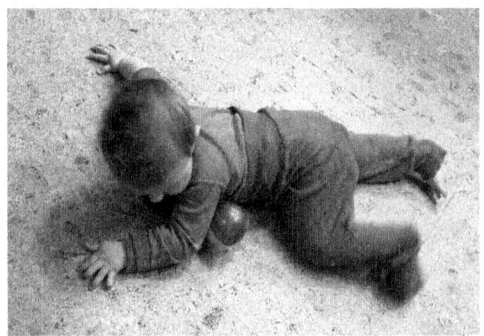 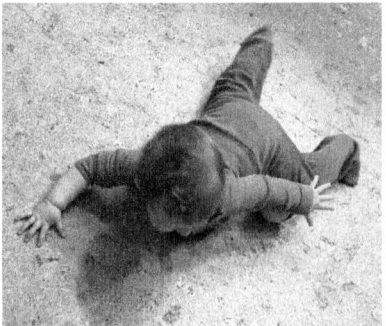 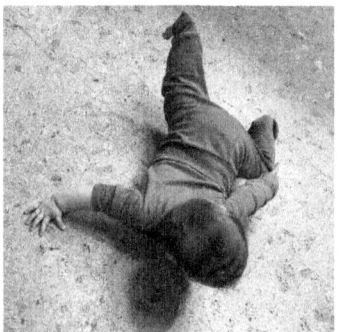

This sequence shows a lovely example of the countermovement during free movement. The child is pushing into the floor and to the right with their right arm. Thus, their body spins around to the left as they reach for the moving toy. Here, they are experiencing the countermovement at an unconscious level, and thus developing their sense of self-movement.

When children are a little older, they often carry around objects of varying weights. During this activity they sense varying degrees of the countermovement. They use their arms to lift the object up, and the weight of the object counters this upward force and pulls the arms down. Another classic stage of play is pouring—children especially like to pour water—from one container to another. This involves a more complex functioning of the sense of proprioception. In pouring, the child's limbs are sensing a changing amount of weight, and thus a changing degree of the countermovement. For skillful movement, the child's limbs must perceive and adjust to the changes.

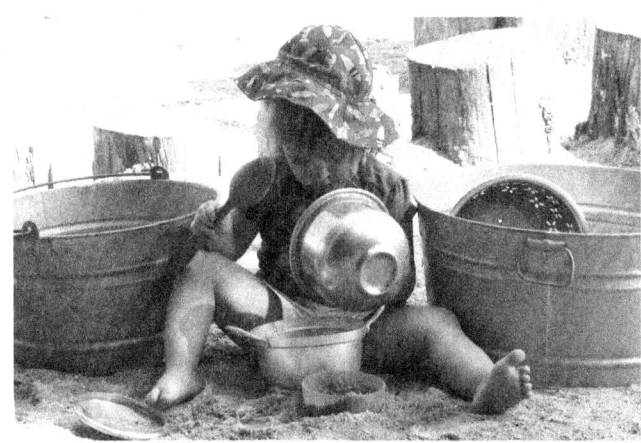

This child has poured sand from one container to another.

The Sense of Proprioception and the Spacial Dynamics Streams

Rudolf Steiner describes the etheric body, also known as the life-force body, as "an extremely delicate and finely-organized vehicle."[26] He says that there are particles in the life-force body that are in continual motion, and he describes these motions as currents. Jaimen McMillan has studied and worked with these life-force currents for decades. McMillan refers to them as streams, and describes them as dynamic paths of movement on and around the body. There are archetypal forms and directions of the streams that are most conducive to health and well-being. However, the form and direction of the streams are not a given. They develop over time and are subject to change. As adults we can learn to perceive our streams, and influence, choose, and change them. This generally takes a movement training, such as the Spacial Dynamics training, where one learns to direct one's own movements first, often in slow-motion, to awaken a perception of their subtle countermovements. Additionally, in the Spacial Dynamics training, one learns therapeutic, hands-on techniques, as well as activities and exercises, in order to support another person to select and modify their streams. (The life-force body and the streams will be more fully discussed in volume 2.)

Many years ago, I learned from Jaimen McMillan that one's proprioceptive awareness is directly related to the direction, dynamic, and form of one's streams. Healthy proprioception exists when the streams are operating in the archetypal direction and form.[27] This knowledge changed my entire way of working with children who had challenges in this sense. When one grasps the enormity of this concept, one can see that in order to support the healthy development of the sense of proprioception, one must support the healthy spatial development of the child, which includes the development of their streams.

How do the optimal directions and forms of the life-force streams get established in the first place, in the developing baby and toddler? There are essentially two ways. The first is through imitation: the child imitates the streams that are living in the adult's space. Hence, it is very helpful for adults to have awareness and facility with their own streams. We are typically unaware of our own streams, yet—as noted above—it is possible to learn to perceive and influence them. The second way is through the baby's free movements during the gross motor sequence. Initially, at the start of life, the directions of the vast majority of the streams are coming in toward the body. We can recognize this in the way the young infant moves their limbs. The young infant's limbs are not oriented to anything out beyond their limbs—they are not peripherally oriented. Rather, they are moving indiscriminately. For example, the arms are not moving intentionally to reach for a toy, or to move a toy on the surface; rather, the arms bat the air randomly, in a chaotic manner.

Over time and under appropriate conditions, the streams reverse course. It is noteworthy that the streams change first, and then the child's movements reflect the changes. As a result of the ordering of the life-force streams, the infant's chaotic movements are tamed, and the limb movements become influenced by the objects that the children want to play with, the structures that they want to climb on, and the surfaces that they are moving on. For example, when a child climbs up onto a rung on the Pikler triangle (see appendix 3), the rungs determine the placement of their hands and feet. Here, the streams move in the opposite direction—out away from the body. The limbs are sensing the rungs. They are moving in relationship to the periphery.

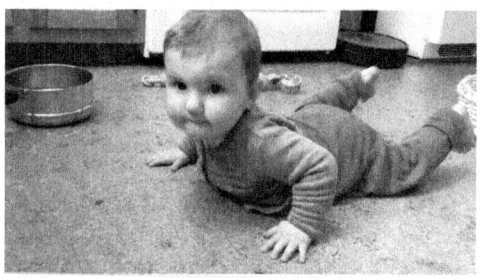

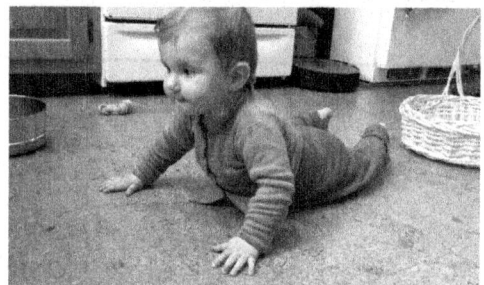

The baby plays on their tummy and pushes down through their arms into the floor, as they rise up off the surface. Here, the arm streams are developing the mature, outward direction.

As development proceeds, then, the directions of the life-force streams, which are initially incoming, change to be directed out and away from the body. This happens gradually, over the first months and years of life—tenuously at first and then more substantively. Another place that we see evidence of this change in the direction of the life force streams to become out and away from the body is when the child pushes down into the supporting surface and their body is displaced upwards. This happens countless times all throughout the gross motor sequence. For example, when the baby stands up from squatting, they push the floor down with their feet, and their body is displaced upwards. In this pushing down activity of the legs, the streams of the legs are outgoing.

In the pushing-down activity of the arms, the streams are also out and away from the body. The streams become well established in the habit body (or the etheric body) because these movements typically happen hundreds and thousands of times when the child has opportunities for free movement.

We can observe that proprioception is developing well when the movements of the limbs are initiated from the periphery—unconsciously—such as when the baby's reach for a toy begins with their seeing it. In contrast, we can observe that proprioception is not functioning well when the person's movement are initiated centrally—consciously—as was the case with Ian Waterman, where he had to think about all of his movements. Therefore, it is optimal if we refrain from verbally instructing a child in how to move, because this asks the child to think about their movement, and then the movement is initiated centrally.

During respectful caregiving activities (see chapter 1 for a deeper discussion of respectful caregiving), which can start on day one of life, the adult engages the child's participation at whatever level the child is capable of. For example, the newborn may simply hold their arm still in order for the adult to pull on the sleeve of the shirt. Engaging the child to move a limb, or hold it still, in relationship to an article of clothing also supports the developing peripheral orientation of the limbs.

Peripherally Oriented Movement of the Limbs

It has been well established for decades that when a person reaches for a glass, their hand forms to the shape of the glass before touching it. Here, the periphery (the glass) dictates the movement of the fingers, so that the fingers are in the correct spatial configuration to pick up the glass. This happens automatically. The person is not body-bound—their movements are not overly tense. Instead, they are present in their body and also out beyond their hand. The person has a simultaneous awareness of the glass, the hand, and the space between them as the hand moves, although this awareness is generally unconscious. In this way, fluid, coordinated movement ensues. When the adult's limbs move in such manner, they are manifesting the archetypal forms and directions of the streams, and healthy fluid movement occurs. Here the adult's movements are qualitatively very worthy of imitation.

There are many other examples of the limbs operating out of a peripheral orientation. One is when an expert woodworker carves a spoon out of a piece of lilac wood. An experienced woodworker will "find" the form of the spoon in the wood. The knots and grain and colors of the wood dictate the movement of the woodworker's hands. The motions of the woodworker's hands are initiated peripherally. Similarly, a master sculptor will "find" the form of their sculpture in the piece of stone. An experienced bread baker knows how long to knead the dough and whether to add more flour, according to the feel of the dough. The activity of the baker's limbs is determined by what is beyond their hands—the dough. Let us also consider a classic game for two kindergarten-aged children. They lie on their backs, feet to feet, with their feet up off the floor, pressing into each other, and performing a bicycling motion. Here the child must sense out beyond their own feet into the partner's feet in order to achieve the motion.

When a new skier comes home from their first day on the slopes, it is not uncommon for them to comment on their day by describing how many bruises they got when they fell down, how well their equipment fit them, and how cold they got. All of these comments are about the person—they are centrally-oriented. When an experienced skier comes home at the end of the day, they often comment on the quality of the snow, the conditions on the slopes, and the weather. All of these comments are about the periphery! This skier is out beyond themself, in the environment.

The Sense of Self-Movement and Perceiving Forms in the Environment

With the sense of self-movement, we perceive the movements of our own body. Rudolf Steiner says that the sense of self-movement also allows us to perceive forms in our environment:

> We are normally not aware of how we perceive when we perceive color and form at the same time. Someone who perceives a colored circle might say, "I see the color, and I see the roundness of the circle or the circular form." However, here two very different things are confused. At first you see only the color through the specific activity of the eye. You see the circular form when you subconsciously use the sense of movement and unconsciously make a circular movement in the etheric or astral body, thus raising it into cognition. When the circle you have apprehended through your sense of movement rises to cognition, it is then joined with the perceived color.[28]

Thus, the development of the sense of self-movement is foundational for proper perception of the forms in our environments. Proprioception allows us to recognize the shape of a circle, a stop sign, or a slow-moving vehicle sign on the back of a tractor. Similarly, the sense of self-movement is also key also for learning to read, as the child must perceive the forms of the letters to distinguish them from each other. I have worked with many children over the years who have struggled with reading. The children were typically also receiving tutoring for reading, so other factors were also likely at play, yet I often observed that the children's reading improved as they refined their sense of proprioception.

How We Perceive Movement in Our Environment

The sense of self-movement allows us to perceive our own movements and also the shapes of objects in our environment. But how do we perceive the movements of other people and of objects in our environment? Let us consider the following anecdote. Early in my career as a physical therapist, I worked on a rehabilitation unit in a hospital, and I specialized in working with patients who had suffered strokes. One time, I was teaching a patient's husband how to transfer her from the toilet to her wheelchair, so that she could go home for the weekend. I demonstrated the transfer, and then asked the husband to try it. The husband looked at me with a blank look, and said, "I don't get it. What do I do?" I responded with an equally blank look, as I honestly didn't know what I had done. We are aware of our thoughts, but I wasn't in my head—I was in my limbs. Additionally, I was also out beyond my limbs, sensing the patient's movements. This is a good example of Rudolf Steiner's assertion that we are awake in our thinking and asleep in our willing—in what our limbs are doing.

My limbs had sensed the patient's muscle tone and knew when she was ready to begin the transfer. My limbs had sensed what direction she was moving in and knew how much I needed to guide her. My limbs had sensed whether her legs were supporting her body weight, and knew how much support I needed to give her. The patient and I had been involved in a limb-to-limb type of communication, of which our intellects had no part. To accommodate the husband, I repeated the transfer, this time translating it step by step to my intellect and verbally describing it to him, and then he was able to do it.

There were other clients with family members who learned directly from my demonstrations, bypassing their heads. These family members did not learn well from verbal cues; in fact, verbal cues even irritated some of them. These family members had a higher degree of "limb intelligence." Their limbs understood without needing to compensate with their intellects. They could imitate me limb-to-limb. I didn't fully understand the significance of this until years later when I studied Spacial Dynamics, but at the time I did recognize that if a family member could learn nonverbally, the transfer was usually more skilled, and the patient was safer than they were with those whose family members who needed verbal instruction.

What was going on here? As was mentioned in chapter 13, Jaimen McMillan characterizes the *spatial gestalt* as the entirety of the shifting forms and dynamics of movement that surround the physical body. This invisible gestalt surrounds, embraces, and enlivens the physical body. It balances out the weight of the physical body with appropriate levity. Included in the *spatial gestalt* are the many individual streams. When the individual streams are ordered and woven together, integrated movements of grace, harmony, and proportion are possible. The spatial gestalt is also commonly known as the *movement body*. It serves as a sensing organ. The development of the spatial gestalt is very significant, and typically not well understood, in the context of child development. It is through the spatial gestalt that we are able to perceive the movements of others and of objects in the environment.

Each of us creates our own unique spatial gestalt—and it may serve us for better or for worse. When the spatial gestalt is operating out of an archetypal form, then one can perceive and follow the movements in one's environment. In the newborn and toddler, the form of the spatial gestalt has not been sufficiently established for the child to fully or consistently follow the movements in their surroundings. It can be very disorienting when we can't perceive and follow the movements of our environment. Therefore, it is helpful for the young child if we slow down, and order our movements so they are predictable and easy to follow. One time, I was setting up a classroom in a Waldorf grade school where I was to teach for three weeks during our Sophia's Hearth summer conference. My son and daughter-in-law were there to help me. They brought along my grandchildren. The two-year-old played happily with objects in the room, as we adults had a lengthy discussion about how to best arrange the room for my teaching. When we started to move the desks out into the hall, the two-year-old cried and insisted on being held. It is my interpretation that she was distressed because she couldn't follow the movements in the room. There were too many movements, they were sudden, they were happening simultaneously in different parts of the room, and they were of a large scale with regard to the size of the room. Not only could she not follow the movements, but they also didn't make sense to her. As soon as we finished moving the desks, she was fine and did not need to be held.

Similarly, some children do well when they arrive at preschool or kindergarten and there are only a few children present, but by the time the whole group has arrived, they may become upset. It can be that the child isn't able to follow the movements of so many children in the classroom. After all, young children don't move in predictable ways. Depending upon the severity of the upset, these children often do better in settings with a smaller number of children.

15: The Sense of Balance

The fourth and final foundational sense is the sense of *balance*. According to Rudolf Steiner, "what the sense of balance conveys to us is our own state of balance."[1] Are we in balance or are we falling out of balance?

The sense of balance gives us information about the position and movement of our head in relation to the three-dimensional space around us. Through this sense we develop spatial awareness and orientation. We ascertain the position of our head—whether it is upside down or right side up, tilted to the right or left, rotated to the right or left, or bent forward or backward—and also whether our head is speeding up or slowing down. For example, we can tell if we are falling. The organs of the sense of balance comprise the vestibular system. These ingenious sensory organs are elegantly designed and are present in mirror-image in each inner ear. They include the three semicircular canals, which perceive rotational movement, and two otoliths, which perceive linear acceleration.

Let us compare the sense of balance with the sense of self-movement. The organs for the sense of self-movement are all throughout the body, in the muscles and joints. They give us information about the positions and movements of our body parts in relationship to each other. As noted in the previous paragraph, in contrast, the organs for the sense of balance are localized in the head. We receive information only about what is happening to our head from the sense of balance. It doesn't give us any information about the rest of our body, even though our limbs and trunk are used in balance reactions. The sense of self-movement comes into play so that the balance reactions are carried out in a coordinated fashion. Here we see the intimate relationship between these two senses.

Our sense of vision also gives us information about the position of our head in space. The visual system is closely tied to and can activate the vestibular system. Parents and teachers frequently report to me that they get dizzy when watching a child spin on a swing, even though they are only watching, not moving themselves. Similarly, if we watch a visual presentation at an Omni theater (using a super-sized, curved screen to engage our full visual field), we may feel as if we are flying in a propeller plane doing loop-de-loops when we are actually sitting still in our seats.

Just like the other foundational senses, our awareness of balance is also largely unconscious. We don't have to consciously direct our balance reactions—we just balance. My four-year-old granddaughter recently explained this to me in her four-year-old way. She had made herself an obstacle course in the living room and was sitting atop one of the living room chairs, balancing, when she told me that she had magic. She said that *she* doesn't balance, instead *her magic* balances her. Additionally, we don't usually pay attention to our balance unless we fall out of balance, or are at risk of doing so.

The Newborn Is Not Adept with Balance

When I graduated from physical therapy school, I took a pediatric job in South Dakota, and there—of all places in the country—I took a scuba diving class. The class began in a swimming pool. I reveled in the feeling of weightlessness—a temporary release from the relentless gravitational forces of the earth. I felt little resistance to my movements, except when I used the flippers in order to go fast. But mostly, I just floated around.

FREE MOVEMENT FROM THE VERY START

The scuba class soon progressed to diving in a lake, where, unfortunately, my equipment malfunctioned on my first dive. My air gauge read that I had plenty of air, however, my tank was empty, and I was thirty feet underwater, at the bottom of the lake. My scuba buddy was nowhere to be found, and I quickly realized that the buddy breathing* that we had learned in the swimming pool for this very situation was not an option. I was on my own. Fortunately, I made it to the surface of the lake and then to shore. As I was walking out of the water onto the beach, I experienced great awkwardness. Here was the resistance of the earth, in great measure! My body felt so heavy and cumbersome, compared to its ease-filled motion under the water. Additionally, I had what seemed like an inordinately large, ponderous tank on my upper back which made me top heavy, and I was also wearing flippers. It was hard to balance. When I got to shore, I took off my equipment and lay down on the beach, flat on my back. At that point, I realized what had happened and that it could have gone badly for me. I was shaken up. I didn't sit in a lawn chair or lie prone—instead, I instinctively chose to lie on my back on the ground. I needed to feel the constancy and certainty of the earth supporting me. This was a very orienting, grounding position for me. It was as if I needed to bond with the earth again after such an upset.

Years later, after I had studied the sensory development of the infant in depth, remembering this event gave me insight into the newborn's state of affairs. I was top-heavy with the scuba tank high on my back, and so is the newborn because of their relatively large, heavy head. Additionally, their ability to balance is essentially nonexistent and their movements are awkward. The combination of these factors is potentially overwhelming to such an inexperienced and immature human being. One can appreciate the incredible wisdom of placing a newborn on their back on a firm, flat, stable surface.

When one is at risk of losing one's balance, it is not uncommon for the person to experience apprehension or even full-blown fear. Dr. Judith Falk speaks about this and puts it in a larger context by which to understand caring for the young infant. She references Donald Winnicott.† He says that the child needs to be "held" in a proper manner, in the larger sense of caring for the child as a whole being: "The right 'holding' protects the child from physical danger, it takes into account the sensitivity of the skin, the sensitivity to sounds, the sensitivity to light, and the fear of falling."[2] When held and carried by the adult, an infant must be protected "with absolute security from the fear of falling, or even of losing balance."[3] Being cared for with competence and sensitivity gives babies a feeling of security, and then they don't react with excessive muscle tension. This is very helpful for the development of the sense of balance, as excessive muscle tension blocks the manifestation of balance reactions.

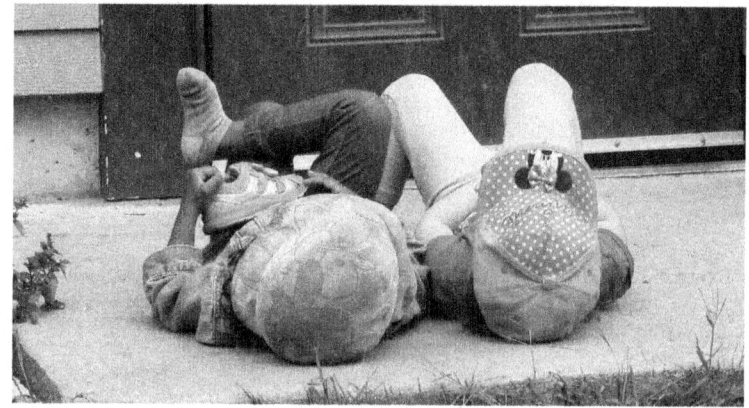

These two preschool children have chosen to lie on their backs during outside play time. The position provides an orienting opportunity with the constancy of the earth underneath them and the open sky above them.

Dr. Falk recommends lifting, carrying, and putting down the infant in a supine position until they themself achieve a vertical position. This makes sense, because until the child takes up the vertical position through their own efforts, they are not fully prepared to balance in that position. The infant needs to be "lifted and carried with the

---

* *Buddy breathing is an emergency measure where two people share the air from one tank by taking turns using the air mouthpiece.
† *Donald Winnicott (1896-1971) was an English pediatrician and psychoanalyst who is well respected in developmental psychology today. He is well-known for his concept of the "good enough parent."

largest possible portion of [their] body being securely supported. When taken into the arms, the entire vertebral column of the young infant must be supported, and [the] head must be protected from even the slightest swaying and swinging, and the balance among the different parts of [the child's] body must be kept."[4] This is a wonderful description of how to hold and carry an infant. In this way, the child is not subject to any perturbations that would result in the child's feeling that they are losing their balance. Please note the adult's attention to the child's head. The adult is preventing any excess movement of the child's head. In addition to supporting balance, this is very helpful for the integration of the Moro reflex and for the establishment of the gesture of a still, quiet head. (The Moro reflex and the significance of the gesture of the still, quiet head will be discussed more fully in volume 2.)

What Can Astronauts Teach Us about the Infant's Developing Relationship with Gravity?

We can better understand the newborn's initial experience of gravity from the research of the space programs over many decades. These programs have studied the effects of weightlessness on human beings while in space as well as their readjustment to gravity when they come home. An article from the European Space Agency offers many interesting observations. For example, after they have made the adjustment to living in space, "Most astronauts find their freedom from gravity exhilarating."[5] However, initially, there are sensory adjustments to be made. "In the absence of gravity, signals from the vestibular system and the pressure receptors[‡] are wildly misleading. The effect usually leads to immediate disorientation: many astronauts suddenly feel themselves upside-down, for example, or even have difficulty in sensing the location of their own arms and legs."[6] Half or more of the astronauts go through a phase of vomiting and nausea, although usually, they adjust over the course of a few days, learning that "In space, 'down' is where your feet happen to be."[7] On the earth, we orient ourselves in space via our perceptions from the vestibular system, the visual system, and the pressure touch part of the tactile system. However, in space, because of the lack of gravity, vestibular and pressure touch input are lacking, and so the astronauts must rely heavily on vision for their spatial orientation.

When the astronauts come back to earth, they must readjust to the forces of gravity—their vestibular and deep pressure touch systems, which have essentially been on holiday when they were in space, must get back to work. The astronauts typically experience difficulty with their balance, initially, "and if they close their eyes, they are very likely to fall over."[8] However, this is usually short lived, lasting only a few days. "There is one re-adaptation that can take somewhat longer to accomplish, although the consequences are more likely to be amusing than crippling. Several long-duration Russian cosmonauts have reported that months after their time in space, they still occasionally let go of a cup or some other object in mid-air—and are quite disconcerted when it crashes to the floor."[9]

From these studies, we can see how profoundly gravity informs the general spatial ordering of life on earth. Here on the earth—unless we have been in space—we adults take it for granted that if we let go of an object in mid-air, it will always fall down. However, the newborn has arrived from the spiritual world, where the forces of the earth are not applicable.[10] It is noteworthy that dropping things is a universal phenomenon in the baby's play. It is one of the ways that children first explore gravity with objects. The baby spends months playing on the floor, dropping a toy, watching what ensues, picking it up, and dropping it again. Babies also universally sit at the table in their high chair or other type of chair and drop spoons and pieces of food, seemingly fascinated that the items fall to the floor. An interesting observation was made at the children's home in Budapest, directed by Dr. Pikler, regarding the "drops and picks up" activity. Although the staff tried to keep as much consistency as possible, the babies who lived there would occasionally have to be moved to a new room in the building. The staff carefully

---

‡ The skin contains two types of touch receptors: pressure touch and light touch. Because of the lack of gravity, there are fewer occurrences of pressure touch in space. When a person sits, lies down, or stands on the earth, the weight of their body presses into the surface and they experience pressure touch. This doesn't happen in space because the astronauts are weightless. For more on the sense of touch, please see chapters 11 and 12.

planned for these moves for weeks in advance, in order to make the move as nondisruptive for the babies as possible. Nonetheless, it still amounted to a significant disruption for the babies. After these moves, whatever was the newest form of play disappeared for approximately a month before it reappeared again. However, the babies never stopped dropping and picking up their toys! In fact, "the frequency of 'drops and picks up' activity was unexpectedly very high and constantly rose in the first 10 days after the room change."[11] Because the babies had been moved to a new room, they were disoriented. However, they could still count on the constancy of gravity. The toy would always fall down when it was dropped, and this gave them security.

Babies progress to other types of play where they can experiment with gravity. In prone (tummy-lying), they place toys atop small platforms and then push the toys off the platform, watching them fall. The platforms can be as simple as a small cardboard box, an overturned basin, a firm cushion, or a low footstool. Stacking blocks and knocking them down is another classic game where children witness the effects of gravity. When babies reach the vertical stages of sitting and pulling to stand, they enjoy "standing up" toys that are taller than they are wide. An empty bottle of dishwashing liquid is a good example of this type of toy. Here, the fine motor activity is mirroring what the child is doing in their body—like the bottle, they are also trying to come into verticality without falling over.

Besides witnessing objects falling down, when their gross motor skills reach a sufficient level, young children will want to experience their own bodies falling down, toward the center of the earth. They will naturally climb up onto various places and jump down. It is my observation that young children are universally drawn to this activity. It mirrors their journey down from the heavens—here they are literally "coming down to earth." It may not be appropriate for them to jump down from certain places, yet it is satisfying for the children if the adults provide them with some places from which jumping down is allowed.

In contrast to being in space, when we are on the earth, no matter where our feet are—whether we are doing a handstand or lying down—down is constant. It is always toward the center of the earth. Every object and person on the face of the earth is being drawn down toward the center of the earth by the force of gravity. In order to achieve verticality, then, we must overcome this constant force of being pulled down. Jaimen McMillan has explored this phenomenon in depth. He relates that we don't *lift* ourselves up off the surface—rather, our bodies are *displaced* up, as a result of our pushing down into the surface. The baby is learning to do this all throughout the entire gross motor sequence. For example, when babies transition from prone with their heads lying on the surface to prone on elbows, they push the floor down through their forearms, and their head and upper body are displaced up off the surface. This pushing down into the floor is also referred to as orienting to the supporting surface. Similarly, when babies transition from squat to standing, they push the floor down, and their bodies are displaced up off the surface into standing. To maintain standing, they must continue to exert a downward force into the surface in order for the body stay upright.

The same is true in sitting. As McMillan observes, we say, "sit up." However, if we want to sit with good posture, we must exert a continual downward force into the chair, so that our trunk and upper body remain vertical. We actually "sit down" in order to "sit up." One thing that is so pronounced about babies who are raised according the Pikler approach is that they have beautifully erect postures when they reach vertical positions. This is because they have learned how to push down into the surface.

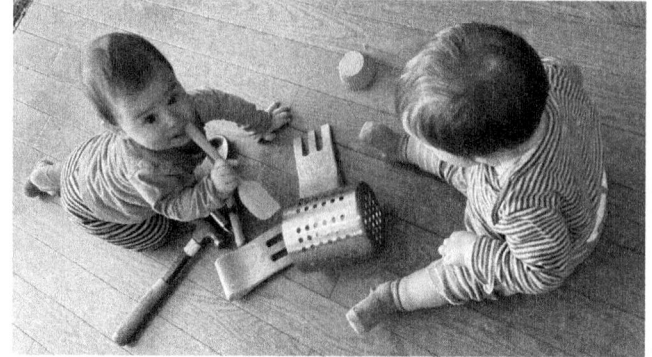

In the child on the right we see the beautifully erect sitting posture of a child who has had self-initiated movement from the very start.

In contrast, when a young baby is placed into sitting before they can get there on their own, they don't know how to push down into the surface, and so they compensate by pulling up off the surface—they tense up, their shoulders elevate, they strain to hold the position, and they don't feel secure.[12]

What Can a Modern Dancer Teach Us about the Infant's Developing Relationship with Gravity?

Modern dancer and choreographer Doris Humphrey (1895–1958) was a pioneer in the American modern dance movement. She was an innovator in dance technique and dance theory. In *The Dance Technique of Doris Humphrey*, author Ernestine Stodelle writes about Humphrey's characterization of the dancer's relationship to the supporting surface, something we typically don't think much about.

> In the Humphrey movement, the sensation of bodily weight change is a vivid experience. Contact with the floor is a positive motion, not necessarily heavy in terms of accented sound but realistically firm. Although the body gives in to the ground (floor) as if pulled magnetically downward, it does this with a deliberate sense of its relationship to the earth. This action becomes a physical and emotional statement, a way of saying simply and unequivocally, "I am." To acknowledge reality was a basic premise of early modern dance. Being rooted meant having power; being rooted meant having identity. "The modern dancer," wrote Doris Humphrey, "must . . . establish [their] human relation to gravity and reality."[13]

At birth, the infant is essentially bound to the face of the earth. Initially, they have no ability to manage and overcome the forces of gravity. In order to achieve mastery of their bodily instrument, they must come into relationship with gravity. This happens gradually, in the first months and years of life. A crucial question (asked at an unconscious level) in this early period of life is, "Where is down?" The child learns where down is by pushing down into the supporting surface, with the subsequent upward displacement of their body, as described above. For example, in supine, when the infant pushes down through the back side of their pelvis, the legs are displaced up into the air. The baby also pushes down in prone through their hands, and their upper body is displaced up off the floor into prone on extended arms.

When the baby can move freely, without being restricted in baby equipment, they will naturally push down into the floor hundreds and even thousands of times. In this way, children develop an inner certainty of where down is. In contrast, if the child is placed into sitting before they can reach the position through their own initiative, they typically compensate by pulling up off the surface. Hence there is an "up and away" gesture, rather than a "down and into" gesture, regarding the surface. With the "up and away" gesture, the child is essentially bracing themselves against any movement, because the position is too difficult for them. They literally can't learn to balance in it. They cannot freely move within the position, nor into and out of the position. They tense up. The muscle tone is higher than is optimal, and there is strain. However, when the child achieves sitting through their own efforts, they sit with a "down and into" gesture, regarding the surface. Here, the posture is optimal, the muscle tone is not excessive, there is no strain, and the challenge to balance can be met when they shift their weight to reach for a toy or to move a toy, for example. It is not too hard for them to balance in a position that they have achieved independently, because they have prepared themselves for the position before they moved into it. As so elegantly described above, Doris Humphrey's dancers used the "down and into" gesture.

In a professional dance performance, one can perceive an almost elastic quality in the dancer's relationship to the opposing forces of gravity and levity. According to Humphrey, the dancer surrenders to the gravitational forces pulling them down to the earth. Simultaneously, the dancer also manifests an airborne mastery of the forces of levity—at times they seem to hover in the air. To me, when I witness such movements of grace and beauty, I relate the dancer's movement to a celebration of the child's motor journey into verticality. It is as if the dancer is "playing" with gravity and levity, just as very young children do, and elevating the activity. Humphrey explains that through the dancer's exploration of these two opposing forces, they gain power and identity, saying, "simply and unequivocally, 'I am.'"[14] In other words, they perceive themself as spirit. In his lecture series *Spiritual Science as a Foundation for Social Forms*, Rudolf Steiner agrees with Humphrey's observation of the dancer's experience of their "I am." Steiner explains that it is through the sense of balance that the human being can perceive themself as spirit.[15]

Here are some related thoughts of Henning Köhler regarding our ability to sense ourselves as spirit through the sense of balance, in which, interestingly, he also speaks about dancing:

> There are physical laws to which human beings would have been fully subjected if there were no souls and egos in their bodies to enable them to stand upright and to move. Walking and standing, we have an experience of our emancipation. And we have no sense of being pulled down, or heaviness, when we dance, or hop on one foot, or balance on a fence. We could not do any of these things without that sensing of inner symmetry and space, of being "up-borne in our soul-space, of being spirits," as Rudolf Steiner described it. . . . We human beings have within us light that enables us to erect and open ourselves to what lies above. That is what the sense of balance makes possible for us to perceive: that inner light, lifting us erect and opening us to the sphere where angels dwell.[16]

Here Köhler speaks of an experience of emancipation from the forces of gravity when we walk and stand. Indeed, the baby certainly seems to have a feeling of emancipation when they take their first steps, and parents commonly speak about the joy exuded from their toddler during their first steps. Young children continue to celebrate their victory over gravity for years, with further accomplishments of hopping, jumping, galloping, and skipping. Indeed, it seems as if a healthy young child cannot simply walk across a room; instead they skip, they dance, and they lilt.

Ego Activity and the Drive for Verticality

In the following passage, Steiner speaks about the infant's acquisition of verticality and relates it to the activity of the ego: "Let us go back to the first thing that the child learns: to walk, learning a balanced posture. There is more connected with this than is usually thought. Connected with it is the bringing about by the ego of a specific physical process which changes [human beings] from a creeping to a walking being. *It is the ego that erects the human being* [emphasis added]."[17]

Rudolf Steiner repeatedly discusses the significance of the human being's attainment of verticality. In a 1910 lecture, he says that of all the creatures on the earth, the human being is the only one who attains the vertical position. This distinguishes humans from animals whose spines are horizontal to the earth; he discounts that apes are erect beings.[18] In another lecture, Steiner says that the vertical position allows the human being to have a relationship with the entire cosmos. Our head is freed to look upward into the cosmos, with attainment of the vertical position. This happened during humanity's evolution as a whole, and the child recapitulates this event during their individual development. Additionally, he says that "the vertical position of the human spine distinguishes human beings as bearers of I-being."[19] (The ego, or "I"-being, is discussed in greater depth in volume 2.)

When we observe babies over time, as they endeavor to achieve verticality in their own unique ways, we can witness this individual ego activity. I once observed a baby as he negotiated his movement journey up into verticality. As a young baby, he was very contented to play on his back and on his side. During these early stages, he seemed to be in no hurry. It was as if he simply wanted to savor the luxurious experiences of these horizontal positions. When he got to belly-crawling, things changed. He seemed to wake up a little more. He belly-crawled all over the house, quickly and adeptly. He also easily spun around 360 degrees in each direction on his belly.

He achieved prone on extended arms and started to get onto hands and knees. He continued to explore prone on extended arms, would stretch out his legs behind him, and raise his body into a plank position.§ Sometimes he wobbled and toppled to either side in the plank position—only to try it again. Soon, he started climbing up and over every possible thing that he could climb onto—such as his relatives' outstretched legs on the floor. His inner drive to reach verticality was tangible, and he seemed truly unstoppable. Over time, he became adept at crawling, pulling to stand, and independent standing. When he took his first steps, it was with a triumphant air. As he practiced stringing more and more steps together, he often plopped down on his bottom, only to stand right back up and try again. It is interesting to note the old saying, "You can't keep a good person down." I would add, "You can't keep a baby with active ego forces down—they simply must achieve verticality."

Where Can We Witness the Development of Balance in the Growing Infant?

In the previous chapters, we have discussed the development of the three other foundational senses: the senses of touch, life, and self-movement. One way we can witness the child's developing sense of touch is in the way they position their entire bodies in order to receive tactile input from various surfaces, objects, and other people. We can watch the child's developing sense of life in their growing ability to co-regulate and self-regulate. We can see the child's developing sense of self-movement in their increasingly fluid and coordinated movement. Where do we see the development of the sense of balance in the infant and young child?

Static Balance

In what positions do we balance? When I have asked this question to adults, most people respond that balance occurs in standing. This makes sense, because most people have suffered a fall when walking. Most have not fallen when they were sitting or lying on their backs, for example. However, during free movement, the child balances within *every* developmental position, including: supine, side-lying, prone, side-lying on elbow, side-sitting on extended arm, sitting, hands-and-knees, kneeling, squatting, and standing (here, sitting means balancing on two sitz bones without using the arms for support). For example, if a baby who is lying on their back with their legs in the air shifts their legs to the side beyond the point of control, they fall down into side-lying.

Balancing within a position is referred to as static balance. With static balance, the child is not moving through space—they are staying in the same position—learning to maintain the position or playing with a toy there. However, the term is misleading, because the child is not static. With every subtle weight shift, such as when they bat their arms, they are constantly adjusting their posture within the position.

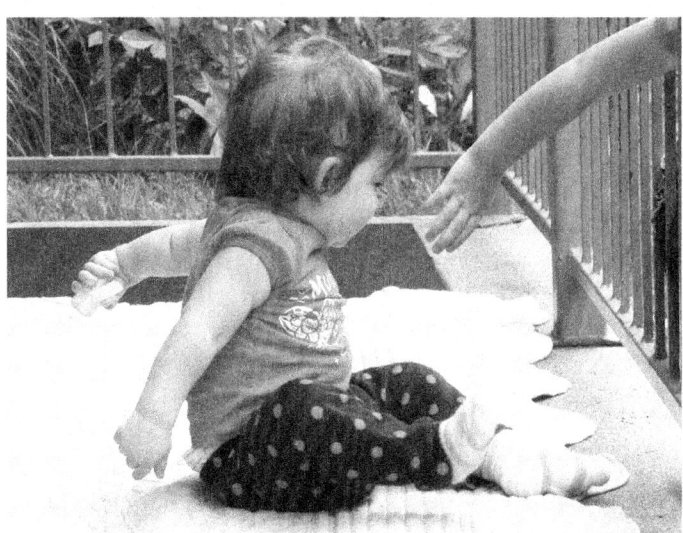

Here is a lovely example of static balance. This child maintained the sitting position when another child tried to take away their toy. They quickly adjusted their posture as they moved the toy behind them. Here we see the relationship between social development and sensorimotor development, as the child's ability to protect the toy is related to their ability to balance.

---

§ In a plank position, the person is supporting themselves on their hands and on the balls of their feet. Their spine is straight and their arms are extended.

Dynamic Balance

A second type of balance is dynamic balance, when the baby is moving through space. Dynamic balance manifests in two ways: when babies are transitioning between the different developmental positions and when they are using movement as a means of locomotion, in order to get somewhere. Let us first look at the development of dynamic balance in transitional movements. In free motor exploration, there are a plethora of transitional movements, including: supine to/from side-lying, supine to/from prone, prone on elbows to/from side-lying on elbows, hands-and-knees to/from sitting, and sitting to/from side-sitting on extended arms. In all of these transitions, the movements are typically performed to the right and to the left. Additional transitions include heel sitting to/from kneeling, kneeling to/from standing, and squatting to/from standing. In these last three transitions, the baby may initially support themselves with their hands on vertical bars or on a surface such as a small bench.

We can support the development of balance by making it a habit—for as long as is appropriate—to place the baby on their back whenever we lay them down in the movement space. When a child has solidly reached sitting or standing, laying them on their back would no longer be appropriate, as they would resist this. However, before a baby reaches independent sitting, we can still place them on their back when we lay them down—even if they will nearly always turn to their tummy right away. In this way, they get an extra opportunity to perform the transitional movement of turning from supine to prone, which is very beneficial for their balance. Similarly, whenever we pick up a baby we can make it a habit to pick them up from the supine position. The details of this might look like this: If we approach a baby to pick them up and they are playing in the prone position, we can tell them that we want to pick them up and ask them to turn onto their back. Initially, we may need to tell them that we are going to pick them up and that first, we will turn them to their back. Very soon they will learn this pattern and will self-initiate turning to their back when we approach them to pick them up. Additionally, when they want to be picked up, they may communicate this to us by rolling to their backs and likely batting their arms and legs and vocalizing in order to get our attention.

Dynamic balance also develops in activities of locomotion, such as rolling, belly-crawling, crawling on hands and knees, climbing, knee-walking, hands-and-feet walking (or bear walking), and walking.

How Can We Witness the Development of Balance in the Growing Child?

Balance can be observed by looking at two factors: the size of the base of support and the height of the center of mass. The center of mass of the adult human body is generally slightly below the belly button, although the location varies with different body types. It is slightly higher in the baby, as the head is proportionally larger than in the adult. The weight of the upper body and that of the lower body are in balance at the center of mass. The base of support is the area defined by the outer edge of the body parts (or extensions of the body parts such as a cane) that are in contact with the supporting surface. Like the center of mass, the base of support is changeable. If a person hangs onto a railing or a piece of furniture, they have increased their base of support. If a baby is supporting themselves on both feet and both hands, as in a bear walking position, they have a relatively large base of support. If a person is lying flat on their back with their arms and legs out to the sides, they have a wide base of support, and a low center of mass. If they are standing on one foot on their tiptoes, they have a relatively small base of support, and a high center of mass. We automatically adjust our base of support and our center of mass, according to the level of challenge to our balance that we are faced with. If we are on a boat, and there are not many waves, we may be able to keep a relatively narrow base of support and a high center of mass—we may stand fully upright with our legs a normal distance apart. If there are heavy waves while we are on a boat, we automatically adjust our posture—we increase our base of support by widening our stance, and we lower our center of mass by hunkering down.

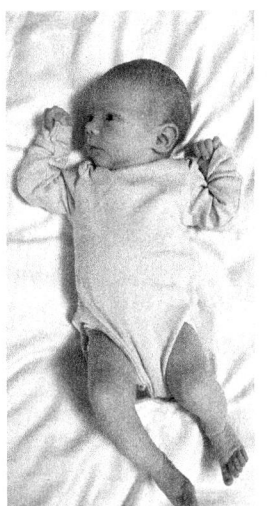 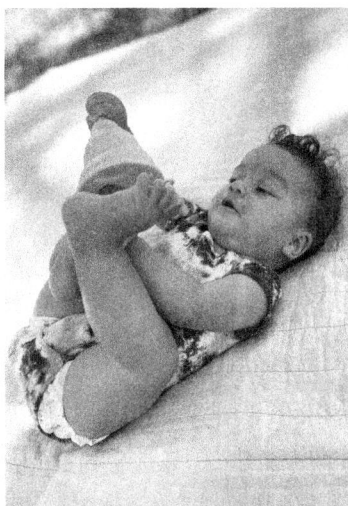 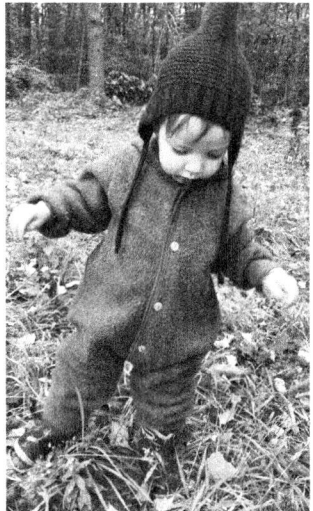 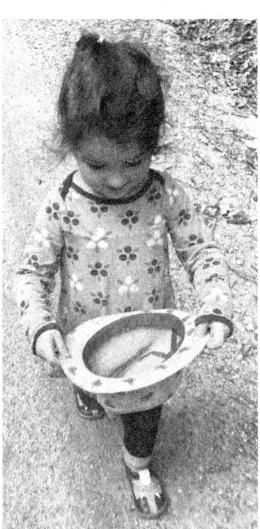

Far left: This week-old baby has a low center of mass and a wide base of support, lying flat on the surface. Second from left: This baby has a higher center of mass and a narrower base of support as they play with a toy with hands and feet up off the surface. Second from right: This toddler is walking on slightly uneven terrain. They have a wide base of support. Far right: This three-year-old has developed more balance in walking and has narrowed their base of support. In this photo they were carrying home a treasure in their hat, found on the walk.

A Progression of Balance

In each developmental position, there is a predictable progression of balance. The infant achieves a new developmental position, and then learns to maintain the position over increasing periods of time. Maintaining the position can be more difficult than one would think, because it requires a finely tuned interplay of muscles. As infants explore being in a new position, they move a little bit—perhaps by waving their arms or legs, reaching, or turning their heads—and with these subtle movements, their center of mass shifts. The infant's body, especially their core, then has to accommodate the weight shift, or else they may fall out of the position—if they reach too far for a toy, for example.

Learning to balance includes losing one's balance, and our bodies go through all manner of gyrations when we lose our balance—with the primary purpose of preventing our heads from hitting the ground, should we fall all the way to the floor. If we start to lose our balance, we may counterbalance by lifting an arm, a leg, and by rotating our trunk. If we perform all of these maneuvers when we start to lose our balance, and they are still not enough to avert the fall, the protective extension reactions, typically, are automatically activated. Here, we extend an arm to keep from hitting our head on the floor. Better to break a wrist than to have a concussion, although we are not thinking about this. We just do it. Balance reactions are automatic, but also can be modified by training and practice, such as learning to roll when falling—and this is a good idea, as it can reduce our injury when we do fall. Many times, when we start to fall, we recover our balance and do not actually hit the floor. Babies do this frequently as they move through each of the gross motor positions.

We can recognize an infant's recent achievement of a new developmental position because they characteristically use a wide base of support in it at first. As their balance develops in that position, we can recognize this too, because their base of support typically narrows. After a while, they may have improved their balance enough to manage playing with toys in the new position. Playing with toys involves still more weight-shifting within the position—especially if they are playing with a relatively heavy toy—which further challenges their balance, and so their base of support may widen again. As they gain more competency with their balance

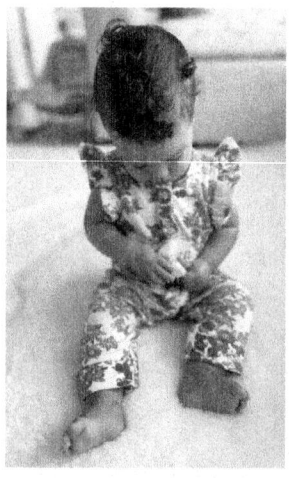 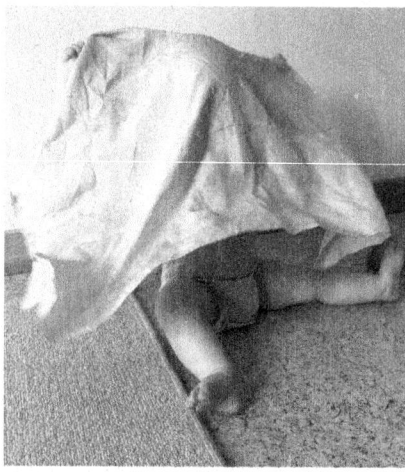

Above, left: Playing quietly with their toy is not challenging this child's balance, and accordingly, they have assumed a narrow base of support. Above, right: Playing more vigorously with a silk has challenged this child's balance, and so they have assumed a wider base of support.

when playing with toys, their base of support again narrows. If one observes a baby over time, one can witness these nuanced changes in the baby's balance.

Please note that we must attend to the manner in which we observe a child, as they are very sensitive to our thoughts and feelings about them. To me, observing a child's progression of balance in a respectful way is one way to enhance my relationship with them. When we can truly see a child and what they are working on, this can lead to a deepening of our reverence for the child.

It is helpful to note that development is not linear! For example, even if a child is crawling and pulling to stand, they may go back down to play on their backs. In fact, even two-year-olds will occasionally lie on their backs, hold a dolly up on their shins and play in that position. It benefits youngsters to freely choose the positions in which they play, because it can be very comforting to go back to "home base" and play there from time to time.

Mining the "Balance Gold" in the Full Gross Motor Sequence

In order to support the child's development of balance from the very start of life, it is helpful to give them opportunities to balance in which they can choose the particular positions that suit them. Progression through the different stages of development is not uniform. The child may linger in certain stages, and pass more quickly through other stages. We can trust that the child's higher Self knows what is best for them. If we try to direct their motor development by teaching them certain skills or placing them in positions before they can get there through their own initiative, they may miss out on certain stages or may not spend as long in a particular stage as they would have without our intervention.

When the child is given the time and space to negotiate the gross motor sequence fully, the child can learn how to fall in the lower horizontal positions of supine, side-lying, and prone, where the chances of injury are relatively small. For example, a baby may "fall" by simply rolling over and landing with a thud. When the baby gets this immediate feedback, they quickly learn how to roll without falling. It usually only takes a couple of little mishaps. We actually want them to have experiences with low-risk falls. It is valuable preparation for later on, when they get to the higher positions of kneeling and standing, where potential falls have higher risk. If a baby has had opportunities to learn nuanced balance reactions and how to fall safely in the lower positions, they are less likely to have injuries to their heads when they reach standing and early walking. Falling safely means, first and foremost, being able to fall without hitting the head. We can easily recognize when someone's balance is not optimal because they have frequent falls where they get hurt, and this often includes hitting their heads. Children with challenges to their balance can also be recognized, for example, by the way they negotiate a balance beam or a stream, in that they typically rush across. It takes more balance to go slowly and carefully from stepping stone to stepping stone in order to cross a stream, and so children who are challenged in balance go quickly, often missing the stones and getting their feet wet.

It is helpful to understand what happens spatially when a person falls and/or when they hit the ground. There can be a slight, subtle separation of the physical body from the finer bodies. (Rudolf Steiner speaks about human beings having bodies that are not physical; included in these finer bodies are the etheric and astral bodies. The finer bodies are explored in volume 2.) It is therefore the shock of this sudden separation that evokes fear or confusion. If a baby or young child has taken a slight tumble, and they are obviously not hurt and not in distress, it may best to take the matter lightly. Exclaiming with surprise, levity, and a smile: "Oopsie daisy!" can make a difference as to whether they take the unexpected descent as a serious insult or as just a little bump on life's rocky road. It can also be a good practice to leave the child to themself for a short period while the finer bodies and the physical body realign themselves—while they "come back to" themselves. If the tumble was physically and emotionally too much for them to handle, going right down to the place where they fell on the ground to surround and embrace them there, at the scene of the crime, can help them recollect themselves, rather than rushing them away before they can reassemble themselves. It goes without saying that if the child is still in danger, or actually injured, removing them to a safe place or favorite comfort spot can work wonders to provide comfort, care, and solace.[20]

Magda Gerber, who was a student of Dr. Pikler and later founder of RIE (Resources for Infants and Educarers), once stated: "Learning to fall, getting up again, and moving on, is the best preparation for life."[21]

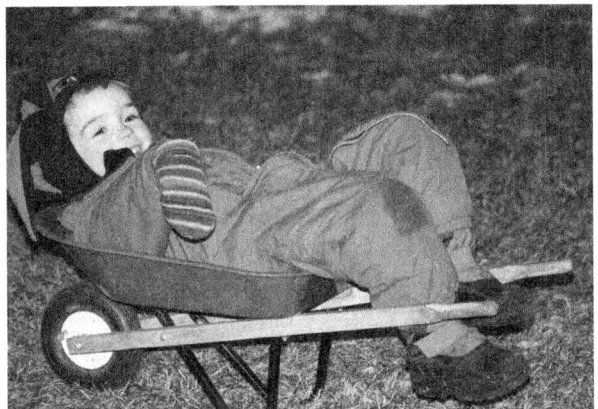
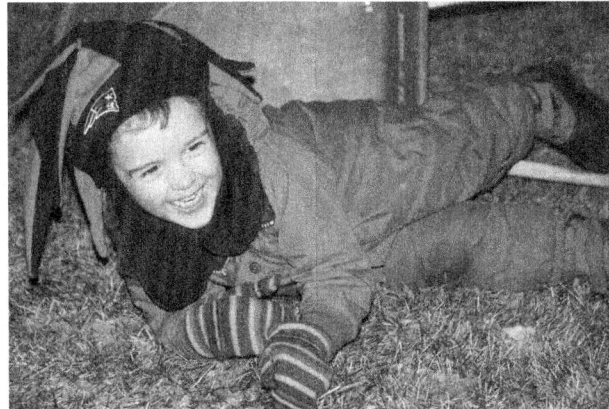

The children heard a story about a farmer who had harvested his pumpkins from the field and headed for the barn with them; on the way he stumbled, and all the pumpkins fell out of his wheelbarrow. The children played out this story for twenty minutes later that afternoon, intentionally falling out of their wheelbarrows over and over!

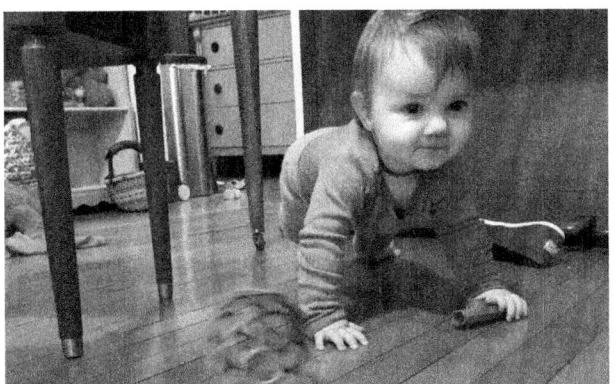
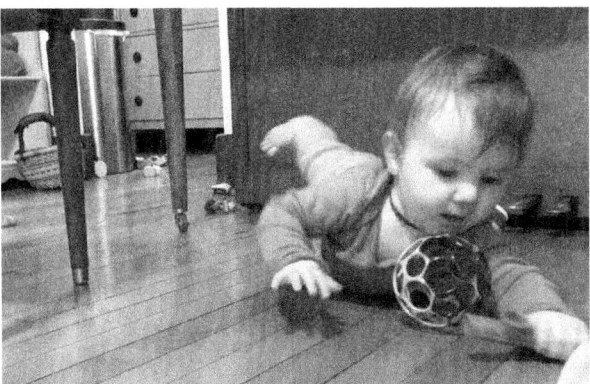

This baby was belly-crawling across the floor. They transitioned up into hands-and-knees and then fell down to the floor. They did not hit their head, and they did not cry. Instead, they paused for a moment, looked around, and then reached for a nearby toy. Learning how to fall and recover is an integral part of learning to balance.

The "Just Right" Balance Challenge

Children need lots of opportunities to develop their balance over the early months and years of life. Particularly helpful are circumstances that give them the "just right challenge" to their balance.¶ If the balance challenge is too difficult, they can't learn to balance, and if it is too easy, it's no good either. The degree of challenge that the baby is willing to undertake varies according to their level of ability. As noted earlier in the chapter, when the child is provided with opportunities for free motor exploration, they will take the next developmental step only after sufficient preparation, and only the child knows—at an unconscious level—when the time is right. If we place a child prematurely in a position that they can't get into by themselves—a position that is above their ability—they won't be able to learn to balance there. To consider an extreme example, imagine being suddenly placed in a precarious position—perhaps up on a high circus platform—and expected to walk a tightrope. This likely would be too difficult for us. It wouldn't help us to develop our balance. It would probably elicit fear, and perhaps even interfere with our relationship with the person who put us in this position.

The degree of challenge that the baby is willing to undertake in their balance also varies according to the moment-to-moment state of the child. Optimally, the child is settled and secure after a respectful, loving caregiving interaction. Factors which may cause a child to decline engaging in balance activities include a certain level of fatigue, hunger, or discomfort, or a combination of such factors. Perhaps they are cutting a tooth or have a soiled diaper. Perhaps there is too much commotion in the room, and they are dysregulated.

When the children get older, they also need opportunities to find the "just right balance challenge." Here is a lovely example of two children exploring their balance. A tree had been cut down in the woods behind their house, leaving a large tree trunk. For the two-year-old, it was enough to climb up onto the fallen tree trunk, momentarily lie on her tummy there, and then climb down. The 4 1/2-year-old wanted to walk the entire length of the trunk over and over. Neither child's hand was held, and neither child was encouraged to do anything. They alone determined their balance explorations. Another child at another stage in their balance development might have crawled along the trunk or simply sat on it.

Supplying older children with raw materials with which to construct obstacles courses is often a very satisfying way for them to find their "just right balance challenge." The raw materials can include wider and narrower boards, stumps, benches, and stepping stones. Pieces of nonskid shelf liner can serve to make the constructions safe, and there may need to be a "construction safety engineer," i.e., the teacher, to make sure the boards don't slip. For some children, simply walking on a wide board on the floor is enough. Other children want to be up off the floor, on a narrower board.

Uninterrupted Time to Balance

It is helpful to give babies long, uninterrupted periods of time to explore, "listen" with their bodies, and "play with" their balance. Time to focus solely on what they are doing is optimal. It is not helpful to draw their attention away from their activity. Consider a time when your balance was at risk. Perhaps you were out hiking, came across a bridge that had washed out, and you needed to cross the stream by stepping from rock to rock while wearing a backpack. This would not have been a good time for someone to strike up a conversation with you. You would have needed to pay full attention to what you were doing. (However, this does not imply that balance is at a conscious level, for our balance reactions occur unconsciously.) Similarly, speaking to young children when they are learning to balance is not helpful. In the following passage, Agnes Szanto-Feder addresses the common practice of adults speaking to children during their movement explorations.

¶ A. Jean Ayres, founder of the sensory integration therapy movement, coined the term the "just right challenge" as a condition which supports and enables the process of sensory integration.

Sometimes adults warn children about some "danger" even though they were calmly going about their business, "Careful! You might fall! You might hit yourself!" In such cases, children might trip and stumble or fall down from where they climbed up to because the adult diverted their attention from whatever they were doing. Especially when starting something new, they need all their attention to "hear" and perceive the *internal* messages and warnings sent by their own body and senses and act accordingly. . . . At other times, the exact opposite may be observed. The children feel they cannot fully control the situation, so they try to be careful or may even get out of the situation. The adults then encourage . . . them, "Don't be afraid!" "You can do it!" even though the children—based on the messages sent by their complex perception system, which is the core of their own security—have drawn the conclusion that the given situation is not suitable for them.[22]

Talking to children in such a situation is counterproductive, because we want the children to trust their senses. When we "talk them through it," they pay less attention to themselves, and so we short-circuit their sensing abilities. "They need internally perceived elements, which are more complex than words, to know where to put their feet in the next moment."[23] Balance is not an intellectual process—it cannot be learned well through verbal instruction. If an adult does see that a baby or toddler is at risk of falling when climbing on the Pikler triangle, for example, rather than instructing them verbally, it is better to approach the child, slowly and calmly, and see if they can figure it out themselves, all the while spotting them as necessary. Often, the adult's close proximity is enough—especially if the adult remains calm and grounded in their own body, as the child will imitate the adult's spatial gesture.

This same approach may be used with older children, although there may be instances where verbal assistance may be called for when dealing with older children. For example, when a kindergarten-aged child who has had less experience with self-initiated movement has climbed up in a tree and is unable to climb down, it might be necessary to "talk them down." If a baby or toddler were to climb up onto something and not be able to get down, the adult would come close and see if their presence was enough for the child to resolve the situation. If not, the adult would orient the child, saying something like, "I see that you are stuck up there and I'm going to bring you down." Then the adult would lift the child down to the ground, without any instruction.

Supporting the Child's Developing Balance—Without Physical Support

It is not helpful to hold a baby or toddler's hand or otherwise support their body in an attempt to help them balance. When we give physical support in these ways, we introduce an outside influence which actually interferes with their ability to perceive their own bodily organization in relationship to the gravitational field and in response to the balance challenge. This makes it difficult for the child to learn to balance, and also to learn how to fall.

Firm Surfaces

We also support the baby's developing balance by providing them with appropriately firm surfaces. Dear reader, please stop for a moment and stand on your non-dominant leg on a firm floor (wooden, linoleum, cork, or bamboo, if possible, rather than thick carpet) for a few seconds. Then get a small pillow or cushion from the sofa and stand on it with your non-dominant leg. Chances are, it was easier on the firm floor. Similarly, this is the case for babies who are just learning to balance.

The Three-Dimensional Nature of Balance

In every position, in order to balance, we must achieve an equilibrium among all three planes of space: above/below, front/back, and right/left. Inherent in the gross motor sequence are opportunities to experiment with balance in each of the three planes of space more specifically. For example, to maintain side-lying, the baby must balance so that they don't fall forward or backward. Here, they are focusing on finding the balance between the spaces in front and in back of the body. One can observe the child's subtle weight shifts and wobbles as they figure this out. Earlier in the chapter, a baby was described as assuming the plank position and then falling to either side, only to try it again. Here, the baby's activity emphasizes finding the balance between the right and left sides of the body. When a baby initially stands and walks, they typically elevate their hands to be up by their shoulders, and their overall appearance is a little "top heavy." Over time, the hands relax down, and later yet, they establish an arm swing. Here they are particularly coming into balance with regard to above and below.

Let us consider the spatial features of balance in more detail. In his book *Our Twelve Senses*, written from his lectures, Albert Soesman discusses this phenomenon. He says that balance is not an internal bodily affair, but rather we can balance because we fill the space outside of us with our being: "The reason that I can stand up here is that my being fills the entire room. I extend up to the ceiling, over to that curtain, over to the door, to the wall, to the lamp. I fill the entire space of this room."[24] He goes on to explain that when we don't fill the surrounding space, we are afraid. It is not uncommon for this to happen when we stand on the edge of a precipice. This is because we feel that we are being pulled forward into the emptiness of the space in front of us that we have not filled, and indeed, we are at risk of falling when our space is not evenly filled out.

Jaimen McMillan has studied and explored the spatial features of balance for decades, and has inspired the discussion in the following sections of this chapter. McMillan has created spatially oriented exercises for his students of Spacial Dynamics. In these exercises, the student always starts by filling the body space. Then, the student can learn to enhance their balance by perceiving the spaces out beyond the body and filling those spaces in equal measure in a dynamically changing, moment-to-moment manner. For optimal balance, the three-dimensional space surrounding the body is filled evenly. For the majority of us, chances are that the spaces surrounding our bodies are not filled evenly. We all typically have dents and cracks in our peripheral spaces, from past experiences that are still impacting us. However, we are often not aware of this. When we encounter a balance challenge, these irregularities in our space become apparent. We can witness this during an activity like walking a narrow balance beam or standing on our non-dominant leg and closing our eyes. Perhaps we have a strong tendency to fall to the left. If we fill the left space in equal measure to the space on our right side, our balance will reflect this, and we will be steadier.

The Fibula Stream, a Determining Factor for Successful Balance

Jaimen McMillan describes the life-force streams as dynamic pathways of movement that weave the spaces on and around the body into a unified whole. In his work with literally tens of thousands of students and clients, McMillan has identified the fibula stream** as being very significant for successful balance. The archetypal form of the fibula stream moves down the outer thigh toward the outside of the knee, circles the knee, continues down the outside of the lower leg (along the fibula), behind and below the ankle bone, and goes along the upper and outside edge of the foot, through the toes. Earlier in the chapter, we discussed the crucial role of orienting to the supporting surface for successful balance; the establishment of the fibula stream is pivotal in one's ability to come into relationship with the supporting surface. Through the fibula stream, we "ground" ourselves.

When I work with children—and with people of any age—who have challenges in their balance, I also find the fibula stream to be invaluable. I once worked with a ninety-year-old woman who had poor balance. Using a hands-on technique, I traced the fibula stream, as described above, on the woman's clothed legs. I followed up with guided movements in order to assist her to incorporate the fibula stream into her walking pattern, and then she was able to carry it out independently. Her balance improved so much that she got rid of her walker!

** The fibula and the tibia are the two long bones of the lower leg. The fibula is the smaller one on the outside.

How Does the Fibula Stream Typically Develop in the Growing Child?

Please note that the fibula stream is an outgoing stream. It travels out and away from the body, so that the person can come into relationship with the ground, and when the stream functions in this fashion it is most conducive for successful balance. At the beginning of life, this archetypal form and direction of the fibula stream has not yet been established. At this stage of life, let us call it the "pre-fibula" stream. Here it travels in the opposite direction, up and back in toward the body. In fact, the vast majority of the streams of the newborn travel in toward the body—with good reason. The newborn needs to fill the space of their body.

As a result of the initial incoming pattern of the pre-fibula stream, primitive movements, known as the primitive reflexes, manifest and dominate the movements of the child's legs. (The primitive reflexes will be further discussed in volume 2). They result in unsophisticated, stereotypical movements in the legs. The kicking reflexes are examples of these types of movements.

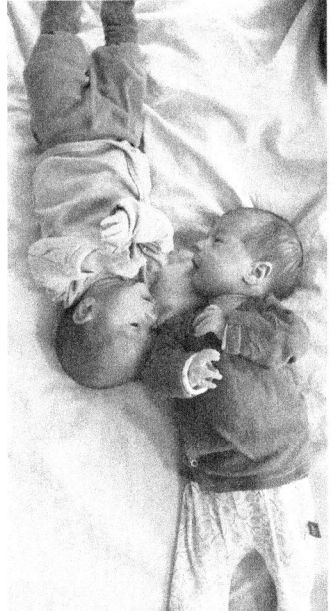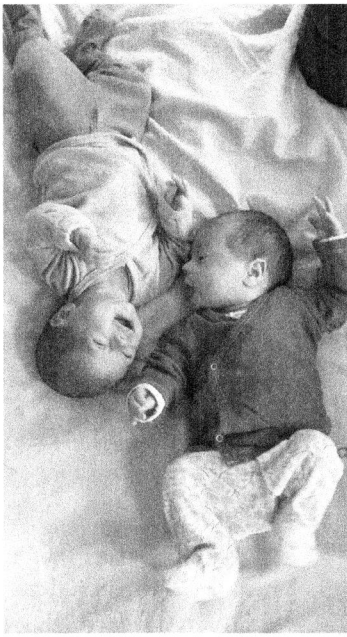

The baby on the right is manifesting a classic reflexive movement of the legs. The legs are initially fully extended. When the flexor withdrawal reflex is triggered, the legs quickly pull up into a fully flexed position. These reflexive movements are stiff, jerky, and without volitional control.

The streams exist in the spaces on and around the body. When the streams are activated, these spaces move, and the body can't help but follow along in the pattern determined by the stream. Hence, we say that a primitive reflex is triggered. Each of the many primitive reflex has its own underlying, incoming "pre-stream."

As the streams are prescriptive of the child's movements, when the streams change, the movements change. When the primitive, incoming leg streams are active, the primitive reflexive gestures are up and away from the periphery and in toward the body. This increases the muscle tone in the legs, the baby feels their legs, and they don't perceive what is out beyond their legs. That the baby feels their legs in this manner is developmentally appropriate—it increases the awareness of the body and helps to build the body scheme. This is an important stage of development. However, in order for development to then proceed, the streams must be transformed.

When the streams are transformed, the movements also transform. The key underlying factor in the development of balance is the transformation of the pre-fibula stream into its mature, healthy, archetypal form. The mature gesture of the fibula stream is out and away from the legs, making possible the ability to perceive and orient to the periphery—to the supporting surface. In this way, balance also becomes possible. We are able to balance because we can evenly fill the space out beyond our bodies, as well as the space inside out bodies—the body space.

Unfortunately, it is not a given that the transformation and reversal of the initial pre-streams will take place during development. The incoming streams are good and necessary at the beginning of life in order to help sense the body space. However, development is hampered if the incoming pre-streams don't reverse course and flow outwards. Fortunately, we can learn to perceive the gestures of the underlying streams and provide the environmental conditions that are most supportive for the streams to transform.

There are two conditions that provide optimal opportunities for the transformation of the primitive streams. The first condition is free movement in the early months and years of life within the context of a loving relationship and a developmentally appropriate and rich physical environment in which the child can find activities of interest. The second condition is that the child have adults who have incorporated the mature, archetypal forms of the streams into their own spatial gestalts. When the mature fibula stream is consistently active in the adults who are routinely in the child's environment, the child will naturally imitate their spatial gestures. It is possible for us adults to learn to wear the mature fibula stream—to weave it into the fabric of our spatial garment that we wear every day. I personally have found the Spatial Dynamics training to be invaluable in this regard.

We can perceive that the streams are changing direction and starting to flow outward when the baby starts to sense out beyond their limbs. For example, babies frequently play in supine, passing objects between their hands and their feet. In order to be successful and not drop the object, they must sense more than just their limbs—they must also sense the object. The photo on the top left is a lovely example.

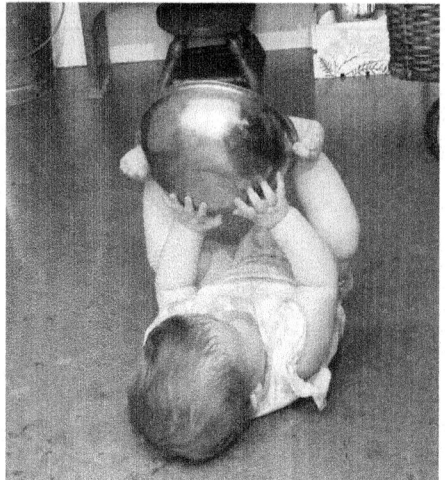

This baby spent an extended period playing on their back with a metal bowl, manipulating it with their hands and feet. In contrast to the above photos, here the movements of the legs are not reflexive; they are volitional, coordinated, and in relationship to the periphery—to the bowl.

Similarly, it is not uncommon for babies to lie prone and play with an object with their feet. The child is not using vision, because they can't see their feet—they are perceiving the object purely through their feet.

The fibular stream is also being transformed from its pre-fibular form into its archetypal form when babies push into the floor with their feet, and this happens countless times during free movement. In this way they are also sensing out beyond their feet, perceiving the supporting surface.

There are additional ways to support the development of the fibular stream. Allowing the child to be barefoot as much as possible helps them to sense out beyond their feet. I once worked with a baby who had been belly-crawling for quite some time. He adeptly pulled his body along with his arms, yet his legs dragged passively behind him. I noticed that he was wearing stiff, high-top shoes, and so he couldn't get a grip into the floor with his feet. When I suggested to his mother that she let him go barefoot, he started pushing into the surface with his toes in no time. Thus, he started to develop the mature fibula stream.

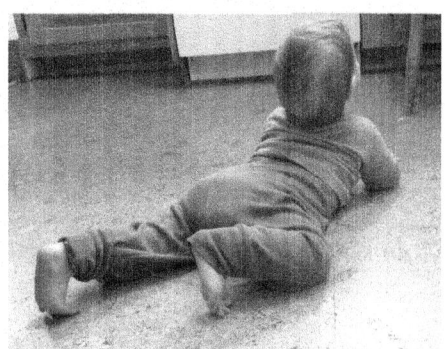

Here is an example of a baby who is orienting to the floor with their feet as they stabilize themself to look up.

Supporting the child's feet with a properly placed footrest when they are sitting in a high chair or other type of chair at the table is also conducive to grounding through the feet. For the older walking child, seated scooters (with four wheels and no pedals) are a lovely means of supporting the raying out through leg and foot that is necessary for balance. Balance bikes (with two wheels and no pedals) also support the development of the fibula stream. Balance bikes are generally appropriate as young as two and a half or three years and up to five or six years, depending on the child.

Tricycles are not as helpful, as the child's feet do not touch the ground, and the feet passively circle back and up toward the body in a hiccup type of gesture. For older kindergarteners and those in grade school, roller skating and ice skating are wonderful activities for the children to continue to develop the healthy raying out gesture through their feet. When I was a child, we had metal roller skates that fastened to our shoes. My sisters and I would spend hours skating around the block. The extra weight of the skates helped us sense our feet, and the alternating motion of pushing down into the sidewalk helped us sense out beyond our feet into the surface.

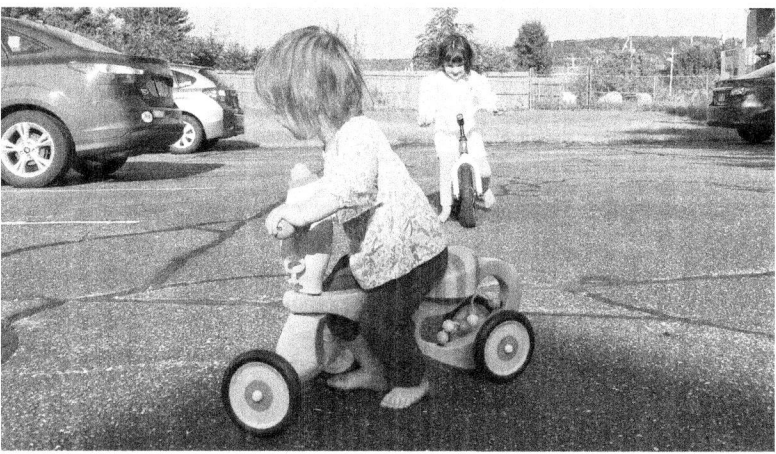

It is especially apparent that the child in the foreground is pushing down and backward into the ground as they propel the scooter forward. The feet have a raying out gesture, further establishing the fibula stream.

Similarly, in cross-country skiing, the child pushes down into the ground. (Technically, the child pushes down and backwards during skating and cross-country skiing. Pushing down into the surface allows the child to stay upright and pushing backwards into the surface allows the child to be propelled forward.) There are wide skis without poles that are appropriate for children as young as three years. Young children sometimes take paper plates (the inexpensive, slick kind) and use them to "skate" indoors on carpet. This is another lovely activity to support the development of the healthy raying out through the feet.

Car sickness is not uncommon in young children. Here, the overriding gesture of the child is "up," and unfortunately, the result is "up-chuck." In my experience, when the child is able to more fully incorporate the "down" gesture into their movements, of which the fibula stream is an important element, the car sickness resolves. I have also observed that babies stop spitting up as much when they start pushing down through their feet into the floor, thus establishing the fibula stream.

In a therapeutic setting, a therapist trained in Spacial Dynamics can teach parents the hands-on technique for the fibula stream. The parent can then incorporate the stream rhythmically into the children's routine, perhaps as an ending to a diaper change or before bed, for example. I have also created artistic renditions of the fibula stream by incorporating it into touching games and into movements put to verses. I have taught these to parents and early childhood teachers with good results. The touching games are especially nice for infants, and the older children can imitate the movement games. As discussed in chapter 12, whenever we touch an infant or a very young child, we must be aware of how the child is responding to our touch. We read the child's non-verbal cues and respond accordingly, so the touch experience is positive.

Identifying a Vestibular Challenge

In order to be comfortable in the world, one must be comfortable in the body. We develop an ease in the body by developing capacities in our four foundational senses. We simply don't feel safe in the world if we do not have a basic competence in our foundational senses, and nowhere is this more true than when we experience a challenge in our sense of balance.

Consider a time when you did not feel secure in your balance. Hopefully the condition didn't last too long. Perhaps you tried to walk a slack line, and the task was simply too hard for you. Perhaps you were walking on ice and couldn't get enough traction in order to orient to the surface. Perhaps you got on a carnival ride, and the ride was more intense than you thought it was going to be, causing you to lose where *down* was. It made you nauseous, and your lunch came *up*.

An adult student of mine once related to me that on one occasion she got caught up in a wave at the ocean and was turned around and around. She said that by the time she got to shore, she had become so disoriented that she literally didn't know who she was! Here, we see the polar opposite of Doris Humphrey's assertion that "being rooted meant having identity." This person was not rooted. She had lost her grounding, and she also lost her identity.

I lived in California for several years and experienced a handful of earthquakes. During the earthquakes, the ground shook, and it shook me up also, as I lost my inner knowing of where down was. People have also reported to me that they lose their grounding when they walk across a bridge whose surface is like a grate—with spaces in it so they can see through it to the river below. This type of bridge is disorienting for some people, making it uncomfortable for them to cross the bridge.

The above situations can give us insight into what it is like to have challenges with our balance. When balance has not developed properly, this can lead to a set of characteristic behaviors in which the child—or person of any age—experiences a high degree of fear in certain situations that typically would not cause concern to other people. Examples include: not wanting to invert one's head, not wanting one's feet to leave the ground (as in climbing or going on an escalator), or not wanting to walk on ice or uneven ground. The term for this is gravitational insecurity. This is a good name for the phenomenon, as the person has not yet come into a secure relationship with gravity. The person is truly frightened, and it is counterproductive to force them into a balancing activity.

In my experience, the most effective way to support a child who has challenges with their balance is to help them reverse the primitive leg streams (that have the pattern of up and in toward the body), as this is not serving them well. Guiding them to establish and incorporate the archetypal fibula stream into their movement habits will help them orient to the supporting surface and thereby come into a healthy relationship with gravity.

APPENDIX 1:
Supporting Free Movement through the Physical Environment

This appendix describes some of the physical attributes of play spaces that are designed to support free movement for infants and very young children. However, an appropriate physical space is only part of what is needed. Respectful, engaged caregiving is equally important.

It is helpful if the baby's play space is distinct from their sleeping space. Edmund Schoorel explains, "Children begin earthly life without memory. . . . Initially the faculty of remembering is bound to external objects such as furniture in the house, objects in the near surroundings, the daily trip to the grocery store, or whatever serves as a marker. The child's consciousness connects to these objects and not to the individual inner experiences."[1] When the child is put down to sleep in a consistent place—be it a bassinet, or a crib—the child can come to associate going to sleep with that place, and the place can trigger the child's going to sleep. Therefore, it is nice to have a designated sleeping space. Another cue that helps babies settle into sleep is a routine of dressing them in sleep sacks before they go to bed. The American Academy of Pediatrics recommends that children under one year old should not sleep with soft objects or loose bedding as a prevention for SIDS.[2] After one year, a comfort toy, such as a small stuffed animal or a cloth diaper, can help them transition into their cribs.

The Size of the Movement Space

The size of the movement space for the infant and youngster should be comfortable from the perspective of the child. If we were to place a newborn in a space the size of a football field, that would obviously be too large a space for them to feel secure. They have been in tight quarters in the womb for many months, and a gradual transition to larger spaces is beneficial. Dr. Pikler established a general rule of thumb for the movement spaces of young infants: the space should be slightly larger than the distance that the child is capable of moving. Thus, the infant has territory to explore while feeling secure in it. High ceilings sometimes affect young children adversely. Going into a large box store with a high ceiling, for example, can be overwhelming for them. If the play space has a high ceiling, it can be helpful to "lower" the ceiling by draping cloths across it. The cloths can also mitigate excessive noise. Thick curtains and perhaps a tapestry on a wall also can help with too much noise.

Protection

The play space should be safe and offer protection for the child. Many times, parents deal with the issue of safety by placing their infants in baby equipment. The babies are generally safe in these devices, but unfortunately, their movements are significantly restricted in them. Thankfully, there is another way! Instead of limiting the child's movements with a device, the child can have free movement within a defined, safe space. Gates are helpful to keep the child away from dangerous items and places with too much commotion—such as where dogs may be running or where older children may be playing. Gates with vertical bars are especially nice when the babies are learning to pull-to-stand and stand, as the bars are good handholds. One can also use pieces of furniture as ways to create a contained space. The space should be made safe so that the adult does not need to unnecessarily supervise or worry about the child when they are playing—if the adult is anxious, the child will perceive this. Outlet covers and other basic safety precautions, such as baby-proofed cabinets where cleaning supplies are kept, are, of course, necessary. Additionally, items in the play space should not have to be protected by an adult. Removing valuable, breakable items from the space helps ensure that the adult can feel relaxed. A rule of thumb is that the space should be so safe that if the parent were to be locked out of the house, the child would incur no physical harm.

It is also helpful to provide a protected play space for an older child when a younger sibling has recently started to belly-crawl and crawl. This prevents conflict because the mobile baby then doesn't interfere with the older one's play scenes. Gates can be used in this situation. Older siblings can also set up their play scenes on a table or bench where the baby can't reach.

To clarify, the child is not left alone during their play time. They continue to be embedded into the loving warmth provided by the adult, but the child is afforded a degree of privacy for their play and motor explorations. However, if the child needs something, the adult will readily and lovingly respond.

Independence

Dr. Pikler describes the children who were reared at Lóczy as having independence. She explains, "They do not expect help from adults either in order to change place or to change postures. As for their play activities, they usually apply the already well-known former performances and not the newest performances they are just learning."[3] She also outlines the nuanced ways in which adult help may be needed:

> This does not mean that these children do not need the help of adults in general. The inexperienced infant exercising new ways of activity or while playing often gets into unexpected situations in which [they] cannot help [themselves.] For instance, [their] clothing may slide down or [they] may meet other unexpected accidents, in which case the child becomes uncomfortable, unhappy and seeks help. The adult ought to give this help as soon as possible, otherwise the child becomes timid and loses the pleasure in being active. But the difference between giving this needed help and having the adults put the child in different positions is that here the need for help is always accidental and the help rendered is limited to putting the child back in the familiar starting position or helping [them] get rid of the unexpected trouble.[4]

Here is a good example of a situation in which a baby needed this type of help: The baby, lying on her back, was barefoot and pushing with her heels, propelling herself backward across the kitchen floor. She pushed herself underneath a pantry cabinet that was against the wall and up off the floor approximately eight inches—a space underneath the cabinet that was open on the front with a support structure on either side. Because she was going backward, she couldn't see where she was going and was unprepared to find herself in this location. She was also unable to move out of this space. Her mother noticed her predicament, came close, explained to her what had happened, where she was, and that the mother would slide her out of there.

The Horizontal Position

It is optimal for infants and young babies to be placed on their backs on a *horizontal* surface. The back-lying position provides the most free movement as well as the largest field of vision for the baby. Indeed, young infants spend considerable time exploring their environments with their vision. They look at objects in the environment, including things we adults do not normally pay much attention to. Back-lying is also the position in which babies have the most possibility to see and connect with the adult who is caring for them.

Looking is one of the first volitional movements of the young infant. Lying on their back on a horizontal surface is the optimal position for the young infant to freely turn their head and look around. This is also the most optimal position for the infant to learn to coordinate holding their head still while looking at a particular object of interest. The stable horizontal surface helps them to stabilize their head, and a stable head provides a stable base off of which the eyes can track and focus—i.e., the eyes learn to move independently from the head. It is helpful to give the child the time and space for this very basic first step of visual control, as—among other things—visual skills are foundational for our ability to attend. Our attention follows our vision.

When we lie flat on the floor, the weight of our body pushes down into the floor, and the floor pushes back up in equal measure. The weight of the body is distributed evenly in the horizontal position. This helps the baby develop their body scheme. (For more on the development of the body scheme, see chapter 11). If a baby is placed in a reclined sitting position, such as in an infant seat, there is more pressure on the lower back and buttocks than on the upper body. This unequal distribution of pressure gives unequal sensory input to the child's body and may interfere with the development of body scheme. Additionally, on the horizontal surface, it is easier for the baby to move their limbs, trunk, and head than it is in a reclined seat.

Moses baskets and wooden playpens provide horizontal surfaces in which newborns and young infants may explore movement. Playpens are not realistic for many families as they may take up too much room in a small apartment or home. In larger homes, playpens with an elevated floor can work well, especially in colder climates, where the floor might be cold, but the floor is also an option. Many times, parents are uncomfortable placing their babies on the floor. A sheepskin on the floor is often more appealing to parents, and the benefits of sheepskins are many. The world is so large for a young baby. Sheepskins create a small, delineated part of the world that is cozy and warm. Repeatedly placing the baby on a sheepskin gives them a place that becomes familiar and comfortable. Sheepskins are easy to transport, and the baby can recognize a safe haven when they are in a new place. Sheepskins that are manufactured without toxins are preferable.

A Pikler crawling box is another option that provides a horizontal surface for a young infant. (The Pikler crawling box is described in appendix 3.) The box can be placed open side up onto a kitchen table, for example. Additionally, a fleece can be placed inside the box for a very young infant. This is a nice alternative to placing a baby in a sling seat on the kitchen counter while the parent is cooking a meal. The Pikler box allows the baby to be in the horizontal, yet they cannot scoot off the end of the table and fall. They are up off the floor and can see the activity in the kitchen.

The Importance of Firm Surfaces for Coordinated Movement

We have a different experience when we push down onto a firm surface (such as a wooden, linoleum, or cork floor) than when we push down into a softer surface (such as a shag carpet or a thick pad), because firmer surfaces give us more proprioceptive feedback—the sensory information from our muscles and joints that tells us the positions of our various body parts. I have lived in California, where the tectonic plates are prone to shifting, in Virginia, where the soil is full of clay, and also in New Hampshire, which is the granite state. When I moved to New Hampshire, I could literally feel my posture becoming more erect, as the granite gave me a significantly firmer surface off of which to push. Simply put, it is easier to achieve an erect posture, and also easier to move, on firmer surfaces. When people walk on the beach at the ocean, they generally walk where the waves come onto the sand, rather than farther back, away from the water. The surface is firmer at the water's edge than farther back, where the sand is dryer. If we walk on the dryer sand, it takes more work, we get tired sooner, and we may not enjoy it as much. Opportunities to move on firm surfaces are helpful to infants, as they are just learning to move, and firm surfaces provide opportunities for movements that are more efficient, successful, and pleasant. Dr. Pikler sums it up adroitly when she says, "We too prefer dancing on parquet floors, to dancing on mattresses."[5]

In order to move effectively and to feel secure in our movements, we need to be able to engage with the surface in a predictable way. An example of when this does *not* happen is when we walk on ice. Our feet do not meet enough resistance from the surface, and we cannot sufficiently push down into the surface. As a result, we may slip and fall, or our movements may be haphazard. This can be unnerving. We may feel anxious because we are not able to "ground ourselves."

Additionally, if we do not adequately orient to the supporting surface, there can be musculoskeletal and perceptual consequences as well. If we do not push down into the surface, what often happens is that we pull ourselves up off the surface—we get "all tensed up." Over time, we may end up with chronically elevated shoulders and painful necks. Different muscle groups are used when pulling up away from the surface than when pushing down into it. Movements characterized by excessive "pulling up" interfere with our ability to perceive and act in the outer world, because our attention comes back to our inner world. For example, we cannot really carry on a conversation when we are walking on ice, because we are concentrating on just trying to not fall down. An example of a surface that was too slippery for babies who were just learning to crawl is presented below.

Surfaces to Support Belly-Crawling and Crawling

The children's home directed by Dr. Pikler in Budapest was in existence for over sixty years, and during this time, except for three children, every baby crawled reciprocally. At one point, the maintenance department put extra coats of varnish on the wooden floor in one of the babies' rooms. This made the floor too slippery, and three babies did not learn to crawl. The adults remedied the situation by subsequently only using one coat of finish on the wooden floors. Additionally, at the Pikler Institute, part of the babies' rooms had wooden floors. Wooden floors have less resistance, and are therefore more conducive to learning to belly-crawling. The other part of the rooms had carpet, which offers more resistance and is better for learning to crawl on hands and knees.

I saw the wisdom of having these two types of surfaces available to infants when I watched my own grandchildren negotiate the motor sequence. Their home has wooden floors throughout the house and a cork floor in the kitchen. There are two moderately sized rugs in the home. My grandchildren belly-crawled for many months, and they became very adept at it, eventually belly-crawling throughout the entire house quickly and easily. When they first started to get up onto hands and knees and crawl, they did this on the rugs, but they would quickly return to belly-crawling on the wooden and cork floors. It was fascinating to watch them switch their form of locomotion according to the surfaces they wanted to travel over. They were not consciously deciding to do this; their bodies simply knew what the most efficient and most comfortable movement for them was, based on the surfaces. After they had mastered hands-and-knees crawling, they easily crawled over both surfaces. I have known other babies who scooted in a side-sitting position on a wooden floor and then crawled on their hands and knees on carpet, switching movements when on the different surfaces. At Sophia's Hearth, we have noticed that grass is a good surface for learning to crawl as it offers a good amount of resistance. There have been several times when our babies began to crawl when they were first outside on the grass in the spring.

Firm Surfaces and Learning

Babies are learning about the world and how it works. In order to do this, they need accurate information. When babies are playing with a toy on a firm surface, they receive more accurate information about the toy than they do when playing with it on a softer surface. For example, if a baby repeatedly drops an object on a wooden floor, the object will move in a consistent way, and it will sound a certain way. One object that is dropped onto the wooden floor will respond significantly differently than another object will, and the child will be able to learn to distinguish the signature characteristics of the different objects. However, objects that are dropped onto softer carpet do not display such degrees of difference. Children love to bang their toys, and these sounds will be muffled on carpet, whereas on a wooden floor, the object's sound is more able to "ring true." Firm surfaces provide sound foundations for learning! When children explore in this manner, they have opportunities to come into a relationship with the underlying order and majesty of the world. This type of relationship with the world can be deeply satisfying and comforting to the growing child, and its effect may be long lasting.

Not only are soft surfaces less advantageous for learning, but the child may not be as successful in their play. For example, on softer surfaces, objects do not stand up as easily, and blocks do not stack as easily. This may negatively affect the child's feeling of agency during play.

Are Firm Surfaces Safe for Babies?

The answer is yes. Firm surfaces, such as wooden, cork, and linoleum floors, are safe for babies. (However, I would not recommend a concrete floor.) Firm surfaces are ideal for the infant to begin to learn to balance. When the baby bumps their head on a wooden floor, for example, they receive immediate feedback. After two or three times, they learn not to bump their head. With padding on the floor, the baby does not receive as much feedback from the bump, and potentially does not learn as much. As a result, they may incur more bumps in the long run, and the bumps that happen later on may be more serious. Firm surfaces provide optimal conditions for the baby to learn to balance and to fall safely. They are also learning judgment—what am I capable of achieving without suffering a bump, and what am I not capable of?

Éva Kálló and Györgyi Balog, in *The Origins of Free Play*, summarize it this way: "A rigid play area floor quickly teaches a child unequivocal lessons about the laws of gravity while [they are] still lying and moving very close to the ground. This far and no farther! Such clarity forces [them] from an early age to fall carefully or to move with enough care that [they do] not fall down in the first place."[6]

Temperature

The room should ideally be a comfortable temperature—warm, but not too hot. The question sometimes comes up about whether a radiant-heated floor is beneficial for babies who will be down on the floor for extended periods. While this idea may sound good, real-world experience has shown that this type of floor is too warm. A simple, unheated cork or wooden floor will come to thermal equilibrium with the air as long as there are not cold drafts.[7] As noted above, placing the baby on a nontoxic sheepskin on the floor can create a warm and inviting space. Intensive care nurseries have used sheepskins in the bassinets of preemies for years, as they have noticed that the babies gain weight more readily when kept warm. At home, putting a wool blanket underneath the sheet in the bassinet or crib will serve the same purpose.

Clothing

Ideal apparel is neither too loose nor too tight, and does not impede the child's movement. For example, dresses are especially difficult for crawling and climbing. Ribbons can get tangled. Hair ties and bows can interfere with movement for babies who are exploring horizontal positions. Dr. Pikler was very attuned to the children's need for nonrestrictive clothing. She paid particular attention to the details of the children's clothing. For example, she saw to it that the straps of the sunsuits buttoned on the sides of the children's shorts—rather than on the back—so that the straps were less likely to fall off the shoulders, which might draw the child's attention away from what they were doing. The children did not wear hoods attached to coats, as hoods impair free movement of the head. Instead, hats were worn. Balaclavas also allow for free movement of the head. Pillows were not used in the children's cribs, as pillows interfere with correct alignment of the head on the spine.

The baby does not yet experience their body as a whole, nor as separate from their environment, and so keeping the baby's body covered with clothing affords a degree of protection and definition, although I do not recommend covering an infant's hands. Similarly, it is beneficial to let the feet be bare, as long as the child is warm enough. (Bare hands and feet are discussed in the following section.) It is helpful to think of clothing as a type of sheathing. Even in warm weather, a thin layer of cotton is beneficial for this purpose, although obviously, one would not want a child to become overheated. In the colder weather, layers of wool or silk next to the skin are optimal. The adult is responsible for determining if the child is too hot or too cold, as young children do not yet have this capacity. My first grandchild was born in the spring, and I bought a wool onesie and wool leggings for her. My daughter-in-law and son were surprised that I had bought wool for her at that time of the year. However, they dressed her in the wool, and observed. They found that she was significantly less fussy when she was dressed warmly. We find the same thing at our childcare at Sophia's Hearth. We recommend to our parents that they dress their children in wool clothing during the colder months. If a baby comes to us without wearing wool, we have a stash of wool clothing that we dress them in while they are with us during the day, and then send them home at the end of the day in their own clothing.

It is also helpful if the babies wear hats during their waking hours, as hats decrease the amount of body heat escaping from the head. As infants' heads are proportionally larger than those of adults, this is especially important. In addition, as it generally takes from twelve to eighteen months for the last of the fontanels to close, dressing babies in hats when awake offers a layer of protection for this vulnerable part of the body.

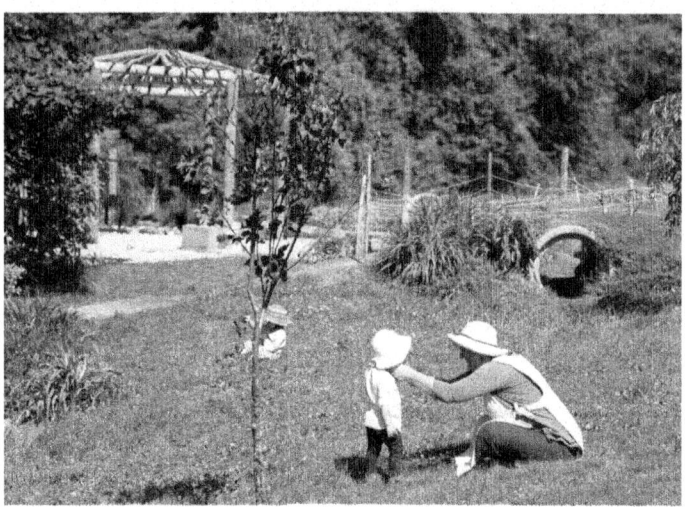

This teacher is tying a child's sun hat, which came off during outside play time.

A new teacher once told me that she couldn't keep hats on the babies because the babies kept taking them off. In this case, repeatedly putting the hat back on the child in a calm, loving manner will remedy the situation. More often than not, the child will become used to the feeling of being ensheathed by their hat, and it will come to feel good to them.

Conserving energy is an important consideration in colder climates, and dressing children in layers helps keep them warm; however, too many bulky clothes can impede their movement! Silk and wool are warmer than cotton. If silk or wool are used instead of cotton, the clothing can be less bulky for the same amount of warmth. Once, I had a baby referred to me for delays in her motor development, and when I observed her, she was quite sedentary. It was a cold winter that year, and she was dressed very warmly in bulky layers. In addition, she wore thick cotton diapers with a diaper cover. I suggested that we heat up the room and take off her clothes, and when we did this, the baby immediately started moving. It was simply a matter of too many clothes. At the children's home directed by Dr. Pikler in Budapest, children spent their "waking time, depending on the weather conditions, with the least necessary clothing."[8]

It is nice when the diaper changing room is warm enough so the infant can be comfortably naked for short periods of time and have an opportunity to enjoy some unhindered movement.

Bare Hands and Bare Feet

Sometimes newborn clothing has hand coverings, so that the infant does not scratch their face. However, this type of garment can negatively affect the child's awareness of their hands. The baby is born without body awareness, and they need opportunities to discover their bodies. One of the first parts of the body that the young infant discovers is their hand—they discover one hand at a time. Initially, the hand simply moves through their visual field, but they don't recognize it as belonging to them. Gradually, they learn to hold the hand still, in a position where they can see it. They learn to focus their eyes on their hand. Then they use a combination of vision and movement to *discover* their hand—they move their hand as they look at it. Over time they begin to realize that their hand is moving, and perhaps that *they* are the one who is moving it. It is *their* hand! It is primarily through vision and movement that the infant takes ownership of their hands. The infant can better see and "find" their hands if they are not covered. Trimming and filing the baby's fingernails can be done while the child is asleep to prevent them from scratching themselves.

It is optimal if babies and toddlers are barefoot during free play. Being barefoot helps prevent slipping and falling. It also serves a more unrecognized purpose, that of supporting the development of the sensing capacities of the foot. Accurate sensing is required for coordinated movement and balance, and more sophisticated sensing abilities allow for more complex motor skills and balance. If we were to wear very thick, rigid platform shoes or to walk on stilts, we may have difficulty perceiving the ground underneath us and be more prone to stumbling and falling. In order to be successful, we would need to sense out beyond the thick sole or the stilt in order to perceive the surface. Babies who are just developing their ability to sense out beyond their feet do better with thinner soles, or without shoes.

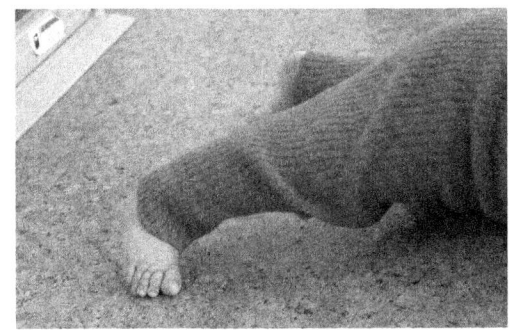

In back-lying, babies often use their feet as if they were hands, holding toys with their feet and passing them back and forth between their feet and their hands. In the same way that we take off our gloves to better find and pick an object out of a backpack, it is optimal for the baby if there is direct skin contact between the feet and the objects. The babies are doing what Rudolf Steiner gave as a remedial exercise for older children who were experiencing developmental challenges—he had these children use their feet like hands! Steiner recommended that they draw pictures with their feet—holding the crayon with their toes.

This baby is wearing wool pants and is active, so their feet are warm. Their primary means of locomotion is belly-crawling. Being barefoot helps them to better push into the floor with the toes, making it easier to incorporate the legs into the belly-crawl pattern.

Sometimes babies lie on their tummies and explore an object behind them without using vision, holding the object between their feet and manipulating it. In this example, especially, we can see the sensing capacities of the feet developing. The baby needs to feel the weight, size, and shape of the object with their feet, in order to successfully hold it and move it. When the baby is doing this, they characteristically become quiet, giving the activity their full attention.

Being barefoot supports the baby in learning many different motor skills. As described in the caption of the previous photo, when the baby is learning to crawl on their belly, being barefoot helps them more efficiently push into the floor with their toes, because they will not slip as much. Similarly, when babies start to climb on the Pikler triangle, they need to feel the rungs on the triangle and perceive the distance between the rungs, in order to coordinate their movement. The sensing capacities of the foot help inform the body how best to proceed. (The Pikler triangle is described in appendix 3.)

The Foot and Leg

It is important that a baby be kept warm enough. Leg warmers on the lower legs help the child stay warm while still being barefoot. Socks with grippers on the bottom of them are also good choices to keep babies warm.

If young children need to wear shoes, it is optimal if the soles of the shoes are thin and flexible. I once observed a relatively new walker who did quite well inside, where she was barefoot, but outside in the snow with thick-soled, stiff winter boots, she crawled over to one of the raised garden beds in the yard, pulled to stand, and did not move. She was certainly capable of walking, but the snow, combined with the properties of her boots, did not allow her to adequately sense, and then negotiate, the ground. When her parents got more flexible, thinner boots, she was able to walk outside on the snow. The following winter, she did well in the more traditional, thicker-soled winter boots, as the sensing capacities of her feet—and hence her balance—had improved by then.

It is helpful for the development of the baby's feet to have plentiful opportunities to move in a variety of ways, as this develops the foot musculature. When the many joints of the foot are allowed to move freely, the muscles can be optimally exercised. One result is the development of the arches, which babies lack at birth. It is very healthy for the baby to go barefoot! Where shoes are needed, the best choices are flexible, thin-soled footwear with low tops to allow full ankle motion. A good fit is important—the foot should not move excessively inside the shoe or slipper.

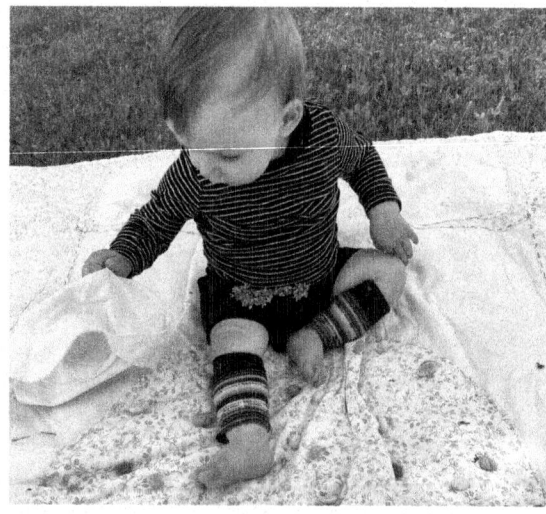

When colorful adult wool socks wear out and get holes in the toes or heels, the tops can be cut off and used as leg warmers for babies. Preschool and kindergarten-aged children also love to use these for dress-up, putting them on their forearms as well as their lower legs. One can also knit leg warmers for the children.

Color

Rudolf Steiner explains that the colors in a child's environment—both seen by the child and worn by the child—have a considerable and, many times, unexpected influence. "The colors in the child's surroundings are important. They exercise quite a different influence upon a small child than upon an adult. Many people think that green has a calming effect upon children. But this is quite wrong. A fidgety child should be surrounded with red and a calm child with green or blue green."[9] This is because the young child experiences the complement of a color. Art therapist Karine Munk Finser explains that "the young child's soul reaches so far into the etheric that they behold and experience the complementary color. We do not know, however, when a red room will begin to appear red to a child and have a red effect. This is an individual transition and the more the child is allowed to remain in a dream consciousness, where the heart unconsciously perceives the etheric, the longer are they experience the complementary color."[10]

When I was just out of college, some friends and I canoed and camped in an area around Lake Powell in the western United States for three weeks. This area of the country has a very reddish landscape. When we returned to civilization, we saw green—the complement of red—for a matter of days. It was an extraordinary visual adjustment for us, and perhaps it gave us a glimpse into the inner experience of color for the very young child.

Lighting

Many people assume natural sunlight is ideal for children, and so it is, but only if the direct glare is avoided. Outside, trees or awnings can provide the needed shade. Inside, translucent window dressings or upward-turned blinds can be used when sunlight is too bright. When artificial lighting is needed, modern LED lights can provide efficient and high-quality light of the desired hue. It is best to avoid direct glare, as with overhead and recessed lights. Instead, lamp shades and light reflected from the ceiling are preferable.

APPENDIX 2:
Toys to Support Free Movement

This appendix is based on my professional and personal insights, gleaned from my study at the Pikler Institute in Budapest and of the work of Rudolf Steiner, tutoring from Anna Ruth Meyer and Dr. Debbie Laurin, and observations of families and children in my care over many years. Anna Ruth Meyer is a Pikler pedagogue and Dr. Debbie Laurin is currently working on her Pikler Pedagogie Thesis. For further information on the topic of toys, I recommend *The Origins of Free Play* by Éva Kálló and Györgyi Balog.[1]

David and Appell discuss the arrangement of toys at Lóczy thus:

> Some objects are always on hand when the children arrive in the play areas, but the totality of the materials is not put at their disposal. New objects are introduced during the play period to rekindle interest as the [caregiver] sees fit. The older children can ask for the games they want. ... The materials for the smaller children are always arranged in the play areas in the same way so that the children can find them quickly when they arrive.[2]

This chapter will explore toys for infants and youngsters, as well as the reasons they are best suited for particular developmental stages. Let us begin with what is recommended for the very young infant.

The Hand

Dr. Pikler identified the hand as the infant's first toy. The newborn does not have much awareness of their body yet, and so it is really quite something when they first discover their hand. This occurs while they are still lying on their back, before they can roll to their side. While the young infant is batting their arms around, they will catch a glimpse of their hand as it hurls through the air. This may happen several times. It piques their interest. The importance of interest must not be underestimated, as interest blazes the trail for the development of coordinated movement. Over time, babies learn to coordinate the muscles of their eyes with the muscles of their arm, so that they can hold their hand in a position suitable for looking at it. This noteworthy accomplishment is often overlooked, yet it is the first milestone of hand-eye coordination, laying the groundwork for what follows. Indeed, Dr. Pikler did not give the baby anything else to play with until they had "found" their hand.

Gradually, the duration of gazing at the hands lengthens. Babies learn to move their hand closer and farther away from the face, rotate their hand, and open and close their fingers. As they integrate their vision with the movement of their hand, they start to perceive that it belongs to them. Initially, they will only be able to look at one hand at a time, off to the side. Gradually, they will be able to bring their hand nearer to the middle of their body and look at it there, and then they will be able to bring both hands to the middle of their body and look at the two hands simultaneously.

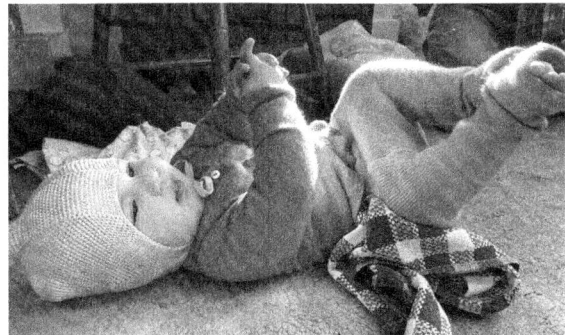

This baby has brought their hands together and is viewing them at the middle of their body.

The Progression of Early Toys

The next toy that Dr. Pikler provided to the infant—who was still in the back-lying stage of development—was a *cotton* cloth, the size of a small dinner napkin. The cotton cloth is lightweight, so that if it falls on the baby's face, it will not hurt them. It is important that the cloth is cotton, and not silk, at this stage of development. A cotton cloth upon on the child's face will not impair their breathing; however, a silk one could, as the lighter-weight silk can be inhaled into the mouth. (However, silks of various sizes and colors are lovely items for older sitting and walking children.) Dr. Pikler's cloths were homemade, characteristically made of polka-dotted fabric, because that is what was readily available. Plain colored fabrics are also nice, because they give the baby the opportunity to perceive the nuanced variations of shading in the napkin. When we were first acquiring materials for our babies at Sophia's Hearth, we could only find napkins with fringed edging, and the babies were very interested in the fringe!

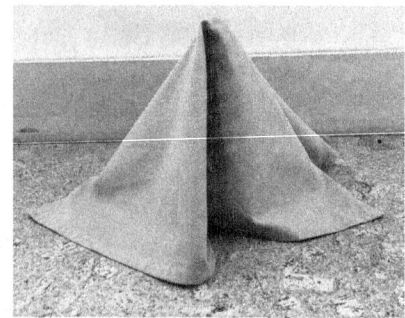

The cotton napkin.

The cotton cloth is placed near the infant, in a sort of teepee shape. The cloth is not put into their hand. This gives the baby the opportunity to self-initiate picking up the cloth—or not. Initially, the baby will typically explore the cloth with their vision. When they try to reach for the cloth with their hand, they may reach too far or not far enough. The baby's accuracy of reaching and grasping will improve with practice. The cloth is ideal for this level of fine motor development, when they are grasping with the pinkie and ring fingers. (See chapter 7 for further description of fine motor development.)

I once had the opportunity to observe a baby playing with a cotton cloth over several weeks. One day, while lying on her back, she inadvertently dropped the cloth on her face. She kicked her legs and batted her arms, with increasing range of movement and velocity. At one point, it appeared as if she would soon start to cry. The cloth was still on her face. Her mother noticed this, and she intervened. However, she did not solve the baby's problem. Instead, the mother came close to the baby and calmly oriented her. She called the baby by her name and told her, "You have a cloth on your face. You dropped it there, and you can take it off if you would like." The baby settled, and, shortly thereafter, pulled the cloth off. The look of success and joy on the baby's face was unmistakable. The mother's actions expanded the child's tolerance for uncertainty and frustration. This is a good example of *co*-regulation. It lays the groundwork for later *self*-regulation by the child.

After the cotton cloth, other small, soft toys can be introduced. With the infant lying on their back, one or two toys can be placed to each side of the infant so they may self-initiate reaching for which ever toy interests them. In the same way that they "find" their hand and spend time looking at it, initially, the back-lying baby will pick up the soft toy and simply look at it while they are turning it around with their hand. It is nice if some of the toys at this stage are asymmetrical, so they will see something different when they turn it around. A classic toy for this age, which grandparents have made for years for their grandchildren, is a cloth giraffe—with a good, long, grabby neck. Other toys include those made of fabric and small kitchen items, such as silicone cups. These toys are

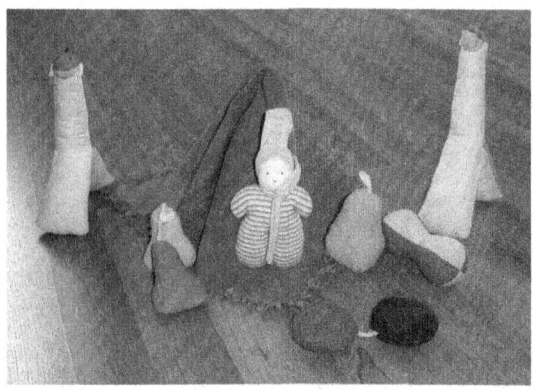

Small, lightweight, soft toys. All of the toys in this photo, except the napkin and the dolly, were purchased from the Pikler Institute in Budapest. Please note that these toys and those in subsequent photos have been grouped together for purposes of displaying them in the photos. They would be arranged differently in an infant classroom or play group, and this is described below.

relatively easy to grasp but are a little more difficult than the cloth napkin is. They are soft and lightweight; if the baby drops such toys on their face, they will not hurt themself. At this stage of development, the baby may be lying on their back, or they may have rolled to their side. As they are not yet mobile, it is best not to give toys that will roll away if they are dropped, as this may unnecessarily frustrate the child.

As the baby develops more coordination, strength, and endurance, they are ready for heavier toys and slightly larger toys. Simple, one-part wooden toys are appropriate. Small wooden rings are a favorite, as are everyday kitchen items, such as wooden spoons and funnels.

Dr. Pikler chose toys that the baby could pick up and manipulate. She specifically did not tie toys to the bars of the baby's crib or hang them from an overhead structure, nor did she use hanging mobiles. When babies are subject to situations where they want to play with an object but cannot because it is out of reach, it may impair their ability to self-regulate. Babies may become very excited when they see a shiny, twirling overhead mobile, but as they are not able to satisfy their impulse to explore it, they may not settle down. If, however, they have toys that are within reach, they may also become initially excited when they see a toy, but they calm down when they pick it up and manipulate it. It is very helpful for the development of the child's autonomic nervous system if they do not stay in a heightened state of arousal for prolonged periods of time, because then that becomes their perception of a "normal" state. It is optimal if the child learns to shift gears back to a comfortable, "middle" level. Whereas looking at a mobile and not being able to interact with it can promote a "spinning your wheels" gesture, freely manipulating an object supports the child in developing more of a sense of agency in the world.

A classic baby toy for this stage of development has movable parts, such as a ring of toy keys. In our childcare at Sophia's Hearth, I have observed that a small wooden book with moveable pages has been a favorite over the years. With these types of toys, the child can ascertain that *they* made the part move and can better understand how this happens, as opposed to a mechanized toy where the child pushes a button. Similarly, toys made from different types of materials that the child can bang together, drop, and wiggle on the floor offer a variety of noises. With these types of toys, the

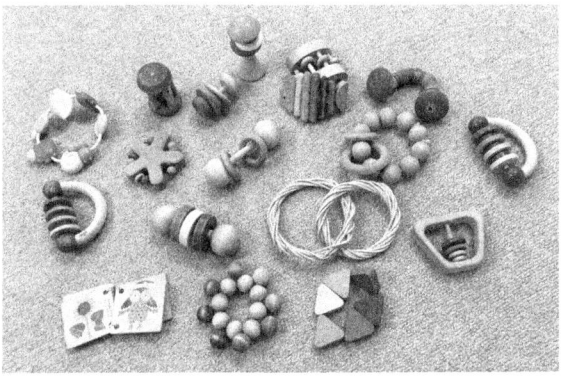

Gradually, toys that have movable parts can be added.

baby can more clearly identify how a particular sound is made and that they were the one who initiated and stopped the sounds. They can also make the noise louder or softer and increase or decrease its frequency. In this way, there are plentiful, nuanced opportunities for the child to develop auditory discrimination.

Progressions of Playing with Toys and Objects

Just as they initially discover one hand at a time, babies will initially play with only one toy at a time. Later, the baby may happen to pick up a toy in each hand. However, as they cannot yet attend to both at the same time, when they look at one of the toys, they will drop the other one. It is, later on, quite an accomplishment when they are able to attend to two toys at once. The typical progression for self-initiated toy and object exploration is as follows: Initially, the baby will play with a single toy by simply holding it in the air, as they lie on their back. Then, while tummy-lying or side-lying, they will play with the toy while it is on the floor. Next, they will play with two toys simultaneously—perhaps bringing them together or placing them side by side or one above the other—and then, with one toy inside the other one. It is a sea change when the baby starts to play with two toys simultaneously, for then they discover and create relationships. For example, they may

FREE MOVEMENT FROM THE VERY START

recognize that one toy is bigger than the other one. One toy is heavier than the other one. One toy is brighter than the other one. Over time, they experiment to find that this toy fits inside that basket, and several toys fit inside a different basket. This object stacks with a similar object. (Cups are nice for this.) This toy sits on top of another toy, and that one falls off. Exploring the relationships between toys indicates a huge cognitive leap for the baby. They are learning fundamental concepts about space. Each particular object exists in only one place in space at a time. The toys are in relationship to each other. The child is empowered because they can change the location of an object in space to influence the relationship between the toys.

At some point, the child discovers that two objects are identical, and this is quite a discovery! The child may carry two of the same objects around, perhaps banging them together, with obvious enjoyment. In order to further support their cognitive development, we can provide larger sets of toys and objects, such as sets of toys that are all the same color, but different sizes, or sets that are all the same size, but different colors.

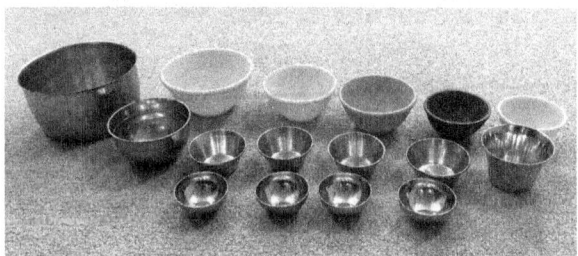 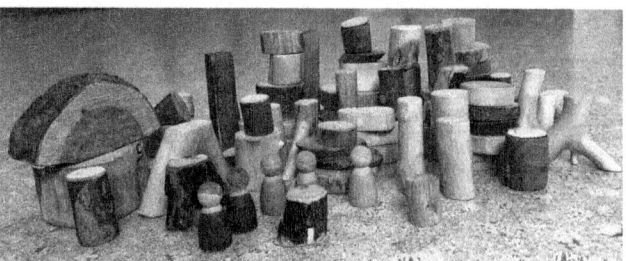

Above, left: Here is a set of bowls. They have different sizes, shapes, colors, and are made of two different materials: metal and silicone.
Above, right: Here is a well-loved set of homemade branch blocks.

Other examples of sets are several cloth ponies, knitted bunnies, or beanbags. Initially, the baby will be interested in finding pairs of items, and later, they may want to gather all the toys of a particular set. This is a typical stage of development. The child is not being greedy. It is natural for human beings to want to create order in their environment. Well-meaning adults often try to make the child share when they start collecting, however, sharing must come from within. Rather than instructions in sharing, the adult can model generosity, and over time the child will come to sharing on their own.

The children progress to selecting subsets from a larger set of toys. For example, they may gather up all the toys of one color or of one size. This type of play lays the groundwork for understanding the "set theory" of mathematics. Later, also, they will select specific items for building projects. For example, they may choose blocks of a certain size and shape to build a particular structure. This is a type of categorizing.

Branch blocks are blocks that are made of assorted sizes of tree branches. They are cut into a few standard lengths and then sanded. However, the bark is left on, knots in the wood are present, and the grain of the wood is very apparent. Branch blocks offer rich opportunities for the development of discernment, as they vary so much in shape, texture, and color of wood. Branch blocks can be made at home.

Kálló and Balog recommend:

> Since we can anticipate that a child of about a year and a half will really start to build in earnest, it is good to have appropriate toys available. A large box of wooden building blocks will serve the purpose, though it can be dangerous if used unsupervised. For most children, building starts already with collection and stacking of smaller or larger blocks, boards, and other elements. Thus, such a box should figure among their playthings.[3]

Slightly before or about the same time they start to place toys on top of each other, they also enjoy lining up toys, such as blocks. This can progress to creating patterns out of blocks and other toys. Older children continue creating patterns, for example, when they string beads in a particular series of colors. Pattern creation and recognition are related to later mathematical functions.

In addition to stringing beads, older children enjoy toys with pieces that can be joined together and taken apart. Train pieces, train tracks, and a tractor with a connection for a wagon behind it are classic toys for this.

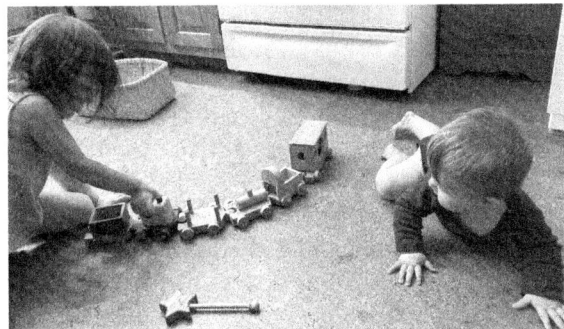

The child on the left is joining together the train cars.

Some children use long strands of finger-knitted cords to connect various things in the house. They can essentially turn a room into a big spider's web with finger-knitted cords. I once entered the bedroom of a kindergartener and a preschooler where they had been quietly playing. They had taken a ball of yarn and completely enclose their bunk bed! Additionally, the children often go through a phase where they want to tie knots, and jump ropes are good for this.

In group settings, enough toys are needed for everyone to find satisfaction, and it is also prudent to have several identical toys. This is especially helpful when one child wants the toy that another child is playing with—the adult may provide the child who is seeking the other child's toy with another one exactly like it. Sometimes, however, there can be too many toys, and the play space can become too crowded and too disordered. Kálló and Balog similarly observe:

> When playing, the children take things from one place to another and leave them lying here and there. At nine months to a year, once they have begun to play in modes which require many smaller-sized items, the floor is often strewn wall to wall with toys. Our experience is that they cannot play as well in the resulting topsy-turvy. The caregiver prevents the chaos by occasionally moving abandoned toys out of the way and by grouping smaller items next to baskets and bowls which are suitable for the put in/take-out mode. [The caregiver] often observes that the children act on the opportunity almost immediately. By recognizing what the children are interested in playing with, [the caregiver] can enhance [the children's] play by adding a few more items which they might need for the game.[4]

When deciding which toys to put aside when the room becomes too disordered, it is helpful for the adult to carefully observe whether the child is finished playing with a toy or not. The child will not take kindly to having something "taken away" from them that they are in the middle of playing with. It is helpful for the toys to be put away at the end of free play periods. In this way, the children can start afresh the next time and experience order in their environment—each toy has its place in the room. It is the adult's responsibility to pick up the toys. The adult does this willingly and without rushing. Some children may find it enjoyable to participate in the picking up. The adult may thank these children, and even ask them to help, if the adult perceives that the children find cleanup pleasurable, however, it should not become a "chore" for them. True to our guiding principle of self-initiated movement, the children are free to help—or not. Dr. Pikler used this same philosophy with children up to six and seven years old.[5]

Children Taking Toys Away from Each Other

Sometimes, in a childcare setting, one baby will take a toy away from another baby, and that baby does not become upset. Therefore, no intervention is needed. Inevitably, however, there will be some conflict when two children want the same toy, and neither one will back down. This is when the art of caring for children comes into play. An in-depth discussion of conflict is beyond the scope of this book. Suffice it to say that, just as with motor development and cognitive development, the adult does not *teach* the child to develop social and emotional skills. Instead, the adult models healthy social interaction and emotional maturity, i.e., the adult works out of imitation, and the child will self-initiate social behavior in their own time. The general guideline is that no one may take a toy away from another child while they are playing with it. If a conflict arises over a toy, the adult will first wait and see if the children can work out the conflict on their own. If the children need help in working it out, the adult may intervene, saying something like, "Jonah, Petra is playing with the toy now. When she is finished, you may play with it." Or "Petra, Jonah would like to play with the toy now. When you are finished, you may put it down and he will have it." The adult must size up the situation and act accordingly so that no one gets hurt—the adult is responsible for the safety of all the children. In dealing with the children, the adult may not use force to take a toy away from a child, as this would be considered a "mini-aggression" as Elsa Chahin and Anna Tardos call these types of occurrences.[6] The adult would not want to impose a mini-aggression upon the child nor model doing this in front of the other children present.

Motor Development and Play

When babies turn to their tummies, they will play with a toy on the floor. They will touch it, stroke it, bat at it, slide it, or roll it. Ideal toys for this stage of development are small metal bowls, which are shiny and make varying sounds when the baby moves them. When the baby bats at them, they wiggle just a little—but they do not move too far away. This may interest the baby enough to scoot on their belly after the toy. Over and over, we can notice that it is the baby's interest that drives their movement. As Dr. Debbie Laurin explains, "Back-lying is a more stable position for play and exploration. It is also a restful position."[7] Therefore, the baby will likely return to back-lying and play with the metal bowl in that position also. By this point in development, they are unlikely to drop it on their face, because their fine motor skills are more developed. Similarly shaped items that are made of different materials can be provided. This will support the child's emerging ability to discriminate. For example, a small metal bowl, a woven basket, and a wooden bowl can all be approximately the same shape and size, yet when a baby bats at them, each one responds differently.

As they gain mastery of grasp and release, babies will intentionally pick up a toy, drop it, and watch what happens. Dropping is a classic type of play, and it serves as one avenue for the child to come into relationship with gravity. When released, the toy always falls toward the center of the earth. This may impart a feeling of constancy and security to a child, especially if they are experiencing a lot of change in their lives. For example, caregivers and parents may come and go. Sometimes parents get divorced or must travel for their work. Caregivers get sick, change jobs, and take vacations. Adults get haircuts and change their clothes. Sometimes they may wear glasses, and sometimes not. In contrast, gravity is constant, unchanging, and predictable. If dropped, the same toy—which is subject to gravity—will always act the same way. The child can depend upon this. Additionally, we can help the child gain a sense of security with predictable daily routines, and in other ways. For example, caregivers at a childcare center can wear the same apron over their clothes every day.

A Word about Plastic Toys

Plastic toys are ubiquitous in Western culture, and there are many points of view from which to consider them. Plastic toys can be a good choice in certain situations—they are often less expensive, and they are readily cleanable. For some parents who might be new to a Waldorf childcare setting or school—where natural toys are plentiful—plastic toys are familiar. However, plastic is far from ideal for the environment. Additionally, plastic toys tend to be lighter weight and monochromatic in color, temperature, and texture. In contrast, natural materials offer more diversity of sensory experiences and, therefore, more opportunities for the development of more refined sensory discrimination. For example, the grain of a wooden toy offers subtle variations of color. Additionally, the baby can feel the ribs of the grain as they move their hands over the wooden toy. Materials that are dyed with natural dyes offer subtle variations in the tones of color. Metal and wooden bowls of similar sizes have different weights, and they also feel slightly warmer or cooler to the touch. The baby's sense organs continue to develop over time after birth. When babies have rich, nuanced sensory experiences, the development of their sensory organs is positively impacted, which can result in more refined sensing abilities.

Firm Cushions and Small Platforms

When babies are reaching for toys and playing with them on their bellies, small platforms (such as upside-down basins) and firm cushions (such as yoga cushions) are interesting items. The foam of a sofa cushion (which is relatively soft) can be removed and replaced with a folded wool blanket (which makes the cushion firmer). Firmer cushions are easier than softer ones for the baby to use in their play.

Babies like to place toys on top of these cushions and then take the toys off, or knock them off. The babies are exploring the concepts of on and off. There is no need for an adult to name these concepts for the baby, for their movements say it all, and at this stage of development the child learns best by doing. Reaching to put toys on the cushions and take them off provides opportunities to develop important diagonal movement patterns, which are foundational for later higher-level coordinated movements. Soon, the baby will belly-crawl over the cushions. Old-fashioned, low-to-the-ground footstools that are sturdy and will not easily tip are other options. Dr. Pikler also placed small inner tubes in the play spaces for the babies in her care. The babies crawl into and out of the inner tubes, and they also place toys inside them and then take them out. This is another lovely opportunity for the baby to develop the diagonal movements that are so important for healthy movement.

Toys for Babies with Increased Mobility

When the baby starts to move through space, e.g., roll across the floor and/or belly-crawl as a means of locomotion, they are ready for more movable toys, such as felted, knitted, or woven balls of various sizes.

They enjoy dropping the balls, watching them roll away, and then retrieving them. The balls can be of assorted sizes—as large as a beach ball, for example. I recall watching a baby lie on his back, playing with a beach ball—holding it with his arms, holding it with his legs, passing it back and forth, and spinning it between his arms and legs. The baby would inevitably drop the beach ball from time to time, and he never seemed to tire of rolling over onto his tummy, belly-crawling after it, and retrieving it—only to start the game all over again. He became very adept at sensing the furniture and other objects and people in the room, and he did not collide with them while he was going after the ball. I remember feeling great respect for the child's spatial awareness when I watched him. He played with the beach ball like this for many weeks, and it was apparent, from the expression on his face, that he experienced immense joy with this game.

About when babies start to crawl, knitted cords are appropriate toys. Children will typically continue to play with these toys for many months.

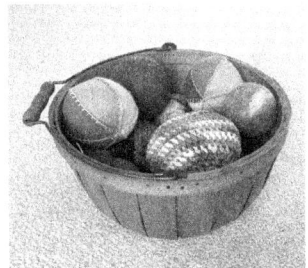
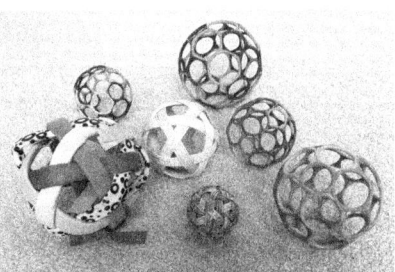
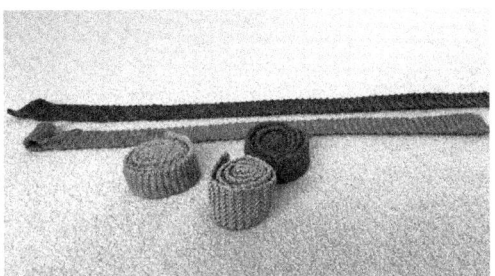

Left to right: Felted, crocheted, and sewn balls; The younger baby can more easily pick up these types of balls; Knitted cords.

At this stage of development, the adult can start placing the toys farther away from the baby, in order that they can roll or belly-crawl over to them to choose what they want to play with. Also, at this stage of development, Dr. Pikler gave the babies ninepins (small wooden toys shaped like bowling pins). These are wonderful toys, because when the baby touches them or bats at them, they move in very interesting ways, and the baby will likely move after them. When babies achieve sitting, pulling-to-stand, and standing for increasing periods of time, they also start to explore verticality with their toys. Stacking blocks is a classic activity for exploring vertical orientation. Babies also enjoy "standing-up" toys, which are longer than they are wide or long. Standing such toys up on end takes more complex hand-eye coordination. The nine pins are a nice object for this type of play, along with items like empty bottles of dishwashing soap. The used dishwashing bottles can also be partially filled with various smaller items—with the lid tightly secured. When my siblings and I cleaned out a relative's home, we found a little wooden toy that was about six inches long. It looked like a cross between a ninepin and a pestle (as in mortar and pestle), and it was labeled as a baby toy of one of our ancestors from the late 1800s!

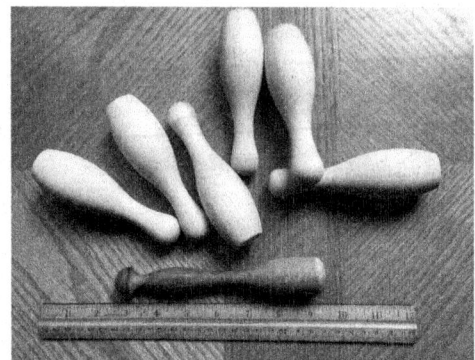 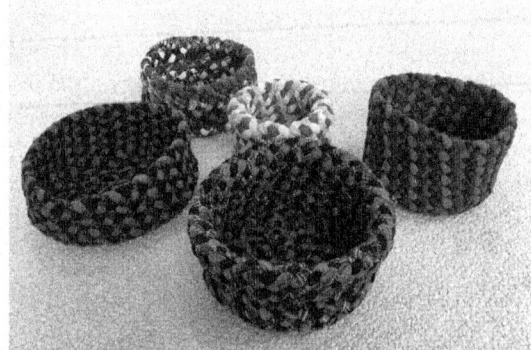

Above, left: Ninepins and antique wooden toy. Interestingly, the antique toy was a favorite of my third granddaughter.
Above, right: This set of braided baskets has been a favorite of the babies at Sophia's Hearth.

Baskets and Containers

Baskets and containers expand the possibilities for playing with toys and objects. The baskets can be of different shapes, sizes, and types, such as cloth-braided baskets, traditional wicker baskets, felted, and knitted baskets.

Containers include basins, nonbreakable bowls, plastic buckets, and little cardboard boxes. Baskets and containers are especially appropriate when babies are collecting and sorting, as described above. Besides their toys, many types of household items and objects from nature can be collected, such as shells and old-fashioned wooden spools (without thread.) Babies love to fill up the baskets and containers with objects and then dump them out. Which basket will hold all of the objects, and which one will not? They pour the items from one container to another. They compare, choose, and try out. If babies are tossing their toys, sometimes this behavior will stop when they are provided with baskets and containers, in order that they may "dump and fill." When they get a little older, early independent walkers love to carry around shopping bags or gift bags. They will fill up the bags with objects of their choosing, walk around, and give the objects to another person, only to take them back again. Small homemade indoor sleds, made of clementine boxes with an attached loop of wide ribbon, also make nice containers into which the children can put objects and then pull around.

It is very helpful if the adult notices which toys the baby is drawn to, when they have outgrown a toy, and when they are entering into a new stage of play, which is then best satisfied by different toys. At about six months, novel toys become interesting to the babies. However, care should be taken so that not too many new toys are added at a time. It is good to keep the old, familiar toys also. If there are too many toys, the play may become superficial. When the child has the same toys over a period of time, they will use them in ever-new ways.

Continuous observations along with continuous adjustments are needed. Decisions come out of understanding development and clearly seeing the child's behaviors. It should be remembered that Pikler's work is an approach, rather than a technique. Nothing should be dogma, and situations with a child are constantly re-evaluated. Kálló and Balog offer specific suggestions for caregivers regarding how to choose the toys for a particular child, based on the adult's observations.

> For instance, if one of the children puts something into a basket, the caregiver should check that there are plenty of suitable potential other containers about. If [the caregiver] sees [the baby] subjecting one item to a mode of repetitive investigation for which another item might be more appropriate, [the caregiver] will place it near [the baby.] If one of the children starts banging an object on the floor, [the caregiver] will offer objects that are most suitable for banging.[8]

Cozy Spaces

Just as babies explore placing items inside baskets and bowls and taking them out, so do crawling babies climb in and out of larger containers and baskets. They love to crawl in and out of small, enclosed spaces. Good old-fashioned cardboard boxes are tried-and-true toys for this type of exploration. Dog beds purchased for this purpose or a bottom cupboard in the kitchen are also favorites. Blankets or silks can be secured with clips to regular pieces of furniture and arranged to create cozy spaces at home. Many variations are possible. Creative use of whatever the environment affords is encouraged!

Babies and youngsters universally seek out cozy spaces. They are learning to inhabit the spaces of their bodies—which are relatively small, compared to the vastness of the spiritual world from which they came. Climbing into tiny spaces mirrors the important activity of coming into their bodies.

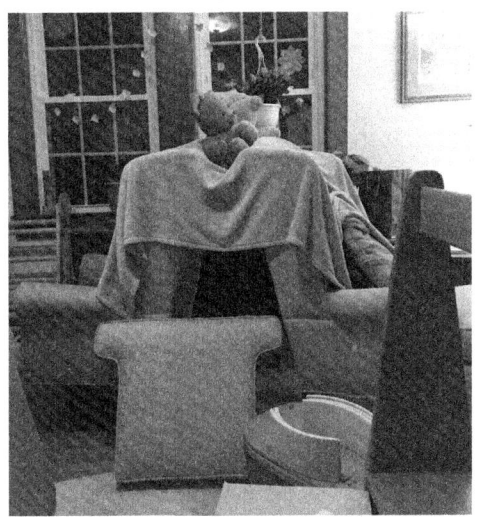

Here, a house has been constructed out of two chairs and a blanket.

Toys for Imaginative Play

The very beginnings of symbolic play can be seen toward the end of the first year. A classic example is that a child will take a cup and pretend to drink from it. When fantasy is just emerging, it is satisfying for youngsters to have objects to help them to imitate the happenings of their day-to-day lives. Little pots with lids, spoons for stirring, and cups and plates are tried-and-true toys for this age. Bean bags and crocheted rounds can be muffins, sandwiches, and eggs. An outdoor set of utensils for cooking with mud, sand, water, leaves, grass, and snow is also suitable. Children like to pretend that they are going to sleep and waking up, and blankets are nice for this. Dolls with accompanying doll beds and blankets, doll buggies, and doll clothes are classic toys for this age. Children like to feed, dress, and *bathe* their dolls, as well as take them for walks in doll buggies. When my siblings and I cleaned out a relative's home, we found a collection of colorful, old-fashioned ladies' hankies and men's handkerchiefs. I have found these to be invaluable items for children's play. Younger children simply enjoy looking at and touching them, stacking them, and moving them around. Older children use them in their "puppet shows" to create scenery, as capes and aprons for standing puppets, and as head scarves and blankets for smaller dolls.

A general principle is that open-ended toys offer more opportunities for the child's inner soul activity than do highly formed toys.

FREE MOVEMENT FROM THE VERY START

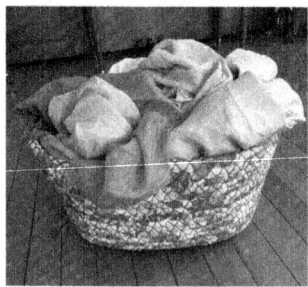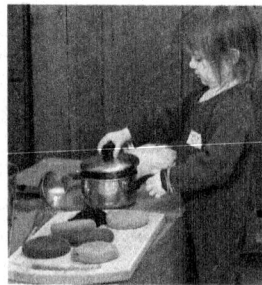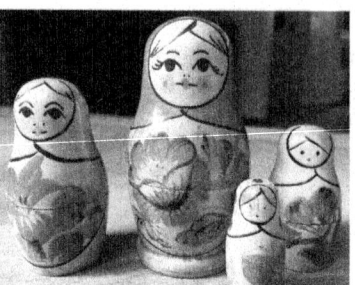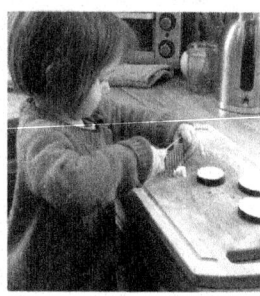

Left to right: Plant-dyed silks are favorite open-ended items for play; This child played for an extended period with a cardboard box, beanbags, and items from a kitchen cupboard. Simple, open-ended items afford the child the opportunity to imagine; nesting dolls are a classic toy for two-year-olds; zucchini is an ideal consistency to chop at this age.

Starting when they can crawl and sit, children will play with silks in a multitude of ways for many years. Initially, they may enjoy simply touching the silks, picking them up and putting them down in a nearby location. Later, they may wrap up their dolls in them and use them as capes. Still later, they may use clips to create little silk houses for their dolls and for themselves. Adults can fold the silks—and handkerchiefs—into knotted dolls and animals. Other examples of open-ended toys are baskets of pinecones, chestnuts, shells, and other natural materials.

Other toys for crawling babies include little cars and trucks and stacking toys. Non-breakable cups are also good for stacking. Walking children are drawn to pull-toys. Two-year-olds enjoy homemade play dough and beads of appropriate size (not too small) for stringing.

Especially for our children today, who are so often in need of protective sheathing, or if a parent is expecting another baby, nesting dolls are suitable.

Youngsters are aware of the events of daily life, and they want to partake of them. When children are two, they may start to want to chop vegetables. Standing at the kitchen counter on an appropriately sized stool and chopping vegetables with a child-sized chopper is typically very satisfying for them.

Children may also want to help hang up socks on a drying rack or put silverware in a tray in a kitchen drawer. It is nice to include the children in these simple activities whenever possible.

Certain children are drawn to play with heavy objects. It is helpful to understand that these children are seeking heavy items for a purpose. Heavy toys elicit extra muscle activation, thereby providing the child with more sensory information from their limbs. This allows the child to better feel and ground themselves in their bodies. These are often the same children who are at risk of throwing heavy items and endangering other children in the room. For these situations, it can be helpful to custom-make heavy sandbags which fit into small woven baskets with handles for the child to carry around, as these items are not conducive to being thrown.

Imagination Continues to Develop

Over time, the child's imagination deepens. Steiner explains the basis for imagination in development:

> As educators, we must respond to the imagination and fantasy of children, which tries to express itself outwardly when they play with toys or join in games with other children. The urge to play between the ages of two and a half and five is really just the externalized activity of a child's power of fantasy. And if we have the necessary ability of observation for such matters, we can foretell a great deal about the future soul life of children merely by watching them play. The way young children play provides a clear indication of their potential gifts and faculties in later life. The most important thing now is to meet their inborn urge to play with the right toys.[9]

Furthermore, children benefit from simple, unfinished dolls, to support their soul activity.

> Give a child a handkerchief or a piece of cloth, knot it so that a head appears above and two legs below, and you have made a doll or a kind of clown. With a few ink stains you can give it eyes, nose, and mouth.... Now the child can add many other features belonging to the doll, through imagination and imitation within the soul. It is far better if you make a doll out of a linen rag than if you give the child one of those perfect dolls, with highly colored cheeks and smartly dressed, a doll that even closes its eyes when put down horizontally, and so on. What are you doing if you give the child such a doll? You are preventing the unfolding of the child's own soul activity. Every time a completely finished object catches their eye, children must suppress an innate desire for soul activity, the unfolding of a wonderful delicate, awakening imagination. You thus separate children from life because you hold them back from their own inner activity.[10]

Johanna-Veronika Picht speaks about the child's "primordial need" for a doll:

> It is a primordial need for the child to have a doll to love, care for and carry around. With it the child can not only carry out through imitation what [they themself have] experienced from the [parent or caregiver], but [they] can also entrust it with all [their] joys and anxieties, yes, it is like a piece of [themself].[11]

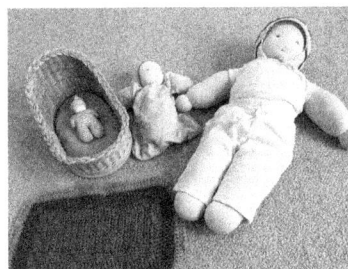 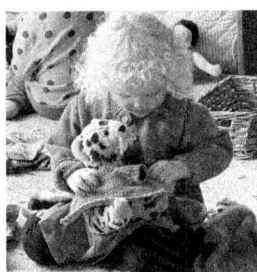

Above, left: Simple dolls support inner activity in children.
Right: This child is dressing a beloved stuffed animal.

In fact, carrying a beloved doll around is one means by which a child may enhance their developing personal space. (For a detailed discussion of the development of personal space, see chapter 13.) Dolls are toys that many children will play with for many years. The child's first doll may be more unformed, perhaps a knotted doll as mentioned above, or a simple handmade sweater doll without individual legs, but just a rounded mass for the bottom portion of the body. For the kindergarten-aged child, a more formed doll "with arms and legs, underwear, clothing, shoes and stockings becomes appropriate,"[12] so the children can dress the dolls.

Picht continues that the doll should not be a caricature: "An exaggerated caricature locks the imagination, and its creative forces remain unstimulated."[13] In other words, this type of doll does not leave the child free. Additionally, the gesture of such a doll may make a deep impression upon the child, in a negative way. Picht relates a classic incident reported by Dr. Alfred Nitschke in this regard:

> The favorite playmate of a very isolated child... was a large rabbit with a grotesque form of very long, thin arms and legs which hung down loosely, a head with extraordinarily large eyes and a very pronounced mouth whose lips the child touched again and again with his fingers. The child, pale and miserable, lay in the same position in his little bed. Nitschke explains, "In this case, the image of the toy animal with its strong expression and its debilitating, tired and dull bearing is thus actually forming extensively the movements and the nature of the child. When the troublesome rabbit had been removed, the child was soon up and about, developed an appetite and no longer bent forward as his rabbit had. The change reached into the depths of this small person. For us, after our long, futile effort, it was almost shocking—for his mother, it was incomprehensible."[14]

Rudolf Steiner recommends children's books, specifically ones "with cut-outs and nicely colored figures that can be moved by pulling strings attached below, so they will do all kinds of things.... These always stimulate children to invent whole stories, and thus they are very wholesome objects of play. Similarly, games with other children should not be too formal but should leave plenty of scope for children's imagination."[15]

APPENDIX 3:
Pikler's Wooden Furnishings

This appendix is based on knowledge derived from my study at the Pikler Institute in Budapest, tutoring from Anna Ruth Meyer and Dr. Debbie Laurin, and observations from my work with childcare providers, families, and children over many years. Anna Ruth Meyer is a Pikler pedagogue; Dr. Debbie Laurin is currently working on her Pikler Pedagogie Thesis.

Dr. Pikler created a variety of wooden structures to support the motor development of the children in her care. She designed them very intentionally to provide inviting possibilities for movement and play—especially for crawling and climbing. Today, only producers that have been certified by Pikler Lóczy are permitted to build furniture and play structures that carry the Pikler registered trademark. There are other wooden products sold on the internet that are similar to Dr. Pikler's furnishings and even use her name. However, if they are not certified, they are not made to the exact specifications of Dr. Pikler's design, and as such, they may be less safe for children. This is especially true of the Pikler triangle. To have sufficiently safe conditions for the children, Dr. Pikler's furnishings are meant to be used in conjunction with the entirety of her approach. This cannot be stressed enough.

The primary wooden structures include the crawling box and its attachment incline, the labyrinth and adjoining cube, the triangle and its climbing ramp, the changing table, the feeding bench, and the stool. These pieces of equipment are all suitable for institutional settings, such as childcare facilities. For the home setting, the climbing box and its attachment incline, the triangle, and the changing table have proven to be very helpful. Some of the other items may be too large or too much of an investment for the home setting. The individual Pikler structures are described below.

The Pikler Crawling Box

This is a piece of equipment that I highly recommend, both at home and in childcare settings. It is meant for babies who have already had some experience with the firm cushions described in appendix 2, on toys. At this stage of development, the baby is repeatedly turning from back to stomach. They may have just started to belly-crawl; however, they are not yet crawling on hands and knees. The crawling box is a shallow wooden box, made in four sizes. It has a bottom and four sides, but no top. Ideally—if space allows—the crawling box should be free on all four sides, and not positioned up against a wall. Initially, the box is placed with the open side up, rather than with the open side down. There is little chance of the baby falling out of the box when it is open side up—that is, when they are lying "in" the box, they can't roll "off." When able, babies will crawl in

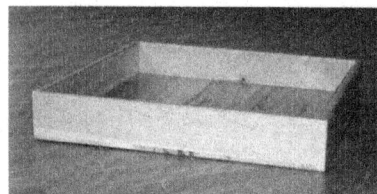 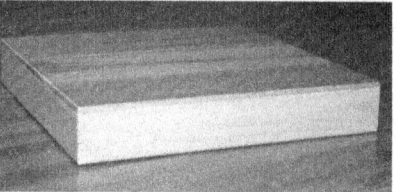 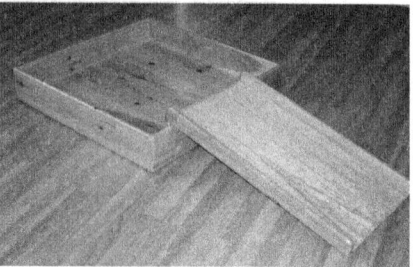

Left to right: The Pikler crawling box with the open side up; The Pikler crawling box, open side down; At right: The Pikler crawling box with accompanying incline.

and out of the box with the open side up. They will crawl headfirst. This is the natural way to carry out this maneuver and is not cause for concern.

Getting into and out of the crawling box is a complex motor task. It requires complicated spatial maneuvering and integrates movement and vision. It is a sophisticated movement that also involves diagonal patterns, which are foundational for later reciprocal crawling and other higher-level coordinated movements. *The benefits of the baby's mastering crawling into and out of the box cannot be overstated.*

Crawling boxes are interesting places to play with toys. Babies put toys inside the box and take them out. They progress to putting toys in the box, crawling in after them, and then crawling out. They may crawl inside the box to get an interesting toy which was intentionally placed there by an adult while setting up the play space. If the adult places a new toy in the box—or anywhere else in the play space, for that matter— it is helpful *not* to point it out to the child, but rather to let the child discover it by themselves—or not.

Later, when children are more accomplished with diagonal movements, the box can be turned over, placing the open side down, and the baby can crawl up on top of the box and crawl off it. This activity supports the development of depth perception. Again, the natural pattern is for the baby to crawl off the box headfirst. Two boxes can be placed next to each other, with one open-side-up and one open-side-down. Additionally, two boxes of different heights can be placed next to each other.

Attachment inclines or ramps can be placed next to the boxes, at one or more sides of the box. The inclines add more options for motor exploration and play with toys. Children love to roll toys up and down the ramps. They are essentially little physicists, exploring the forces of gravity, velocity, and trajectory. They experience and experiment with these same forces in their own bodies when they negotiate the inclines. The arrangement of the various pieces can be changed as needed.

Interestingly, Jaimen McMillan, founder and director of the Spacial Dynamics Institute, also built a crawling box for his own children. This box was used in his living room for many years. McMillan did not know about Pikler's crawling box—the idea for the box came independently to him, and the dimensions of McMillan's box were slightly larger. It was used to climb onto, or, when inverted, to climb into. When in its "closed" position, it also served as a place where the toys could be stored out of sight, and out of the way, till the next day.[1]

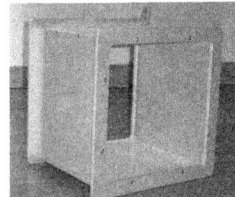

The Pikler cube

The Cube

The babies often belly-crawl through the cube when they are at this stage of development. Later, several cubes can be placed together and the older children climb across the top of them. They can also be turned with an open side up, like a chimney, so the children can climb inside.

The Labyrinth

The labyrinth is a mazelike structure, more complex than the crawling box, meant to be used with one or more wooden cubes. It can be set up in a variety of ways—initially, without turns, and then later, with turns. To negotiate the structure, children who have passed the stage of belly-crawling may have to get back down and belly-crawl through it. It is also full of opportunities for climbing, which is a wonderful activity to integrate the arms with the legs, the front of the body with the back, and the right side of the body with the left. Children

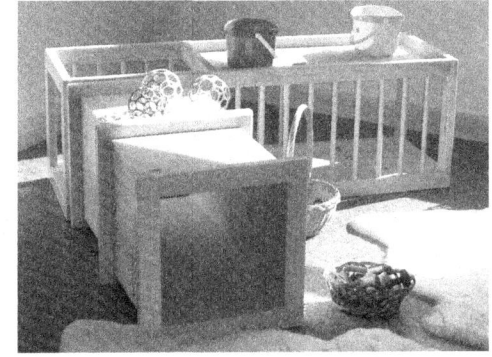

The Pikler labyrinth with wooden cubes.

like to roll round stools through it and crawl in after them, or simply crawl in and lie down to explore what it is like inside the space. Walking children may use it as a surface for their standing play.

The Triangle

The Pikler triangle is aptly named, as it is a triangular structure; the two climbing sides are set with evenly spaced rungs. It is meant for children who have already explored the climbing box, and can be introduced around ten months—babies can explore this piece of equipment in many ways before they use it for climbing. Babies may crawl through it, crawl into its base, lie down, place their legs on the rungs, and place their toys in and out of the bottom space. They typically start to climb it when they are knee-walking or standing up. If the child has not had previous free motor exploration when they encounter the triangle, the adult needs to be close by to spot them, as

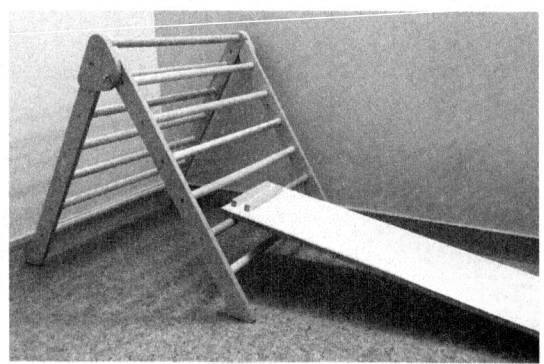

The Pikler triangle with attached incline.

necessary. When children start to climb the triangle, they do not cross over the peak at first; instead, they will climb up and then down the same side. *After* they are adept at climbing it, the incline or ramp can be added. The ramp must be securely attached to be safe—initially to the bottom rung—and then, later, it can be moved up to a higher rung. The ramp can be used with one triangle or can be used to connect two triangles.

The Changing Table

A hallmark of Dr. Pikler's approach is respectful caregiving (including feeding, dressing, bathing, diapering, etc.), in which the child actively participates and has free movement. For example, when a newborn's diaper is changed, this will occur with the baby lying on their back, because that is the scope of their movement possibilities at that stage of development. However, diapering for the older baby looks quite different. An older child's diapering requires a larger, squarer, and more protected space than a traditional changing table affords. The Pikler changing table is 37 inches (94 cm) in width and 28 inches (72 cm) in depth. Compare this with the standard changing mat used most often in the United States today (where most people do not use changing tables). The standard changing mat, usually set atop a dresser without surrounding rails, typically measures 32 inches (81 cm) in width and 16 inches (41 cm) in depth.

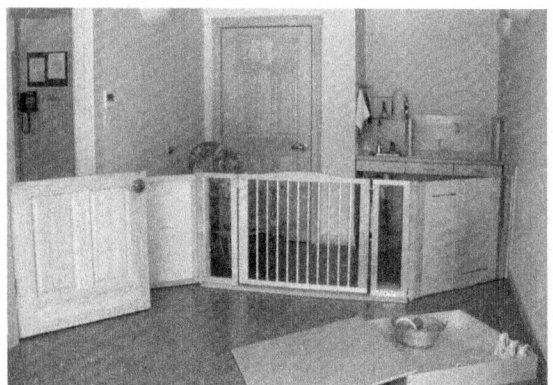 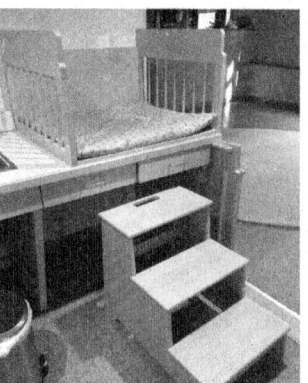 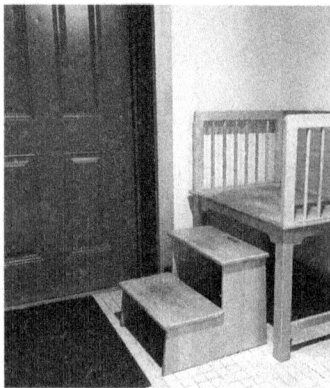

Above, left: This photo shows the gated-off area at Sophia's Hearth where the babies are fed on the caregiver's lap and where they are changed. Center: The walking babies use a set of stairs to climb up onto the changing table. Right: This changing table is in a bathroom with a door leading directly to the play yard. This makes it easy for the children to come in from outside to get their diapers or clothes changed.

With the Pikler approach to diapering, the older baby is more mobile on the changing table. The baby is free to assume whatever position they choose and also to move between positions during diapering. The caregiver responds accordingly to the child's choice of position—be it in back-lying, side-lying, tummy-lying, hands-and-knees, or standing. When the baby changes position or otherwise moves during diapering, the caregiver understands that the baby is not resisting or avoiding participation. Indeed, the baby needs to move *in order* to participate in the diapering. It takes a lot of attention to participate in the diapering activity, and the primary means that the child has to self-regulate is by moving. The Pikler changing table, which is designed to allow and *promote* movement by the child, provides the conditions where cooperation between caregiver and child may occur, and indeed, where a budding relationship between them may develop and flourish.

Dr. Pikler designed her changing table with a railing and vertical bars on three sides. The railings provide safety for the child and allow the adult to stay relaxed. The child may pull to stand and hold on to the railing during diapering. The changing table is open in the front, where the adult stands. Obviously, for safety reasons, the child is never left alone on the changing table. It gives the child a feeling of emotional security if the adult's standing height is at or above the child's height, and so a short caregiver may need to stand on a platform step to achieve the appropriate height. The changing table can be purchased with or without the base. In the latter case, the top part can be secured to the top of an existing chest of drawers in the home.

Pikler changing tables are very appropriate for the home setting. One family, for example, initially placed a Pikler changing table on the top of a dresser bureau, and all went well with this arrangement. However, when their child started walking, she would scream whenever they lifted her up onto the changing table. This perplexed the parents, because using the changing table had previously been such a pleasant experience for all concerned. The child was attending Sophia's Hearth's childcare. The parents inquired and discovered that at Sophia's Hearth, the teachers had changed the routine so that their child had started climbing up onto the changing table by herself. The parents responded by taking the changing table off the dresser bureau and securing it to the top of a cedar chest, which was much lower. With a sturdy stool, the girl could then easily climb up onto the cedar chest by herself, and there was no more crying. The parents sat on another stool while they were changing her so they didn't have to bend over.

The Feeding Bench

The feeding bench is a small wooden table with two benches that are all attached to a platform-like bottom board. The table, benches, and bottom constitute one connected piece of equipment. The infants in Dr. Pikler's care were initially bottle-fed and then also spoon-fed while sitting on the adults' laps. (When the children's home first opened, there were also wet nurses who breastfed the infants.) The following sequence of feeding continues today at the Pikler childcare center in Budapest. When the babies can independently climb into and out of the feeding bench, they progress to eating there. In childcare environments, the feeding bench is used as a transition between lap feeding and eating at a larger table with other children. Initially, an adult sits next to the feeding bench and attends to one child, who sits on one of the two attached benches. When the child is comfortable with this setup, another child joins them, sitting on the other attached bench opposite them. The feeding bench is designed for the child's feet to be on the floor, and the height of the table is such that they can eat without leaning forward. The feeding benches can also be used by older children for drawing or other projects, and it is noteworthy how much the children often grow to love them. They offer security because the seat does not move, and they are interesting places to climb into and out of.

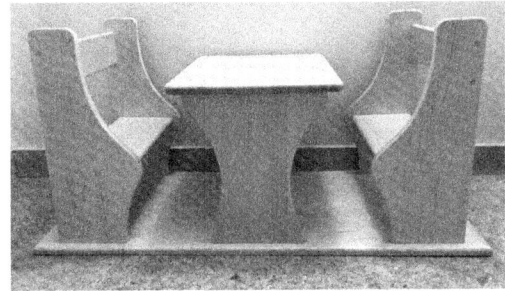

The Pikler feeding bench.

Most parents use high chairs at home. The kind that fit right up to the table—without trays—and where the child can eventually climb up and down by themselves, are nice. These types of chairs allow the child to be at the table with other members of the family, whereas the trays on traditional high chairs give a degree of separation from the others at the table. The child's feet should be supported with a footrest at the appropriate height.

Wooden Stools

When children at Lóczy were developmentally ready to sit at a table with a group of children for meals, Dr. Pikler used individual benches—as opposed to a long bench where several children would sit together. This way, the children have enough space between them. Additionally, using benches without backs builds core strength and promotes good posture, as there is nothing for the child to lean back on.

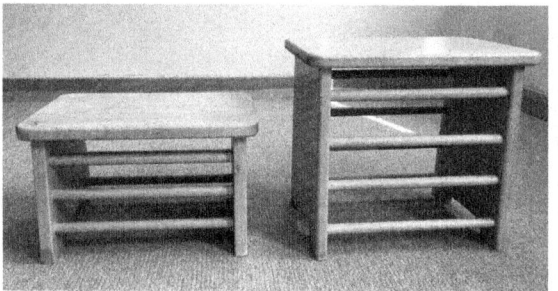
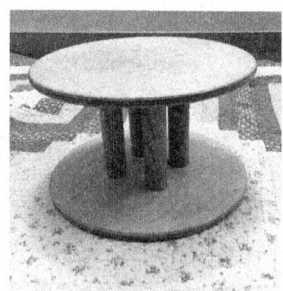

Above, left: Stools for taller and smaller children. Above, right: Round stool.

The stools are used in many additional ways. Children use them to pull to stand and as stepping stones in obstacle courses. They are great for sitting on when donning and doffing outdoor clothing and footwear. The children turn the stools over and use them as containers, putting toys inside them, and pushing them around on the floor. Adults can tie cords to them in the upside-down position, and the children can pull them around like sleds, with their dollies and stuffed animals inside. They also push the round ones around and roll them.

The rest of the items below were not created by Dr. Pikler, but we have found them useful for children before their third birthday at Sophia's Hearth.

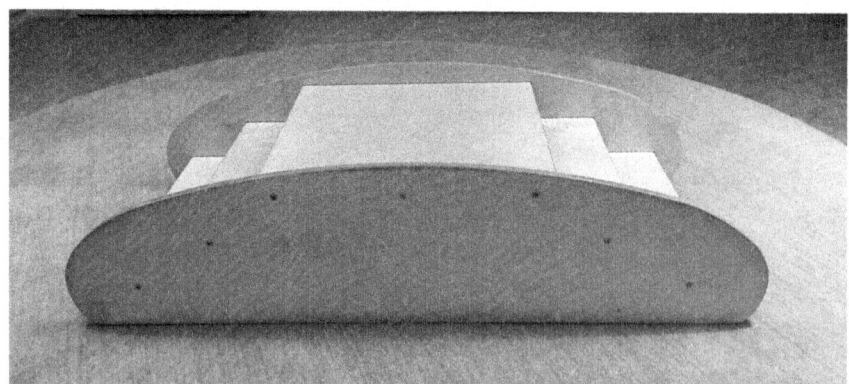

A traditional rocking boat with the open side down.

Other Wooden Items

Rocking boats are traditional wooden structures that youngsters have loved for decades. With the open side down, there are two steps on either side, with a small platform in the middle. Older children can negotiate the stairs in standing, and crawling babies like to crawl or bear-walk up and over them. With the open side up, up to four children can sit comfortably and rock back and forth.

Cloth Hammocks

Cloth hammocks are used in Waldorf parent-child classes and childcare facilities. They are recommended over net hammocks, which can potentially catch buttons or buckles, and which do not give as much deep pressure touch input. Additionally, the hammocks should have no cross bars at the ends, as this can make them tippy. The hammocks can be in a corner of a room, fastened with carabiners into hooks securely placed into studs in the walls. They should be hung so they are low to the ground, and they should be adjustable to different ages and abilities in different classes. There should be no sharp corners around the hammock, and the floor underneath should be appropriately padded with fleeces or a gymnastic mat. The hammock should be easy to put up for certain portions of the class time and then taken down.

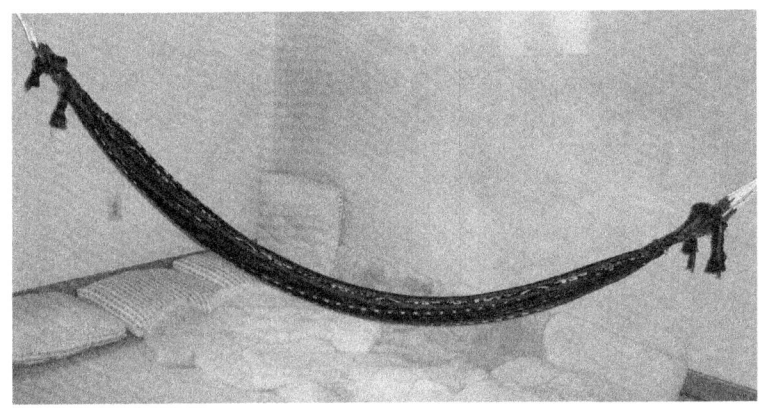

A cloth hammock.

Katherine Scharff, director of teacher education at Sophia's Hearth, shares a story about an early walker who attended her parent-child class with his mother. The child tried for weeks to climb into the hammock—feet first—but to no avail. No one assisted him or instructed him to try it a different way. Then, one day, he went in headfirst. Katherine and the other parents in the room all silently watched, aware that this boy was approaching a major achievement. Soon, they saw one and then the other of his hands appear on the sides of the hammock. Lastly, his face emerged, beaming with the unmistakable joy of accomplishment. The adults inwardly shared his joy, yet no one said a thing.[2] No one cheered, "Yay!", and no one said, "Good job!" There was no need to speak. The child's expression said it all. If the child had looked at his mother or the teacher in a manner showing that he expected a response, they could have smiled warmly and acknowledged the child's activity with something like, "Yes, I see you climbed in," but praise was not necessary.

Safety Concerns for Children of Different Abilities

Frequently, there are infants and young children who have different movement abilities in the same childcare class or parent-child class. This is not unusual, because children develop at different rates. However, in addition to having differing abilities, the children frequently have different awarenesses of their abilities—resulting in different capacities of judgment. Unfortunately, the children who have not yet developed sound judgment are not as safe when exploring the furnishings mentioned in this chapter.

Agnes Szanto-Feder discusses the development of judgment at length in her wonderful book, *Moving with Pleasure from the Beginning*. She explains that there are two categories of children: those who have previous experience with autonomous movement and those without it. Children who are allowed to move freely from day one display certain characteristics in their movements. One of the key characteristics is that when the children are playing, they "can avoid situations *that may be dangerous for them at their current stage of development. This is tangibly proven by observing the children's steady motion, as well as the harmony and smoothness of their movements* [emphasis added]."[3]

In contrast, Szanto-Feder describes the situation for children who have not experienced free motor exploration: "They are inevitably less active than those who were able to move around freely; furthermore, they were only able to hold themselves in forced positions," which frequently resulted in strain and retained reflexes. As a result, in these situations, coordination can be negatively impacted. Szanto-Feder continues, "These children do not know themselves well; they are less . . . aware of their own abilities and limits; and consequently, they cannot look after themselves properly. Their inattentiveness is not deliberate; they are simply unable to decode the 'messages' received via their senses."[4]

It can present a challenging situation for the adult to simultaneously provide opportunities for joyful, pleasant, and freedom-filled movements for both groups of children in a safe way. Szanto-Feder recommends that the adult should stay near the children who have not yet developed sufficient judgment, and "be always available if the children need them. They should notice if the children have overestimated their own possibilities and give them a helping hand. At the same time, however, the adults should not interfere excessively in the children's business." Szanto-Feder continues that "what is also important is for the adults to be able to be happy about the children finding joy in their own activity."[5]

It is not helpful to tell children who have decreased judgment to "be careful," or to "watch what you're doing." Children who have not yet developed judgment need most to learn to sense their movements. When we speak to children in this way, we are distracting them from doing what they need to be doing to be safe—sensing their movements. Unless there is an underlying neurological condition, these children *can* learn to sense their movements and therefore to move in new ways if given the right circumstances. Tact is important in our approach with these children and with their parents. It is not helpful to make a parent feel guilty if their child was not given free motor exploration in the past. Children are resilient, and over time their judgment will improve.

One day, during a parent-toddler group at Sophia's Hearth, a boy was negotiating an incline that was placed between two Pikler triangles. This was a new and challenging motor activity for the boy, and it took all his concentration to accomplish it. He was doing well, until his mother noticed him and started praising him. This drew the boy's attention away from what he was doing, and his movement faltered. The facilitator very adeptly engaged the mother in conversation, gradually turning her own body so that the mother ended up facing away from the boy. With this astute intervention by the facilitator, the mother stopped praising, and the boy's movements returned to their previous, ease-filled state.

APPENDIX 4:
The Outdoor Space

This appendix describes various aspects of outdoor spaces, along with outdoor toys and structures which are developmentally appropriate for children under three years.

Simply Spending Time Outside

Similar to Waldorf early childhood educators—as well as many others—Dr. Pikler believed that time outside was beneficial for infants and young children, and those in her care at the children's home spent considerable time outside. The Hungarian government gave Pikler a home in a residential neighborhood that she remodeled for the children's home. The second floor was converted into classrooms for the babies, and Pikler built decks off of each classroom so that the babies could be outdoors. For each deck, she made fenced, spacious enclosures with awnings for sun protection. During the warm months, she tied containers about the size of window flower boxes to the edges of the outdoor playpens. She filled these containers with water so that the babies could belly-crawl over and stick their hands in the water to play. In the backyard play space, Pikler also devised several other types of structures for water play for the older children in her care. In the backyard behind the children's home, the children played, ate, and had their diapers changed. In alignment with the European custom, the children slept outside for their naps, but not at night.

The Movements of Nature

Most experts believe that it is healthy for young children to be outside in nature, and indeed, nature is filled with life forces that support health. If we look at this phenomenon a little closer, we can recognize another, perhaps less obvious, benefit of being outside. Being outside in nature is profoundly supportive for motor development. As Jaimen McMillan so astutely observed, "The movements of nature are second to none."[1] Archetypal movements and gestures abound in nature, and infants and young children take them in very deeply. Within the trunk of a tree, a sunflower, a tendril of a vine, and a pinecone are the gestures of the spiral.

Grace and majesty abound in the curved movements of a soaring bird, a scampering squirrel, and blowing clothes on a clothesline. Ever upward, outward, expanding gestures exist in mist rising in the morning, in shoots breaking through the ground in the garden, and in flowers opening. I was observing the babies at Sophia's Hearth one warm, windy day. They were happily playing with their toys and

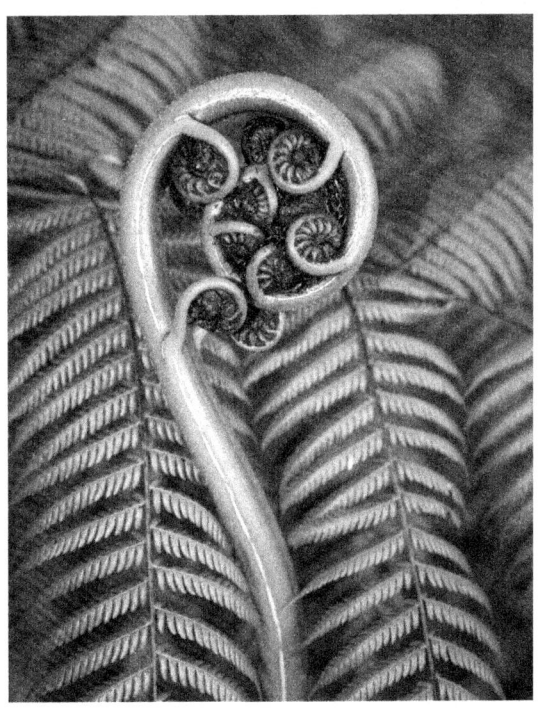

Here, we see the spiral in a new fern shoot.

rolling outside on our covered porch. When a gust of wind would blow a nearby clump of tall grasses in the yard, the babies all stopped what they were doing, looked, and were mesmerized. It is not uncommon for a fussy baby to quiet when taken outside and placed on their back in a fully reclining stroller or on a blanket under a tree.

Young children are attuned to movement in general, and they are especially at home with movements arising from nature, which manifest in the gestures of the etheric world—a world of ever expanding, constantly morphing, pure life forces. The younger the child, the more familiar they are with these types of movements, because they are not yet separate from the etheric world. (The etheric will be further discussed in volume 2.)

Water

The movements of water are especially familiar for the young child, because water is the element which serves as the bearer of the etheric or life forces, and the young child has a direct relationship with these etheric forces. As Dr. Michaela Glöckler states, "The adult's relationship to water is not insignificant to the young child."[2] If we notice the life-filled movements of water, and cultivate a reverence for them, the young child will sense that we have a window into their world. As children are finely attuned to our thoughts and feelings, our attitude toward water can positively impact our relationship with the child.

The water in a river or stream does not travel in straight lines; instead, it meanders and bends. In the eddies of a stream, the water turns in on itself and goes round and round. It emerges from the eddy rejuvenated, and then cascades over, around, and between the ensuing rocks—meeting every new and unexpected turn with life-filled vitality. The movements of young children are akin to the life-filled movements of water. Young walkers do not walk in straight lines. Instead, they swerve and curve—pausing for a moment of full exploratory immersion into whatever draws their attention before flowing on to the next object of interest.

When youngsters are lucky enough to play around small streams and natural bodies of water—at the seashore, the lake, or even in puddles that form after a rainstorm or from garden hoses—they are often deeply immersed in their play, and it can be very satisfying and soothing for them. Most of us have seen and marveled at the joy of children when they play in water: splashing in a puddle, pouring water from bucket to bucket, watering plants in the yard, washing rocks around a flower bed, playing in a backyard wading pool, and mixing up mud.

As adults, many of us choose to go to the ocean when we need to rest and rejuvenate. For young children, however, a little goes a long way, and a kitchen sink or a bathtub can serve the same purpose. When they are out of sorts, it can be very calming for youngsters to stand at the kitchen sink and "wash the dishes," or to get into a tub and take a bath.

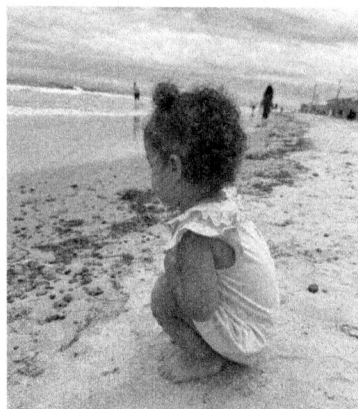

This child is immersed in the sensory experiences of the ocean.

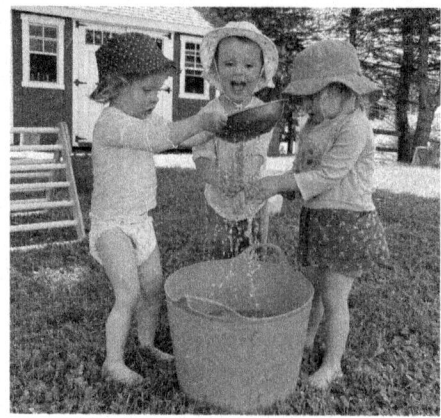

These children are "in their element."

Puppetry and the Movements of Nature

The gestures of puppets can be another way to support healthy motor development. I recently watched Janene Ping, master early childhood puppeteer, perform a simple puppet vignette in which she portrayed a nature sprite.[3] The movements of the sprite elegantly capture the qualities of the life-force gestures of the natural world. These slow, buoyant, levity-filled, not quite predictable, yet very followable, playful, and enlivening gestures were a joy to behold. Ping explains, "The puppeteer is inspired by the study of nature and the gesture of elemental forces, plant life, and animals, with the goal of bringing a resonance with the beauty of the natural world to the child."[4]

Sand

My husband gave our goddaughter Freya Jaffke's classic book *Toymaking with Children*. She has an eighteen-month-old boy. Her husband saw the book lying on the coffee table, and he opened it to a random page. On that page it read, "For outdoor play, the most important item is the sandbox. It should not be too small or too shallow."[5] The next day, the child's grandfather built a large sandbox (five feet by ten feet, eleven inches deep), where the boy has happily played daily for extended periods ever since. The parents say that they can "barely get him to come out of the sandbox!"

I have also found sand tables to be especially valuable, as some children do not like to play in a sand pit, especially in wet weather, but they will enjoy playing at a sand table, where just their hands touch the sand. (Other children want to sit down in the sand pit and bury their whole legs in the sand.)

Sand tables are especially supportive for fine motor development, as the arms work better, biomechanically, when we are standing. This is because the core is more active in standing, and the trunk is the foundation from which the arms and hands work. Indeed, many cooks chop vegetables while standing at the counter rather than sitting at the kitchen table. (For more on fine motor development, see chapter 7.)

It is very nice if the sand pits have a plentiful amount of sand, so that it can be made into a mound. The teacher can rake the sand pit every morning into a fresh little hill, which can be very inviting to the children. The youngsters respond by breaking down the mound, redistributing the sand, packing spoonfuls of it into little crevasses, and building up new forms with their buckets. There is a deeper meaning, too, in the adult's mounding the sand every morning. It mirrors the underlying physiological process, which only happens during the first seven years, of tearing down the hereditary body and building up the individualized body. (The process of incarnation will be discussed in depth in volume 2.)

Young children will naturally take a spoonful of sand and carry it nearby in the play yard to dump it. This is developmentally appropriate. Children do not have a sense of boundaries. The world is one to them, and the world is theirs! It is helpful if the adults plan ahead for this inevitable occurrence and strategically place the sand area, so that the areas nearby will not be adversely affected by any sand that will very likely be carried there by the children. Better to plan ahead for this than to constantly tell young children not to carry sand and dump it. In our

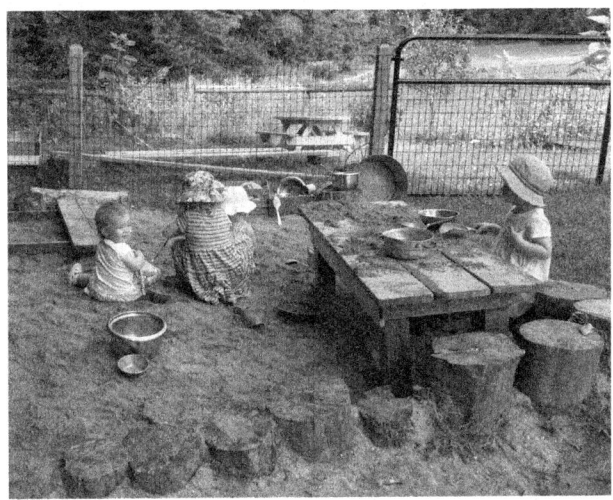

Here, children have the option to sit down and play in the sand, or to play at the table.

FREE MOVEMENT FROM THE VERY START

outdoor play space at Sophia's Hearth we have created two sand pits, as the toddlers love to fill up their wheelbarrows with a load of sand, push them to the other sand pit, and dump them. This way they dump the sand in the other sand pit, rather than in random locations in the yard. Similarly, areas of small rocks or gravel used in the yard as a landscaping feature are very enticing for the children to carry around and deposit into other areas of the lawn. This can be a problem, as one does not want a lawn mower to be throwing out rocks. Therefore, one may want to consider removing the landscaping rocks, so as not to have to supervise the children and impose what, to them, is an arbitrary rule. The ideal is to give the children free movement within a defined space.

It is very helpful for little ones to be barefoot outside in the play yard. The baby's foot is born without an arch, and these environments are especially beneficial in developing the foot musculature—even more so than being barefoot inside, because the various surfaces give more resistance to the movements of the foot.

Outdoor Toys and Tools

Outdoor items for large motor play include child-sized tools such as garden and snow shovels, rakes, hoes, brooms, and wheelbarrows. If the children are ramming the wheelbarrows into each other, this behavior is often remedied with extra weight in the wheelbarrows, so that the children can better sense how to manage them correctly. In the winter, child-sized, wooden snowplows are a popular item for older two-year-olds as well as for preschool and kindergarten children.

Snowplows encourage children to extend all the way out through their limbs, as they push against the resistance of the snow with their legs and guide the plow with their arms. A few years ago, several high school seniors, who had attended Sophia's Hearth's childcare when they were infants and young children, returned to perform a community service project. Over lunch with the staff, they reflected on their experiences as young children at Sophia's Hearth. One young man said that what he remembered most were the snowplows. He commented that, to him and his friends, they were doing real work—they really were plowing the snow. They took their jobs very seriously, and it was very satisfying for them.

A dirt pit or dirt pile in the yard, or an open area in the garden, with hand rakes, buckets, and scoops may be especially interesting for some children who are more drawn to the earth element. I once worked at a public school that had brand-new, expensive outdoor play equipment, and where were the preschool and kindergarten children? They were happily playing at the corner of the yard, climbing up a big leftover pile of dirt.

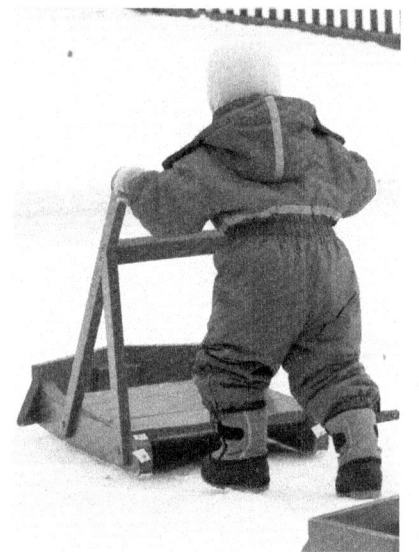

Here is a child pushing a snowplow across a snowy yard.

Independent walkers who have developed to the point that they are steady on their feet enjoy taking their dollies and teddy bears on walks in doll buggies, child-sized shopping carts, and pushcarts. It should be cautioned, however, that these devices are only appropriate when the child is already an accomplished walker. I do not recommend giving them to typically developing children *in order* to help them learn to walk—for that is not self-initiated movement. In self-initiated movement, the child achieves a new motor skill entirely out of their own efforts—without the assistance of a device or an adult. When a child is prematurely given a pushcart, the child will lean on its handle. Children do this because the activity is too difficult for them—they do not yet have sufficient balance for the activity. As a result, their alignment is negatively affected—their heads are in front of their hips, their shoulders are likely elevated, and their weight is on the balls of their feet. This activity actually works against the child's achieving a proper gait pattern, with

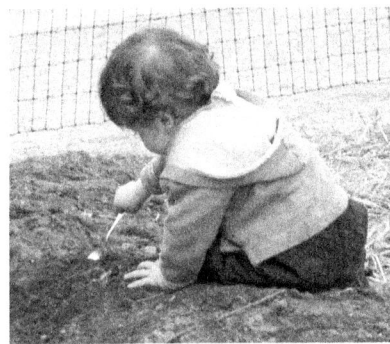 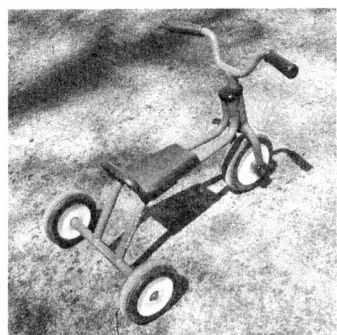 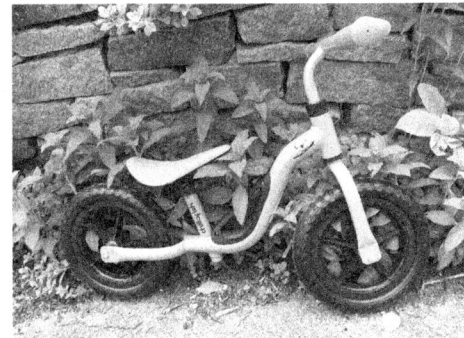

Left to right: This child is digging in the garden bed with a spoon; Seated scooter; Balance bike.

the heels securely down on the ground. In contrast, when children self-initiate their movements, their alignment is appropriate.

Later, when children become well-established walkers, seated scooters (with four wheels and no pedals) offer a new mode of locomotion. True to the principles of self-initiated movement, the child is not helped to get on or off the scooter, nor taught how to use it.

For older children, balance bikes (two-wheeled bicycles without pedals) are lovely pieces of equipment. I have seen typically developing children as young as two and a half years up to five or six enjoy them. Balance bikes are aptly named. They are a means by which the child can explore and enhance their balance. They support the development of the midline between the right and the left sides of the body, and they help establish the important pattern of the legs orienting to the supporting surface (pushing down into the ground.) Tricycles, with pedals, are not as beneficial. With tricycles, the child's feet do not make contact with the ground. Instead, the gesture of the legs when riding a tricycle is like a hiccup—the legs are passively lifted up off the ground by the revolving pedals, especially if the seat is inclined backward. By contrast, with the seated scooters and the balance bikes the legs actively push down into the ground.

Outdoor Structures

Outdoor structures also include those for climbing, crawling, and walking—over, around, under, and through. A rock or a fallen tree trunk, with some of its accompanying branches, makes a good climbing structure. Three-dimensional rocks are developmentally appropriate at this age. Climbing walls are better suited to middle and high schoolers. A slightly complex natural structure can be made by taking a tree trunk, sawing it in half the long way, and securing it slightly above the ground, with the flat side up. Two or three of these can be arranged in an interesting pattern in the yard, and they can be of slightly different heights and widths. A long, wide board can be attached to it, serving as an incline for the children to negotiate. Dr. Pikler created many outdoor climbing structures for the children at Lóczy—for example, a metal arch with rungs.

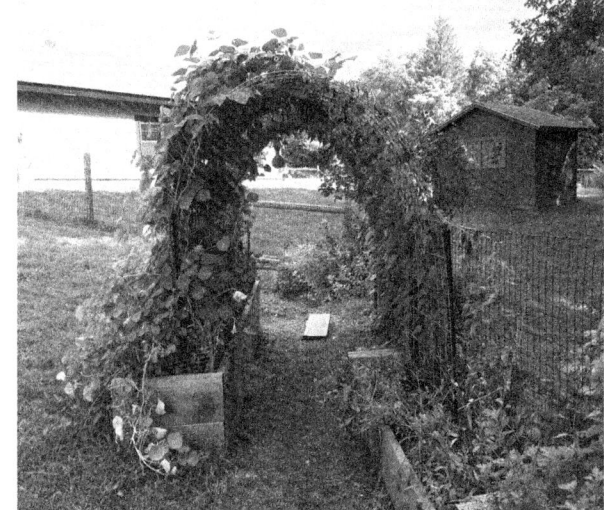

The children enjoy walking through this archway and pushing their wheelbarrows through it. The arch is made of a sturdy type of fencing called "cattle fencing."

FREE MOVEMENT FROM THE VERY START

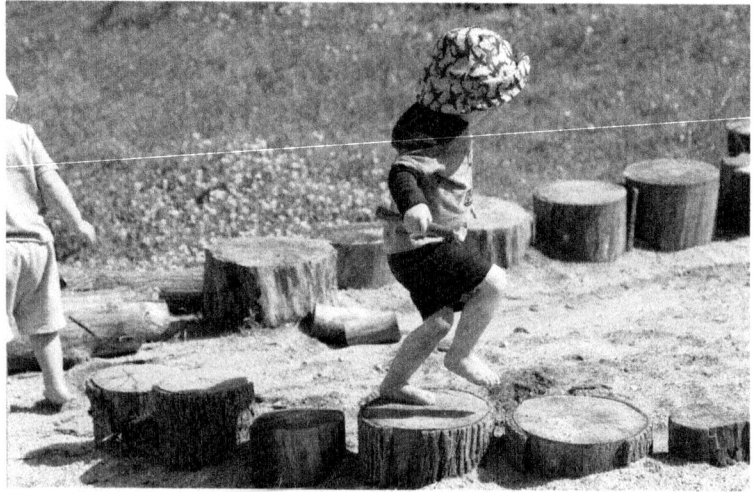

Logs around the edge of a sand pit not only help contain the sand but also are interesting places for the children to walk on and jump down from.

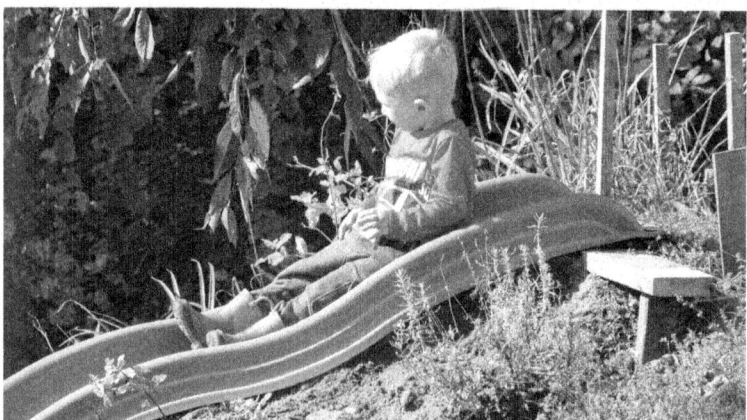

Plastic slides can be placed on the side of a hill.

Walking on different surfaces—such as grass, sand, inclines, and uneven ground—and negotiating curbs and platform steps are big accomplishments for young children. A gently sloping hill offers challenges for crawlers and walking babies. A hill with a steeper slope increases the challenge to their balance. Simply standing on a surface which is up off the ground a few inches can be a noteworthy experience. Stepping stones can be placed, and walkways can be delineated by vegetation.

Like dock pilings, wooden logs can be buried vertically, partway into the ground, so they are sturdy for walking on. The log tops can be the same height above the ground, or slightly varied, or stair-stepped.

Placing slides on the side of a hill eliminates the need for a ladder on the slide. This increases safety and decreases the need for excessive supervision. For a group of children, placing two slides near to each other can also eliminate the need for excessive supervision, as one slide can be used to go down, and the other one for going up. Also, a wide slide can be built to accommodate three or four children abreast. The goal is to not have to overly supervise children, whether due to safety concerns, in order that they take turns, or get them to perform an activity in a predetermined way. Teeter-totters are also classic outdoor structures. They can be made to be low to the ground for the younger children.

Outdoor Vegetation

Garden and flower beds, shrubs, bushes, and trees (including fruit trees) can add beauty and color to the play yard. They bring birds, butterflies, autumn leaves, and healthy food. Strawberry beds are a favorite. In the early summer, young children at home delight in going outside every morning to look for the ripe strawberries. Stepping stones can be placed throughout the strawberry patch. Gourds are lovely plants for children to watch grow. In the fall, the gourds often become "babies" that are played with outside. Velvety plants, such as lamb's ear and mullein, can provide rich textures for the children to explore. Raised garden beds can be used. One family left one of their garden beds unplanted, because their one- and two-year-olds loved to climb into it and explore the soil! Children also like to stand at the edge of a garden bed and play in the soil. Of course, care should be taken that there are no plants with poisonous leaves or berries in the yard.

Vegetation can also offer cozy spaces for youngsters outside. A teepee can be fashioned out of long sticks, with pole beans, peas, or morning glories planted to grow upon it. Trees with branches that grow downwards, such as weeping cherry trees, create lovely sheltering spaces. Bushes such as rhododendrons can be pruned to make little cave-like enclosures.

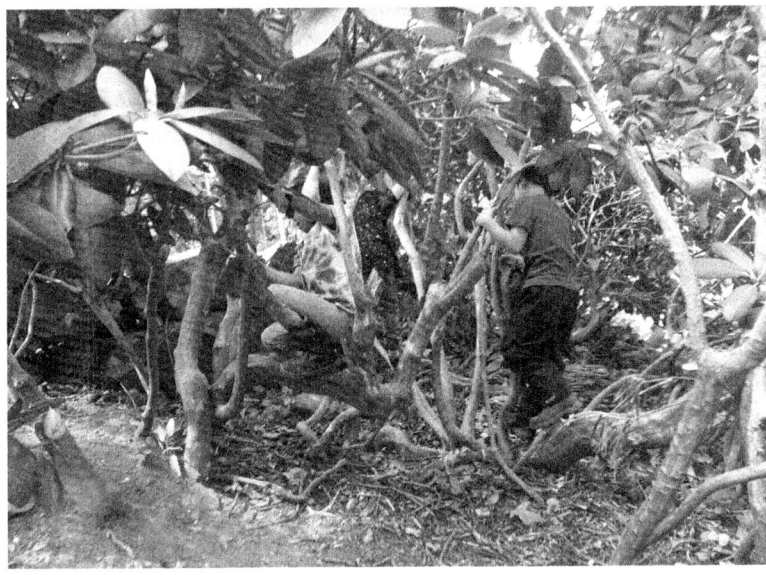

This is a well-established rhododendron patch. It is a very popular spot for climbing.

Trellises, awnings, and canvases can be placed to protect against the sun. They also serve to make a large, open area less overwhelming and more inviting to young children. When I was a child, we would visit our great aunt's house. She had a magical flower garden with special little places to walk along, little inclines, and an open grassy lawn in the backyard, bordered by beautiful bushes and trees, giving the space a cozy, safe feeling. She would bring out old, sturdy, wooden chairs, which were painted a light green, a pile of old white sheets, clothespins, and a large basket of long ribbons. My sisters and I would be occupied for hours, creating and decorating our sheet houses. My aunt would sit on the back step, shelling peas from the garden, and watch us. We would come and join her and later enjoy the peas at supper.

Outdoor Fine Motor Toys

Dr. Pikler believed that infants and young children should have the full scope of free movement both indoors and out. In other words, running is not just for outside! Additionally, fine motor activities are not just for inside. Toys for outdoor fine motor activities include cooking utensils for mud and sand, as well as buckets, pitchers, and containers for pouring various things such as sand and soil. The children especially like to pour water. Cookie cutters and spatulas are nice for snow play. Small wooden dolls and gourds can be provided for doll play outside. Pinecones, corncobs, acorns, and shells are lovely raw materials for outside play. Older children love to create "fairy houses" with these items and little sticks. Sometimes children use the corncobs for "sawing" old stumps.

Outdoor shelves, cabinets, or a shed serve as places to store outdoor toys, gardening tools, balance bikes, snowplows, and so on. Restoring order at the end of outdoor play time is the responsibility of the adults; the children are free to imitate. The manner in which the adults care for the space is something that the children take in deeply—this can orient the children and help give them a sense of security. It has been my observation that children play differently (in that they are more able to engage in their play) if the space has been attended to and prepared for them.

Endnotes

CHAPTER 1:
THE LIFE AND WORK OF DR. EMMI PIKLER

1. Anna Tardos, "Introducing the Piklerian Developmental Approach," 1–5.
2. "It seemed that the children who enjoyed the freedom to roam, run and play where they liked were more alert, more physically capable, and were able to fall without hurting themselves. By comparison, the children of well-to-do families were over-protected, their movements were limited and they did not know their own physical capabilities or limits." Clare Caro, "The Genius of Emmi Pikler."
3. Ibid.
4. Ibid.
5. Caro, "Genius of Emmi Pikler."
6. Ibid.
7. Ibid.
8. Ibid.
9. Judit Falk MD, "Forty Years of Lóczy," 39.
10. Ibid.
11. Ibid.
12. Falk, "Forty Years of Lóczy," 41.
13. Anna Tardos, "From the Hands of the Caregiver," 57.
14. "Self" is used here in reference to the child's developing identity with *self* in relation to *other*—essentially, the I/You relationship. In psychological literature, the capitalization of Self often helps distinguish it from the use of "self" in the everyday, colloquial sense. Examples include Carl Jung's description of the Self as a key archetype, representing the unification of the conscious and unconscious mind; similarly, in humanistic psychology, the Self is central to understanding personal growth and self-actualization.
15. Dr. Myriam David and Geneviéve Appell, *Lóczy*, 39.
16. Judit Falk MD, "When We Touch the Infant's Body," 11.
17. Anna Tardos, "Two-Week Intensive."
18. Falk, "When We Touch the Infant's Body," 7–8.
19. Maria Vincze, "The Meaning of Cooperation During Care," 16.
20. Elsa Chahin with Anna Tardos, *In Loving Hands*, xxiii.
21. Falk, "When We Touch the Infant's Body," 7.
22. David and Appell, *Lóczy*, 38.
23. Tardos, "Two-Week Intensive."
24. Anna Ruth Myers, personal correspondence with author, fall 2023. Anna Ruth Myers is a Pikler pedagogue.
25. Ibid.

CHAPTER 2:
SELF-INITIATED GROSS MOTOR DEVELOPMENT

1. Emmi Pikler MD, "The Competence of the Infant," 187.
2. Emmi Pikler MD, "Learning of Motor Skills on the Basis of Self-Induced Movements," 56–58.
3. Ibid., 60.
4. Ibid., 56.
5. Ibid., 60–62. Note that I've revised "crawl" to "belly-crawl" and "creeps" to "crawl"; in the Pikler literature, what we call belly-crawling is referred to as "crawling," and what we call crawling—on hands and knees—is referred to as "creeping." I will use belly-crawling and crawling throughout this text.
6. Pikler defines sitting as balancing on the two sitz bones without the support of the arms.
7. Pikler, "Learning of Motor Skills," 62.
8. Ibid., 61.
9. Ibid., 68.
10. Ibid.
11. Pikler, "Learning of Motor Skills," 62.
12. Ibid., 69.
13. Anna Tardos, "Two-Week Intensive."
14. Ibid.
15. Pikler, "Learning of Motor Skills," 69.
16. Ibid.
17. Sit-ups for adults are currently a point of contention in the literature, as they are a source of potential low back and neck injury, especially when performed incorrectly. There are safer ways to strengthen the core besides sit-ups, such as planks, where the person assumes prone on extended arms, straightens their legs, and supports the body on the balls of their feet. Planks can also be performed in prone on elbows, rather than in prone on extended arms.
18. Ibid.
19. Ibid.
20. Tardos, "Two-Week Intensive."
21. Ibid.
22. Pikler, "Learning of Motor Skills," 62.
23. Ibid.
24. Ibid., 79.
25. Agnes Szanto-Feder, *Moving with Pleasure from the Beginning*, 29.
26. Ibid., 34.
27. Ibid.
28. Pikler, "Competence of the Infant," 190.

29 Henry David Thoreau, *Autumn*, 222.
30 Emmi Pikler MD, "Emmi Pikler's First Book," 17.
31 Tardos, "Two-Week Intensive."
32 Michaela Glöckler and Wolfgang Goebel, *A Guide to Child Health*, 210–211.
33 Ibid., 208–209.
34 Ibid., 209.

CHAPTER 3:
QUALITATIVE MOVEMENT FINDINGS FROM PIKLER'S RESEARCH

1   Emmi Pikler MD, "Learning of Motor Skills on the Basis of Self-Induced Movements," 69–72.
2   Ibid., 69.
3   Ibid.
4   Ibid., 75.
5   Agnes Szanto-Feder, *Moving with Pleasure from the Beginning*, 31.
6   Pikler, "Learning of Motor Skills," 72.
7   Deb Dana, *The Polyvagal Theory in Therapy*, 22.
8   Szanto-Feder, 30.
9   Ibid.
10 Ibid., 26.
11 Ibid., 136.
12 A. Jean Ayres, *Sensory Integration and the Child*, 85.
13 Szanto-Feder, 31.
14 Ayres, 85.
15 Emmi Pikler, "From Emmi Pikler's First Book: Excerpts from *Peaceful Babies—Contented Mothers*."
16 Pikler, "Learning of Motor Skills," 76.
17 Szanto-Feder, 217.
18 Ibid.
19 Szanto-Feder, 219.
20 Ibid.
21 Mayo Clinic Staff, "Infant and Toddler Health."
22 Ibid.
23 Szanto-Feder, 276.
24 Ibid., 32.
25 Ibid., 220.
26 Judit Falk MD, "Why Should We Lay the Infant in the Prone Position?", 6.
27 Anna Tardos, "Two-Week Intensive."
28 Falk, "Why Should We Lay the Infant in the Prone Position?", 7.
29 Ibid., 6.
30 Falk, "Why Should We Lay the Infant in the Prone Position?", 11.
31 Ibid.
32 Ibid.
33 Szanto-Feder, 277.

CHAPTER 4:
FREE MOVEMENT AND OPPORTUNITIES TO DEVELOP SELF-REGULATION

1   Dr. Myriam David and Geneviéve Appell, *Lóczy*, 81
2   Ibid., 83.
3   Ibid., 58.
4   Tardos, "Two-Week Intensive."
5   David and Appell, 58.
6   David and Appell, 59.
7   Ibid., 59.
8   Ibid., 39.
9   Elsa Chahin with Anna Tardos, *In Loving Hands*, 82.
10 Ibid., 82
11 Ibid., 83.
12 Ibid., 82.
13 Anna Tardos, "From the Hands of the Caregiver," 61.
14 Ibid.
15 David and Appell, *Lóczy*, 39.
16 Ibid., 40.
17 Ibid., 42.
18 Ibid., 54.
19 David and Appell, 54.
20 Ellyn Satter, *Child of Mine*, 3.
21 Ibid., 474.
22 Ibid., 474–475.
23 Ibid., 475.
24 David and Appell, *Lóczy*, 50.
25 Judit Falk MD, "When We Touch the Infant's Body," 11.
26 David and Appell, *Lóczy*, 53.
27 Deb Dana, *The Polyvagal Theory in Therapy*, 4.
28 Mary Sue Williams OTR/L and Sherry Shellenberger OTR/L, *How Does Your Engine Run?*, 1–5.
29 Edward Luker, "Are Video Games, Screens Another Addiction?"
30 Rudolf Steiner, *Education and Instruction*.
31 Ibid.
32 David and Appell, *Lóczy*, 42.
33 Emmi Pikler MD, "Data on Gross Motor Development of the Infant," 307.
34 Agnes Szanto-Feder, *Moving with Pleasure from the Beginning*, 147.
35 Emmi Pikler MD, "Competence of the Infant," 190.
36 Ute Strub, personal correspondence with the author, July 2008.
37 Magda Gerber and Allison Johnson, *Your Self-Confident Baby*, 145.
38 Judit Falk MD, "Forty Years of Lóczy," 18.

CHAPTER 5:
ASPECTS OF SELF-INITIATED MOVEMENT

1. Citing Jean Piaget's classic quote, Magda Gerber writes, "I think Jean Piaget said it beautifully: When you teach a child something, you take away forever [their] chance of discovering it for [themself.]" Magda Gerber, *Dear Parent*, 12.
2. Emmi Pikler MD, "Some Contributions to the Study of the Gross Motor Development of Children," 27–39, 32.
3. Ibid., 33.
4. Ibid.
5. Ibid., 37.
6. Pikler, "Some Contributions," 37.
7. Emmi Pikler MD, "Emmi Pikler's First Book: Excerpts from *Peaceful Babies—Contented Mothers*," 6. This article from the *Sensory Foundation Bulletin* collects this and other excerpts from Emmi Pikler's *Peaceful Babies—Contented Mothers*.
8. A. Jean Ayres, *Sensory Integration and the Child*, 15.
9. Rudolf Steiner, "Children Before the Seventh Year."
10. Rudolf Steiner, "Lecture One," in *Spiritual Guidance of the Individual and Humanity*.
11. Rudolf Steiner, *Self-Education in the Light of Spiritual Science*, 10–11.
12. Pikler, "Emmi Pikler's First Book," 23.
13. Ibid., 12.
14. Ibid.
15. Emmi Pikler MD, "Emmi Pikler's First Book," 12.
16. Ibid.
17. Michaela Glöckler and Wolfgang Goebel, *A Guide to Child Health*, 125–126.
18. Renate Long-Breipohl, *Under the Stars*, 52.
19. Marie Steiner, "Foreword," in Rudolf Steiner, *Education*.
20. Long-Breipohl, 53.
21. Ibid.
22. Rudolf Steiner, *Soul Exercises*, 417.
23. Ibid.
24. Rudolf Steiner, "Lecture 1," in *From Jesus to Christ*, 17.
25. Long-Breipohl, 53.
26. Ibid.
27. Peter Selg, *The Child as a Sense Organ*, 41.
28. Rudolf Steiner, "Lecture Three, Bern, April 15, 1924," in *The Roots of Education*, 36.
29. This phenomenon of the child's "going out and coming back" is a basic hallmark of the Pikler approach. Interestingly, three clinicians, Kent Hoffman, Glen Cooper, and Bert Powell, independently developed a similar "going out and coming back" framework for adults to better understand how to build relationships with young children. It was developed over a thirty-year period and is based on decades of attachment research. Hoffman, Cooper, and Powell call their approach the "Circle of Security." Kent Hoffman, Glen Cooper, and Bert Powell, *Raising a Secure Child*.
30. Bernard Golse MD, "Observation, Application, and Research," 15.

CHAPTER 6:
THE COMPLEXITY OF BABY EQUIPMENT

1. A. L. Abbott and D. J. Bartlett, "Infant Motor Development and Equipment Use in the Home," 295–306.
2. American Academy of Pediatrics, "Tips for Keeping Infants Safe During Sleep from the American Academy of Pediatrics."
3. CanDo Kiddo, "What Parents Need to Know about Baby Gear."
4. Agnes Szanto-Feder, *Moving with Pleasure from the Beginning*, 216.
5. Rudolf Steiner, "Lecture XI: Rhythm in Education," *The Renewal of Education*, 193.
6. Ibid.
7. Jaimen McMillan, personal correspondence with author, January 10, 2025.

CHAPTER 7:
THE INTERPLAY BETWEEN FINE AND GROSS MOTOR DEVELOPMENT

1. The Neurodevelopmental Treatment (NDT) Approach began in England for patients with neuromuscular challenges, including cerebral palsy and stroke. It was originated by Berta Bobath (1907–1991), physiotherapist, along with her husband, Karel Bobath MD. I took my two-month NDT pediatric certification course in 1986.
2. Anna Tardos, "The Researching Infant," 11.
3. Ibid., 14.
4. Frank Wilson, *The Hand*, 276.
5. Rudolf Steiner, "Lecture 4, August 25, 1919," in Rudolf Steiner, *Practical Advice to Teachers*, 51.
6. Emmi Pikler MD, "From Emmi Pikler's First Book," 6.
7. Agnes Szanto-Feder, *Moving with Pleasure from the Beginning*, 29.
8. Ibid., 290.
9. Nicolas Chevalier et al., "Myelination Is Associated with Processing Speed in Early Childhood: Preliminary Insights."
10. Neuro Restart, "Primitive Reflexes," accessed November 19, 2024, https://www.neurorestart.co.uk/primitive-reflexes/.
11. Pikler, "From Emmi Pikler's First Book," 7.
12. Ibid.
13. Ibid., 8.
14. Rudolf Steiner, "Lecture II, 17 March, 1921, Stuttgart," in *Anthroposophy and Science*.
15. Rudolf Steiner, *Practical Advice for Teachers*, 99.
16. Ingun Schneider, "Supporting the Development of the Hand."

CHAPTER 8:
AN INTRODUCTION TO THE TWELVE SENSES

1. Rudolf Steiner, *The Book of Revelation and the Work of the Priest*, 63. From conversations and question-and-answer sessions in Dornach from September 5–22, 1924, reconstructed from notes taken by the participants.

2. Rudolf Steiner, "Lecture III: The Twelve Human Senses, 20 June 1916, Berlin," in *Toward Imagination*.
3. Karl König, *A Living Physiology*, 156.
4. Ibid., 104.
5. Ibid.
6. Rudolf Steiner, "Lecture VIII, 13 August, 1916, Dornach," in *The Riddle of Humanity*.
7. Gerald Karnow, "Living and Working With So-Called Difficult Children, Part I," summary by Nancy Blanning, in Johanna Steegmans and Gerald Karnow (eds.), *Cradle of a Healthy Life*, 125.
8. Rudolf Steiner, "Lecture I, 22 July, 1921, Dornach," in *Man As A Being of Sense And Perception*.
9. Rudolf Steiner, *Foundations of Human Experience*, 143.
10. Ibid., 142.
11. Steiner, "Lecture VII," *The Riddle of Humanity*.
12. Ibid.
13. Ibid.
14. Ibid.
15. Steiner, "Lecture VII," *The Riddle of Humanity*.
16. Rudolf Steiner, "Lecture III, 8 August, 1920, Dornach," in *Spiritual Science as a Foundation for Social Forms*.
17. Peter Selg, *Karl König's Path into Anthroposophy*, 81.
18. Steiner, "Lecture III," in *Spiritual Science as a Foundation*.
19. Quoted in Lisa Romero, *The Inner Work Path*, chapter 1.
20. Ibid.
21. Rudolf Steiner, "Lecture 2: Supersensible Processes in the Activities of the Human Senses, 25 October, 1909, Berlin," in *Wisdom of Man, of the Soul, and of the Spirit*.
22. Ibid.
23. Rudolf Steiner, "Lecture I, 22 July, 1921, Dornach," in *Man As A Being of Sense*.
24. Steiner, *Foundations of Human Experience*, 145.
25. Rudolf Steiner, "Lecture 1: The Position of Anthroposophy in Relation to Theosophy and Anthropology: The Human Senses, 23 October, 1909, Berlin," in *Wisdom of Man, of the Soul, and of the Spirit*.
26. Steiner, "Lecture VII," in *The Riddle of Humanity*.
27. Rudolf Steiner, "Lecture XIV, 2 September, 1916, Dornach," in *The Riddle of Humanity*.
28. Steiner, "Lecture VII," in *The Riddle of Humanity*.
29. Ibid.
30. Steiner, "Lecture III," in *Spiritual Science as a Foundation*.
31. Peter Selg (ed.), *Karl König's Path*, 134–136.
32. Rudolf Steiner, "Lecture 1: Theosophy and Rosicrucianism, 6 June, 1907, Kassel," in *Theosophy and Rosicrucianism*.
33. Karen A. Smith PhD and Daren R. Gouze PhD, *The Sensory-Sensitive Child*, 240.
34. Ibid.
35. Steiner, "Lecture I, 22 July, 1921, Dornach," in *Man As A Being of Sense*.
36. Ibid.
37. Rudolf Steiner, *A Psychology of Body, Soul, and Spirit: Anthroposophy, Psychosophy & Pneumatosophy*, 78–79.
38. Steiner, "Lecture I, 22 July, 1921, Dornach," in *Man As A Being of Sense*.
39. Ibid.
40. Rudolf Meyer, *The Wisdom of Fairy Tales*, 118.
41. Steiner, "Lecture I, 22 July, 1921, Dornach," in *Man As A Being of Sense*.
42. Ibid.
43. Jaimen McMillan, personal correspondence with author, February 2010.
44. Jaimen McMillan, personal correspondence with author, April 2014.
45. I came to the ideas in this paragraph largely through personal correspondence with Jaimen MacMillan, April 4, 2024.
46. Norton Smith, "One Speech," 74.
47. Sheila M. Frick OTR and Sally R. Young PhD, *Listening with the Whole Body*, 16.
48. Jaimen McMillan, personal correspondence with author, October 2018.
49. Rudolf Steiner, "Lecture VIII, 29 August, 1919, Stuttgart," in *The Study of Man*.
50. Steiner, *The Foundations of Human Experience*, 145.
51. Ibid.
52. Johannes W. Rohen, *Functional Morphology*, 28.

CHAPTER 9:
DEVELOPMENTAL ASPECTS OF SENSING

1. Freye Jaffke, "The Significance of Imitation and Example for the Development of the Will," in Joan Almon (ed.), *A Deeper Understanding of the Waldorf Kindergarten*, 15.
2. Rudolf Steiner, "Lecture 2, Torgquay, August 13, 1924," in *The Kingdom of Childhood*, 23.
3. Rudolf Steiner, *A Psychology of Body, Soul, and Spirit*, 17.
4. Georg Kühlewind, *From Normal to Healthy*, 142.
5. Ibid.
6. Ibid., 46.
7. Rudolf Steiner, "Lecture III. Spiritual Disciplines of Yesterday and Today, 18 August, 1922, Oxford," in *Spiritual Ground of Education*.
8. Rudolf Steiner, "Lecture VI. Walking, Speaking, Thinking, 10 August, 1923," in *Education*.
9. Peter Selg, *The Child as a Sense Organ*, 29.
10. Ibid.
11. Rudolf Steiner, "Lecture VII. 12 August, 1916, Dornach," in *The Riddle of Humanity*.
12. Rudolf Steiner, "The World of Spirit or Devachan, Berlin, Feb. 4, 1904."
13. Ibid.
14. Ibid.
15. Stephen Spitalny, *Connecting with Young Children*, 28.

16 Rudolf Steiner, "Lecture IX: Evolution, Involution and Creation out of Nothingness, Berlin, 17th June, 1909," in *The Being of Man and His Future Evolution*.
17 Terri Mauro and Sharon A. Cermak, *The Everything Parent's Guide to Sensory Integration Disorder*, 2.
18 A. Jean Ayres, *Sensory Integration and the Child*, 15.
19 Ibid., 7.
20 Paul Emberson, *From Gondhishapur to Silicon Valley*, volume 2, 920–921.
21 Rudolf Steiner, *The Philosophy of Spiritual Activity*.
22 Ibid., 169.
23 Ayres, *Sensory Integration and the Child*, 6.
24 Ibid., 6–7
25 Ibid., 7.
26 Ayres, *Sensory Integration and the Child*, 5.
27 Ibid.
28 Karl König, *A Living Physiology*, 105.
29 Ibid.
30 Ibid., 202.
31 Ibid., 218.
32 König, *A Living Physiology*, 157.
33 Ibid.
34 Ibid., 158; "To walk upright, to speak and to learn to think are three achievements which are not due to our effort alone for their attainment is beyond our reach."
35 Karl König, "The Human Soul VI: The Twelve Senses of Man."
36 Ibid.
37 König, *A Living Physiology*, 158–159.
38 Ibid., 159
39 Karl König, *The First Three Years of the Child*, 92–93.
40 Steiner, *A Psychology of Body, Soul, and Spirit*, 64.
41 Ibid.
42 König, *A Living Physiology*, 160.
43 Ibid.
44 Ibid.
45 Ann-Marie Widström et al., "Skin-to-Skin Contact the First Hour after Birth."
46 Ibid.
47 Ibid.
48 Ibid.
49 Widström et al., "Skin-to-Skin Contact."
50 Ibid.

CHAPTER 10:
NOURISHING THE YOUNG CHILD'S SENSE ORGANS

1 Rudolf Steiner, "Lecture 6: The Upbringing of Children; Karma, 27 August, 1906," in *At the Gates of Spiritual Science*.
2 Bert Hellinger with Bunthard Weber and Hunter Beaumont, *Love's Hidden Symmetry*, 12.
3 Neal Kennerk and Jennifer Kennerk, *Out of the Garden and into the Desert*, 43–44.
4 David Luke (ed.), *Goethe*, 277.
5 Rudolf Steiner, *A Psychology of Body, Soul, and Spirit*, 58.
6 Helle Heckmann, *Nøkken*, 109.
7 Steiner, "Lecture 6," in *At the Gates of Spiritual Science*.
8 Ibid.
9 Rudolf Steiner, "The Education of the Child in the Light of Spiritual Science," 18.
10 World Health Organization, "Episode #108—How Can You Protect Your Child's Vision?"
11 Ibid.
12 Catherine Jan et al., "Prevention of Myopia, China."
13 International Myopia Institute, "Myopia Is Growing Around the World."
14 Michaela Glöckler, personal correspondence with author, May 10, 2024.
15 Stephen Spitalny, "The Senses as Doorways of Relating," 9.
16 Peter Lang, "Salutogenic Approach to Education in Early Childhood," 50, citing Manfred Spitzer (2005).
17 Jacques Lusseyran, *And There Was Light*, 18–19.
18 Ibid.
19 Ibid.
20 Ibid.
21 Ellyn Satter, *Child of Mine*, 475.
22 Ibid.
23 Ibid.
24 Rudolf Steiner, *Life Between Death and Rebirth*, 34.
25 Rudolf Steiner, "Lecture 2: On the Forming of Destiny, November 18, 1915, Berlin," in *The Forming of Destiny and Life after Death*.
26 Edmond Schoorel, *The First Seven Years*, 125.
27 Rudolf Steiner, "Lecture III. Dornach. 8 August, 1920," in *Spiritual Science as a Foundation for Social Forms*.
28 Henning Köhler, *Working with Anxious, Nervous, and Depressed Children*, 83.
29 Ibid.
30 Ibid., 53.
31 Ibid., 49.
32 David Brooks, *The Social Animal*, 43.
33 Steiner, "Lecture III," in *Spiritual Science as a Foundation*.
34 Köhler, *Working with Anxious, Nervous, and Depressed Children*, 25.
35 Steiner, "Lecture III," in *Spiritual Science as a Foundation*.
36 Köhler, *Working with Anxious, Nervous, and Depressed Children*, 86.

37 Ibid., 97.
38 Ibid., 97–98.
39 Emmi Pikler, "From Emmi Pikler's First Book: Excerpts from *Peaceful Babies—Contented Mothers*," 12.
40 Steiner, "Lecture III," in *Spiritual Science as a Foundation*.
41 Michaela Glöckler, "Forces of Growth and Forces of Fantasy: Understanding the Dream Consciousness of the Young Child," in Joan Almon (ed.), *A Deeper Understanding of the Waldorf Kindergarten*, 36.

CHAPTER 11:
THE FORMING OF THE BODY IMAGE

1 A. Jean Ayres, *Sensory Integration and the Child*, 23.
2 Karl König, *Being Human*, 35.
3 Gay Lloyd Pinder, NDT course, 1984.
4 Judit Falk MD, "When We Touch the Infant's Body," 6.
5 Rudolf Steiner, *The Child's Changing Consciousness and Waldorf Education*, 145.

CHAPTER 12:
THE SENSE OF TOUCH

1 Rudolf Steiner, "Lecture III, 8 August, 1920, Dornach," in *Spiritual Science as a Foundation for Social Forms*.
2 Rudolf Steiner, *Man as a Being of Sense and Perception*.
3 Henning Köhler, *Working with Anxious, Nervous, and Depressed Children*, 56.
4 Ann E. Bigelow and Michelle Power, "Mother-Infant Skin-to-Skin Contact."
5 Ann-Marie Widström et al., "Skin-to-Skin Contact the First Hour after Birth."
6 Bigelow and Power, "Mother-Infant Skin-to-Skin Contact."
7 Widström et al., "Skin-to-Skin Contact the First Hour after Birth."
8 Ibid.
9 See, for example, the gesture games books published by the Waldorf Early Childhood Association of North America, in addition to a book I authored with Nancy Macalaster and Susan Weber of Sophia's Hearth, *Singing and Speaking the Child into Life: Songs, Verses, and Rhythmic Games for the First Three Years* (Spring Valley, NY: Waldorf Early Childhood Association of North America, 2017).
10 Anna Tardos (ed.), *Bringing Up and Providing Care for Infants and Toddlers in an Institution*, 56
11 Rudolf Steiner, "Lecture III: The Twelve Human Senses, 20 June 1916, Berlin," in *Toward Imagination*.

CHAPTER 13:
THE SENSE OF LIFE

1 Karl König, *A Living Physiology*, 106–107.
2 Ibid., 117.
3 Henning Köhler, *Working with Anxious, Nervous, and Depressed Children*, 22.
4 Ibid., 23.
5 König, *A Living Physiology*, 188.
6 Ibid.
7 Ibid., 203–204.
8 Köhler, *Working with Anxious, Nervous, and Depressed Children*, 28–29.
9 Thomas S. Cowan with Sally Fallon and Jaimen McMillan, *The Fourfold Path to Healing*, 396.
10 Ibid.
11 König, *A Living Physiology*, 114.
12 Laurie Kelly McCorry PhD, "Physiology of the Autonomic Nervous System."
13 Ibid.
14 Deb Dana, *The Polyvagal Theory in Therapy*, 22.
15 Dr. Gerald Karnow, "Developing the Eyes to See," summary by Nancy Blanning, in Johanna Steegmans and Gerald Karnow (eds.), *Cradle of a Healthy Life*, 145.
16 Dana, *The Polyvagal Theory in Therapy*, 6.
17 Ibid., 22.
18 Ibid.
19 Ibid., 23.
20 Dana, *The Polyvagal Theory in Therapy*, 23.
21 Deb Dana, *Anchored*, 151.
22 Ibid., 10.
23 Heidemarie K. Laurent, Kathryn S. Gilliam, Dorianne B. Wright, and Philip A. Fisher, "Child Anxiety Symptoms Related to Longitudinal Cortisol Trajectories and Acute Stress Responses: Evidence of Developmental Stress Sensitization."
24 M. A. Kranowitz and Carol Stock, *The Out-of-Sync Child*, 60.
25 Stephen W. Porges PhD, "Play as a Neural Exercise: Insights from the Polyvagal Theory."
26 Ibid.
27 Ibid.
28 Jaimen McMillan, Level IV Spacial Dynamics module, January 28, 2023.
29 Jaimen McMillan, personal correspondence with author, January 30, 2023.

CHAPTER 14:
THE SENSE OF SELF-MOVEMENT

1. Oliver Sacks, "Foreword," in Jonathan Cole and Ian Waterman, *Pride and a Daily Marathon*.
2. Cole and Waterman, *Pride and a Daily Marathon*.
3. Ibid., 15.
4. Ibid., 12.
5. Ibid., 34.
6. Cole and Waterman, 22.
7. Ibid., 56.
8. Ibid., 57.
9. Henning Köhler, *Working with Anxious, Nervous, and Depressed Children*, 97.
10. Rudolf Steiner, "Lecture III, 8 August, 1920, Dornach," in *Spiritual Science as a Foundation for Social Forms*.
11. Cole and Waterman, *Pride and a Daily Marathon*, 58.
12. Ibid., 69.
13. Karl König, *Being Human*, 22.
14. Ibid.
15. Ibid.
16. Cole and Waterman, *Pride and a Daily Marathon*, 84.
17. Ibid., 178.
18. Ibid., 58.
19. Ibid., 59.
20. Cole and Waterman, 124.
21. Hiroko Matsukawa, personal correspondence with author, May 23, 2024.
22. Rudolf Steiner, "Lecture 2: Supersensible Processes in the Activities of the Human Senses, 25 October, 1909, Berlin," in *Wisdom of Man, of the Soul, and of the Spirit*.
23. Jaimen McMillan, Level 3D Spacial Dynamics module, May 6, 2023.
24. Jaimen McMillan, Level IV Spacial Dynamics training module, January 8, 2022.
25. Marita Tulloch, personal correspondence with author, May 30, 2024. Marita is a Waldorf School Teacher and a Master Somatic Movement Educator and Therapist in the discipline of Spacial Dynamics.
26. Rudolf Steiner, "The Constitution of the Etheric Body."
27. Jaimen McMillan, Level I Spacial Dynamics training, August 2000.
28. Rudolf Steiner, *The Foundations of Human Experience*, 143–144.

CHAPTER 15:
THE SENSE OF BALANCE

1. Rudolf Steiner, *Man as a Being of Sense and Perception*.
2. Judit Falk, "When We Touch the Infant's Body," 9.
3. Ibid.
4. Ibid., 10.
5. European Space Agency, "Living in Space."
6. Ibid.
7. Ibid.
8. Ibid.
9. European Space Agency.
10. Rudolf Steiner, *The Spiritual Guidance of the Individual and Humanity*, 59–60.
11. Anna Tardos, "The Researching Infant," 13.
12. Jaimen McMillan, personal correspondence with author, November 2011.
13. Ernestine Stodelle, *The Dance Technique of Doris Humphrey and Its Creative Potential*, 24.
14. Ibid.
15. Rudolf Steiner, "Lecture III, 8 August, 1920, Dornach," in *Spiritual Science as a Foundation for Social Forms*.
16. Henning Köhler, *Working with Anxious, Nervous, and Depressed Children*, 110.
17. Rudolf Steiner, "The Waking of the Human Soul and the Forming of Destiny, 28 April 1923, Prague."
18. "Concerning the oft-mentioned similarity of the human skeleton to that of the ape, the erect gait of the ape has been botched. The ape tried to raise himself up but did not succeed"; Rudolf Steiner, "The Etheric Vision of the Future."
19. Rudolf Steiner, *Soul Economy*, 323–325.
20. Jaimen McMillan, personal correspondence with author, February 2025.
21. Magda Gerber, in RIE Approach, "RIE WEB Clips *See How They Move*," minute 1:16–17.
22. Agnes Szanto-Feder, *Moving with Pleasure from the Beginning*, 142–143.
23. Ibid., 143.
24. Albert Soesman, *Our Twelve Senses*, 47.

APPENDICES

Appendix 1:
SUPPORTING FREE MOVEMENT THROUGH THE PHYSICAL ENVIRONMENT

1. Edmond Schoorel, *The First Seven Years*, 252.
2. American Academy of Pediatrics, "Safe Sleep and Your Baby."
3. Emmi Pikler MD, "Learning of Motor Skills on the Basis of Self-Induced Movements," 72.
4. Ibid., 76.
5. Éva Kálló and Györgyi Balog, *The Origins of Free Play*, 74.
6. Ibid., 41.
7. Roy Swain, mechanical engineer, personal correspondence with author, December 6, 2023.
8. Emmi Pikler MD, "Some Contributions to the Study of the Gross Motor Development of Children," 27–39, 30.
9. Rudolf Steiner, "Lecture V: Metamorphoses of Our Earthly Experiences in the Spiritual World, into New Capacities for Our Next Life, Kassel, 20th June 1907," in *Theosophy and Rosicrucianism*.
10. Karine Munk Finser, personal correspondence with author, November 25, 2024. Karine is an art therapist and the director of Kairos Institute. She directs the Renewal courses at the Center for Anthroposophy and is the director of Transdisciplinary Studies in Healing Education at Antioch University.

Appendix 2:
TOYS TO SUPPORT FREE MOVEMENT

1. Eva Kálló and Györgi Balog, *Origins of Free Play*.
2. Myriam David and Geneviéve Appell, *Lóczy*, 57–78.
3. Kálló and Balog, *Origins of Free Play*, 52.
4. Ibid., 35–37.
5. Anna Tardos, "Two-Week Intensive."
6. Elsa Chahin with Anna Tardos, *In Loving Hands*, 82.
7. Debbie Laurin, personal correspondence with author, December 7, 2023.
8. Kálló and Balog, *Origins of Free Play*, 34.
9. Rudolf Steiner, "Children before the Seventh Year, December 29, 1921," in Rudof Steiner, *Soul Economy*, 113–114.
10. Rudolf Steiner, "Lecture Four, Dornach, April 18, 1923," in *The Child's Changing Consciousness and Waldorf Education*, 73.
11. Johanna-Veronika Picht, "Dolls and Animals in the Child's Room," in Joan Almon (ed.), *An Overview of the Waldorf Kindergarten*, 15.
12. Ibid., 18.
13. Ibid.
14. Ibid.
15. Rudolf Steiner, "Children before the Seventh Year," in *Soul Economy*, 115.

Appendix 3:
PIKLER'S WOODEN FURNISHINGS

1. Jaimen McMillan, personal correspondence with author, April 4, 2024.
2. Katherine Scharff, personal correspondence with author, October 24, 2023.
3. Agnes Szanto-Feder, *Moving with Pleasure from the Beginning*, 135.
4. Ibid., 137.
5. Ibid., 145.

Appendix 4:
PIKLER'S WOODEN FURNISHINGS

1. Jaimen McMillan, personal correspondence with author, August 28, 2023.
2. Michaela Glöckler, personal correspondence with author, February 21, 2023.
3. Jane shares a lovely video of this vignette online: WAPASA, "A Winter Wish," Vimeo video, December 22, 2022, https://vimeo.com/783831219.
4. Janene Ping, personal correspondence with author, January 3, 2023.
5. Freya Jaffke, *Toymaking with Children*, 21.

Bibliography

Abbott, A. L., and D. J. Bartlett. "Infant Motor Development and Equipment Use in the Home." *Child: Care, Health, and Development* 27, no. 3 (2001).

Almon, Joan (ed.). *An Overview of the Waldorf Kindergarten: Articles from the Waldorf Kindergarten Newsletter 1981 to 1992*, vol. 1. Silver Spring, MD: The Waldorf Kindergarten Association of North America, 1993. https://www.waldorflibrary.org/online-library/ebooks/ebooks/an-overview-of-the-waldorf-kindergarten-ebook.

———. *A Deeper Understanding of the Waldorf Kindergarten: Articles from the Waldorf Kindergarten Newsletter, 1981–1992*, vol. 2. Silver Spring, MD: The Waldorf Kindergarten Association, 1993. https://www.waldorflibrary.org/online-library/ebooks/ebooks/a-deeper-understanding-of-the-waldorf-kindergarten,-volume-2-ebook.

American Academy of Pediatrics. "Safe Sleep and Your Baby: How Parents Can Reduce the Risk of SIDS and Suffocation." June 29, 2022. https://doi.org/10.1542/peo_document088.

———. "Tips for Keeping Infants Safe During Sleep from the American Academy of Pediatrics." Accessed August 23, 3024. https://www.aap.org/en/news-room/news-releases/aap/2020/tips-for-keeping-infants-safe-during-sleep-from-the-american-academy-of-pediatrics.

Ayres, A. Jean. *Sensory Integration and the Child*. Los Angeles: Western Psychological Services, 1995.

Bigelow, Ann E. and Michelle Power. "Mother-Infant Skin-to-Skin Contact: Short- and Long-Term Effects for Mothers and Their Children Born Full-Term." *Frontiers in Psychology* 11 (Aug. 28, 2020). https://doi.org/10.3389/fpsyg.2020.01921.

Brooks, David. *The Social Animal: The Hidden Sources of Love, Character, and Achievement*. New York: Random House, 2011.

CanDo Kiddo. "What Parents Need to Know about Baby Gear." Accessed August 23, 2024. https://www.candokiddo.com/news/baby-gear.

Caro, Clare. "The Genius of Emmi Pikler." The Pikler Collection. Accessed Aug. 1, 2024, https://thepiklercollection.weebly.com/history.html.

Chahin, Elsa, with Anna Tardos. *In Loving Hands: How the Rights for Young Children Living in Children's Homes Offer Hope and Happiness in Today's World*. N.p.: Xlibris, 2017.

Chevalier, Nicolas, et al., "Myelination Is Associated with Processing Speed in Early Childhood: Preliminary Insights," *PLOS ONE*, October 6, 2015, https://doi.org/10.1371/journal.pone.0139897.

Cole, Jonathan, and Ian Waterman. *Pride and A Daily Marathon*. Cambridge, MA: The MIT Press, 1995.

Cowan, Thomas S., with Sally Fallon and Jaimen McMillan. *The Fourfold Path to Healing: Working with the Laws of Nutrition, Therapeutics, Movement, and Meditation in the Art of Medicine*. Washington, DC: NewTrends Publishing, 2007.

Dana, Deb. *Anchored: How to Befriend Your Nervous System Using Polyvagal Theory*. Boulder, CO: Sounds True, 2021.

———. *The Polyvagal Theory in Therapy: Engaging the Rhythm of Regulation*. New York: W. W. Norton & Company, 2018.

David, Myriam, and Geneviéve Appell. *Lóczy: An Unusual Approach to Mothering*. Translated by Jean Marie Clark; translation revised by Judit Falk. Budapest: Hungarian Pikler-Lóczy Society, 2001.

Emberson, Paul. *From Gondhishapur to Silicon Valley*, volume 2. Scotland: Etheric Dimensions Press, 2014.

European Space Agency. "Living in Space." Accessed September 5, 2024. https://www.esa.int/Science_Exploration/Human_and_Robotic_Exploration/Astronauts/Living_in_space.

Falk, Judit, MD. "Forty Years of Lóczy: A Talk Given at Lóczy in 1986, on the Occasion of Its Fortieth Anniversary." *Sensory Awareness Foundation Bulletin* 14 (Winter 1994), "Emmi Pikler 1902–1984."

———. "When We Touch the Infant's Body." In *Bathing the Baby: The Art of Care* by Dr. Judit Falk and Mária Vincze. Budapest: Pikler-Lóczy Society for Small Children, 2006.

———. "Why Should We Lay the Infant in the Prone Position?" *Gyermekgyógyászat* [*Child and Youth Medical Journal*], Supplmentum A (May 2011).

Frick, Sheila M., OTR, and Sally R. Young PhD. *Listening with the Whole Body: Clinical Concepts and Treatment Guidelines for Therapeutic Listening*. Madison, WI: Vital Links, 2009.

Gerber, Magda. *Dear Parent: Caring for Infants with Respect.* Joan Weaver (ed.). Los Angeles: Resources for Infant Educarers, 1998.

Gerber, Magda, and Allison Johnson. *Your Self-Confident Baby: How to Encourage Your Child's Natural Abilities—from the Very Start.* New York: John Wiley & Sons, 1989.

Glöckler, Michaela, and Wolfgang Goebel. *A Guide to Child Health.* Hudson, NY: Anthroposophic Press, 1984.

Golse, Bernard, MD. "Observation, Application, and Research." *The Signal: Newsletter of the World Association for Infant Mental Health* 18, no. 3–4 (July–Dec. 2010).

Heckmann, Helle. *Nøkken: A Garden for Children.* Spring Valley, NY: Waldorf Early Childhood Association of North America, 2015.

Hellinger, Bert, with Bunthard Weber and Hunter Beaumont. *Love's Hidden Symmetry: What Makes Love Work in Relationships.* Phoenix, AZ: Zeig, Tucker & Co., 1998.

Hoffman, Kent, Glen Cooper, and Bert Powell. *Raising a Secure Child: How Circle of Security Parenting Can Help You Nurture Your Child's Attachment, Emotional Resilience, and Freedom to Explore.* New York: The Guilford Press, 2007.

International Myopia Institute. "Myopia Is Growing Around the World." Accessed February 12, 2025. https://myopiainstitute.org/myopia/.

Jaffke, Freya. *Toymaking with Children.* Edinburgh: Floris Books, 1988.

Jan, Catherine, et al. "Prevention of Myopia, China." *Bulletin of the World Health Organization* 98, no. 6 (Apr. 28, 2020): 435–37.

Kálló, Éva, and Györgyi Balog. *The Origins of Free Play.* Budapest: Pikler-Lóczy Társaság, 2021.

Kennerk, Neal and Jennifer. *Out of the Garden and into the Desert: The Nine-Year Change Through the Stories of the Third Grade Curriculum.* N.p.: Published by the authors, 2015.

Köhler, Henning. *Working with Anxious, Nervous, and Depressed Children: A Spiritual Perspective to Guide Parents.* Fair Oaks, CA: Association of Waldorf Schools, 2000.

König, Karl. *A Living Physiology.* Camp Hill, PA: Camphill Books, 1999.

———. *Being Human: Diagnosis in Curative Education.* Translated by Catherine Creeger. Hudson, NY: Anthroposophic Press, 1989.

———. *The First Three Years of the Child: Walking, Speaking, Thinking.* Edinburgh: Floris Books, 2016.

———. "The Human Soul VI: The Twelve Senses of Man." *The Cresset: Journal of the Camphill Movement* VIII, no. 3 (Easter 1962). Published on behalf of the Camphill Movement by the Camphill-Rudolf Steiner-Schools, Aberdeen (Scotland).

Kranowitz, M. A., and Carol Stock. *The Out-of-Sync Child: Recognizing and Coping with Sensory Processing Disorder.* New York: The Penguin Group, 2005.

Kühlewind, Georg. *From Normal to Healthy: Paths to the Liberation of Consciousness.* Translated by Michael Lipson. Great Barrington, MA: Lindisfarne Press, 1988.

Lang, Peter. "Salutogenic Approach to Education in Early Childhood." In *Education—Health for Life: Education and Medicine Working Together for Healthy Development*, edited by Michaela Glöckler, Stefan Langhammer, and Christof Wiechert. Spring Valley, NY: Waldorf Early Childhood Association of North America, 2019.

Laurent, Heidemarie K., Kathryn S. Gilliam, Dorianne B. Wright, and Philip A. Fisher. "Child Anxiety Symptoms Related to Longitudinal Cortisol Trajectories and Acute Stress Responses: Evidence of Developmental Stress Sensitization." *Journal of Abnormal Psychology* 124, no. 1 (Feb. 2015): 68–79. https://doi.org/10.1037/abn0000009.

Long-Breipohl, Renate. *Under the Stars: The Foundations of Steiner Waldorf Early Childhood Education.* Gloucestershire, UK: Hawthorn Press, 2012.

Luke, David (ed.). *Goethe.* New York: Penguin Books, 1986.

Luker, Edward. "Are Video Games, Screens Another Addiction?" *Speaking of Health*, Mayo Clinic Health System, July 1, 2022. https://www.mayoclinichealthsystem.org/hometown-health/speaking-of-healthcare-video-games-and-screens-another-addiction.

Lusseyran, Jacques. *And There Was Light.* Translated by Elizabeth R. Cameron. Novato, CA: New World Library, 1963.

Mauro, Terri, and Sharon A. Cermak. *The Everything Parent's Guide to Sensory Integration Disorder.* Avon, MA: Adams Media, 2006.

Mayo Clinic Staff. "Infant and Toddler Health." Mayo Clinic, March 10, 2022, https://www.mayoclinic.org/healthy-lifestyle/infant-and-toddler-health/in-depth/healthy-baby/art-20045964.

McCorry, Laurie Kelly, PhD. "Physiology of the Autonomic Nervous System." *American Journal of Pharmaceutical Education* 71, no. 4 (Aug. 15, 2007): 78. https://pubmed.ncbi.nlm.nih.gov/17786266/.

McMillan, Jaimen. Level I Spacial Dynamics training, August 2000.

———. Level IV Spacial Dynamics training module, Janaury 8, 2022.

———. Level IV Spacial Dynamics module, January 28, 2023.

———. Level 3D Spacial Dynamics module, May 6, 2023.

Meyer, Rudolf. *The Wisdom of Fairy Tales*. Edinburgh: Floris Books, 2001.

Munch, Edvard. *The Scream* (1893). National Gallery of Norway. Accessed May 27, 2025. https://commons.wikimedia.org/wiki/File:The_Scream.jpg

Pikler, Emmi, MD. "The Competence of the Infant." *Acta Paediatrica Academiae Scientiarum Hungaricae* 20 (1979).

———. "Data on Gross Motor Development of the Infant." In *Early Child Development and Care*, vol. 1, edited by Alice Herman and Sandor Komlósi. London: Gordon and Breach Science Publishers Ltd., 1972.

———. "From Emmi Pikler's First Book: Excerpts from Peaceful Babies—Contented Mothers." *Sensory Awareness Foundation Bulletin* 14 (Winter 1994), "Emmi Pikler 1902–1984."

———. "Learning of Motor Skills on the Basis of Self-Induced Movements." Chapter 4 in Jerome Hellmuth (ed.), *Exceptional Infant: Studies in Abnormalities*, vol. 2. New York: Brunner/Mazel, Inc., 1971.

———. "Some Contributions to the Study of the Gross Motor Development of Children." *Journal of Genetic Psychology* 113 (1968).

Pinder, Gay Lloyd. Neurodevelopmental Treatment (NDT) course, 1984.

Porges, Stephen W., PhD. "Play as a neural exercise: Insights from the Polyvagal Theory." Olive Branch Counseling and Training. Accessed September 4, 2024. https://olivebranchsa.com/portfolio-view/play-as-a-neural-exercise-insights-from-the-polyvagal-theory.

RIE Approach (Resources for Infant Educators). "RIE WEB Clips See How They Move." YouTube video, July 1, 2013. https://youtu.be/JIjBhZPNOPM.

Rohen, Johannes W. *Functional Morphology*. Hillsdale, NY: Adonis Press, 2007.

Romero, Lisa. *The Inner Work Path*. Great Barrington, MA: SteinerBooks, 2014.

Sacks, Oliver. "Foreword." In *Pride and A Daily Marathon* by Jonathan Cole. Cambridge, MA: The MIT Press, 1995.

Satter, Ellyn. *Child of Mine: Feeding with Love and Good Sense*. Palo Alto, CA: Bull Publishing Company, 2000.

Schneider, Ingun. "Supporting the Development of the Hand." *Gateways* 41 (Winter 2001). https://www.waldorflibrary.org/journals/98-gateways/1040-fallwinter-2001-issue-41-supporting-the-development-of-the-hand.

Schoorel, Edmond. *The First Seven Years: Physiology of Childhood*. Fair Oaks, CA: Rudolf Steiner College Press, 2004.

Selg, Peter. *The Child as a Sense Organ*. Great Barrington, MA: SteinerBooks, 2017.

———. *Karl König's Path into Anthroposophy: Reflection from His Diaries*. Edinburgh: Floris Books, 2006.

——— (ed.). *Karl König: My Task, Autobiography and Biographies*, translated by Irene Czech and Regina Erich. Edinburgh: Floris Books, 2008.

Smith, Karen A., PhD, and Daren R. Gouze PhD. *The Sensory-Sensitive Child: Practical Solutions for Out-of-Bounds Behavior*. New York: Collins, 2004.

Smith, Norton. "One Speech," *Time Magazine* 182, no. 9 (Aug. 26–Sept. 2, 2013).

Soesman, Albert. *Our Twelve Senses: How Healthy Senses Refresh the Soul*. Translated by Jakob M. Cornelis. Stroud, England: Hawthorn Press, 1990.

Spitalny, Stephen. *Connecting with Young Children: Educating the Will*. Fair Oaks, CA: Chamakanda Press, 2012.

———. "The Senses as Doorways of Relating." *Gateways* 59 (Fall/Winter 2010).

Steegmans, Johanna, and Gerald Karnow, eds. *Cradle of a Healthy Life: Early Childhood and the Whole of Life*. Spring Valley, NY: Waldorf Early Childhood Association of North America, 2012.

Steiner, Rudolf. *The Book of Revelation and the Work of the Priest: Eighteen Lectures* Translated by J. Collis. London: Rudolf Steiner Press, 1998.

———. *The Child's Changing Consciousness and Waldorf Education* by Rudolf Steiner. Hudson, NY: Anthroposophic Press, 1988.

———. "The Constitution of the Etheric Body." In *Initiation and Its Results*, GA 10. Translated by Clifford Bax. Rudolf Steiner Archive. https://rsarchive.org/Books/GA010/English/MAC1909/GA010b_c01.html#Chapter%202.

———. *Education*, GA 307. H. Collison (ed.), no translator listed. Rudolf Steiner Archive. https://rsarchive.org/Lectures/GA307/English/RSPC1943/Educat_index.html.

———. *Education and Instruction, 15 September 1920, Stuttgart*, GA 302a. Translator unknown. Rudolf Steiner Archive. https://rsarchive.org/Lectures/GA302a/English/Singles/19200915a01.html

———. "The Education of the Child in the Light of Spiritual Science." In *The Education of the Child* by Rudolf Steiner. Translated by George and Mary Adams. Hudson, NY: Anthroposophic Press, 1996.

———. "The Etheric Vision of the Future." Lecture 8 in *The Reappearance of Christ in the Etheric*, GA 118. No translator listed. Rudolf Steiner e.Lib. https://wn.rudolfsteinerelib.org/Lectures/GA/GA0118/19100510p01.html.

———. *Foundations of Human Experience*. No translator listed. Hudson, NY: Anthroposophic Press, 1996.

———. "Lecture 1." In *From Jesus to Christ: Eleven Lectures Given in Karlsruhe between 4 and 14 October, 1911*. Forest Row, UK: Rudolf Steiner Press, 2005.

———. "Lecture II, 17 March, 1921, Stuttgart." In *Anthroposophy and Science*, GA324. Translated by Walter Stuber and Mark Gardner. GA 324. Rudolf Steiner Archive. https://rsarchive.org/Lectures/GA324/English/MP1991/19210317p01.html.

———. "Lecture 2: On the Forming of Destiny, November 18, 1915, Berlin." In *The Forming of Destiny and Life after Death*, GA 157a. No translator listed. Rudolf Steiner Archive. https://rsarchive.org/Lectures/GA157a/English/APC1927/19151118p01.html.

———. "Lecture II—On Language: The Oneness of Man with the Universe, 22 August, 1919, Stuttgart." In *Practical Course for Teachers*, GA 294. Translation authorized by Harry Collison. Rudolf Steiner Archive, https://rsarchive.org/Lectures/GA294/English/RSPC1937/19190822n01.html.

———. "Lecture 2, Torgquay, August 13, 1924." In *The Kingdom of Childhood*. Original translation by Helen Fox. Revised. Rudolf Steiner Press, 1982; revised, Anthroposophic Press, 1995.

———. "Lecture III, 8 August, 1920, Dornach." In *Spiritual Science as a Foundation for Social Forms*, GA199. translated by Maria St. Goar. Rudolf Steiner Archive. https://rsarchive.org/Lectures/GA199/English/AP1986/19200808p01.html.

———. "Lecture III. Spiritual Disciplines of Yesterday and Today, 18 August, 1922, Oxford." In *Spiritual Ground of Education*, GA 305. No translator listed. Rudolf Steiner Archive. https://rsarchive.org/Lectures/GA305/English/APC1947/19220818p01.html.

———. "Lecture 4, August 25, 1919." In *Practical Advice to Teachers* by Rudolf Steiner. Great Barrington, MA: Anthroposophic Press, 2000.

———. "Lecture 6: The Upbringing of Children; Karma, 27 August, 1906." In *At the Gates of Spiritual Science*, GA 95. Translated by E. H. Goddard and Charles Davy. Rudolf Steiner Archive. https://rsarchive.org/Lectures/GA095/English/RSPAP1986/19060827p01.html.

———. "Lecture III: The Twelve Human Senses, 20 June 1916, Berlin." In *Toward Imagination*, GA 169. Translated by Sabine H. Seiler. Rudolf Steiner Archive. https://rsarchive.org/Lectures/GA169/English/AP1990/19160620p01.html.

———. "Lecture VIII, 29 August, 1919, Stuttgart." *The Study of Man*, GA 293. Translated by Daphne Harwood and Helen Fox. Rudolf Steiner Archive. https://rsarchive.org/Lectures/GA293/English/RSP1966/19190829a01.html.

———. "Lecture IX: Evolution, Involution and Creation out of Nothingness, Berlin, 17th June, 1909." In *The Being of Man and His Future Evolution*, GA 107 (section 19). Translated by Pauline Wehrle. Rudolf Steiner Archive. https://rsarchive.org/Lectures/GA107/English/RSP1981/19090617p01.html.

———. "Lecture Three, Bern, April 15, 1924." In *The Roots of Education* by Rudolf Steiner, translated by Helen Fox and Frederick Amrine. Great Barrington, MA: SteinerBooks, 2019.

———. *Life Between Death and Rebirth*. Hudson, NY: Anthroposophic Press, 1987.

———. *Man as a Being of Sense and Perception*, GA 206. Translated by Dorothy Lenn. Rudolf Steiner Archive. https://rsarchive.org/Lectures/GA206/English/APC1958/ManBei_index.html.

———. *The Philosophy of Spiritual Activity*. 2nd edition. Translated by Professor and Mrs. R. F. Alfred Hoernlé. Translation edited by H. Collison. London: G. P. Putnam's Sons, 1922. https://www.gutenberg.org/cache/epub/55761/pg55761-images.html.

———. *Practical Advice for Teachers*. Translated by Johanna Collis. Great Barrington, MA: Anthroposophic Press, 2000.

———. *A Psychology of Body, Soul, and Spirit: Anthroposophy, Psychosophy & Pneumatosophy*. Translated by Marjorie Spock. Hudson, NY: Anthroposophic Press, 1999.

———. *Renewal of Education*. Great Barrington, MA: Anthroposophic Press, 2001.

———. *The Riddle of Humanity*. GA 170. No translator listed. Rudolf Steiner Archive. https://rsarchive.org/Lectures/GA170/English/RSP1990/RidHum_index.html.

———. *Self-Education in the Light of Spiritual Science*. Translated by Alan Mullen. Spring Valley, NY: Mercury Press, 1995.

———. *Soul Economy: Body, Soul, and Spirit in Waldorf Education*. Translated by Roland Everett. Great Barrington, MA: Anthroposophic Press, 2003.

———. *Soul Exercises, 1903–1924*. Great Barrington, MA: SteinerBooks, 2014.

———. *Spiritual Guidance of the Individual and Humanity*. Translated by Samuel Desch. Hudson, NY: Anthroposophic Press, 1991.

———. "Spiritual Science, Freedom of Thought, and Societal Forces, Stuttgart, December 19, 1919." In *Freedom of Thought and Societal Forces: Implementing the Demands of Modern Society* by Rudolf Steiner, translated by Catherine E. Creeger. Spencertown, NY: SteinerBooks, 2008.

———. *Theosophy and Rosicrucianism*, GA 100. Rudolf Steiner Archive. https://rsarchive.org/Lectures/GA100/English/ANS1942/19070620p01.html.

———. "The Waking of the Human Soul and the Forming of Destiny, 28 April 1923, Prague." Lecture 1 in *The Waking of the Human Soul and the Forming of Destiny*, GA 224. No translator listed. Rudolf Steiner Archive. https://rsarchive.org/Lectures/GA224/English/SBC1970/19230428p01.html.

———. *Wisdom of Man, of the Soul, and of the Spirit*, GA 115. Translated by Samuel and Loni Lockwood. Rudolf Steiner Archive. https://rsarchive.org/Lectures/GA115/English/AP1971/WisMan_index.html.

———. "The World of Spirit or Devachan, Berlin, Feb. 4, 1904." In *Concerning the Astral World and Devachan* by Rudolf Steiner. Great Barrington, MA: SteinerBooks, 2018.

Stodelle, Ernestine. *The Dance Technique of Doris Humphrey and Its Creative Potential*. 2nd edition. Princeton, NJ: Dance Horizons/Princeton Book Company, 1978.

Szanto-Feder, Agnes. *Moving with Pleasure from the Beginning: The Importance of Observation in Early Childhood*. N.p.: Xlibris, 2020.

Tardos, Anna. "From the Hands of the Caregiver." In Anna Tardos (ed.), *Bringing Up and Providing Care for Infants and Toddlers in an Institution*, translated by Alexandra Sargent, Alex Kajtár, Ágnes Zádor, and Linda Kunos. Budapest: Hungarian Pikler-Lóczy Society, 2007.

———. "Introducing the Piklerian Developmental Approach: History and Principles." *The Signal—Newsletter of the World Association for Infant Mental Health* 18, no. 3-4 (July-Dec. 2010).

———. "The Researching Infant." *The Signal: Newsletter of the World Association for Infant Mental Health* 18, no. 3–4 (July–Dec. 2010).

———. "Two-Week Intensive." Author's notes from a two-week intensive, 2007.

Thoreau, Henry David. *Autumn: From the Journal of Henry D. Thoreau*. H. G. O. Blake (ed.). Houghton, Mifflin, and Co., 1893; Elibron Classics Series, Adamant Media Corporation, 2004.

Vincze, Mária. "The Meaning of Cooperation During Care." In *Bathing the Baby: The Art of Care* by Dr. Judit Falk and Mária Vincze. Budapest: Pikler-Lóczy Society for Small Children, 2006.

Weber, Susan, Nancy Macalaster, and Jane Swain. *Singing and Speaking the Child into Life: Songs, Verses, and Rhythmic Games for the First Three Years*. Spring Valley, New York: Waldorf Early Childhood Association of North America, 2017.

Widström, Ann-Marie, et al. "Skin-to-Skin Contact the First Hour after Birth: Underlying Implications and Clinical Practice." *ACTA Paediatrica* 108, no. 7 (2019). https://doi.org/10.1111/apa.14754.

Williams, Mary Sue, OTR/L, and Sherry Shellenberger OTR/L. *How Does Your Engine Run? A Leader's Guide to the Alert Program for Self-Regulation*. Albuquerque, NM: Therapy Works Inc., 1996.

Wilson, Frank. *The Hand: How Its Use Shapes the Brain, Language, and Human Culture*. New York: Vintage Books, 1998.

World Health Organization. "Episode 108—How Can You Protect Your Child's Vision?" *No Excuse Podcast*, Nov. 30, 2023. https://www.who.int/podcasts/series/science-in-5/episode--108---how-can-you-protect-your-child-s-vision.

About the Author

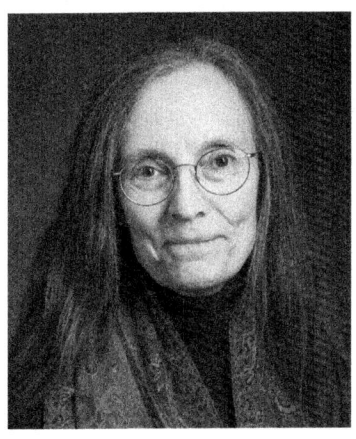

JANE SWAIN is a pediatric physical therapist, movement therapist, and adult educator in the field of Waldorf education, who has published in several American and international journals. She is an associate director of the Early Childhood Teacher Education Center at Sophia's Heath in Keene, New Hampshire, and a core faculty member there; she is also a Senior Therapeutic Trainer for the Spacial Dynamics® Institute in Mechanicville, New York. She has studied at the Pikler Institute in Budapest, Hungary. She is certified in Bothmer Gymnastics, Sensory Integration Praxis Testing, and in Bobath/Neuro-Developmental Treatment for children with cerebral palsy and other neurological conditions. Jane taught movement education for the early grades at her local Waldorf school, and has spent decades working with children and their parents and consulting in classrooms.